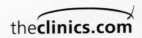

theclinics.com

SLEEP MEDICINE CLINICS

Sleep and Disorders of Sleep in Women

Guest Editor
HELEN S. DRIVER, PhD, RPSGT, DABSM

March 2008 • Volume 3 • Number 1

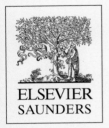

ELSEVIER
SAUNDERS

An imprint of Elsevier, Inc
PHILADELPHIA LONDON TORONTO MONTREAL SYDNEY TOKYO

W.B. SAUNDERS COMPANY
A Division of Elsevier Inc.

1600 John F. Kennedy Boulevard • Suite 1800 • Philadelphia, PA 19103-2899

http://www.sleep.theclinics.com

SLEEP MEDICINE CLINICS Volume 3, Number 1
March 2008, ISSN 1556-407X, ISBN-13: 978-1-4160-5871-7, ISBN-10: 1-4160-5871-0

Editor: Sarah E. Barth

Sleep Medicine Clinics (ISSN 1556-407X) is published quarterly by W.B. Saunders Company, 360 Park Avenue South, New York, NY 10010-1710. Months of publication are March, June, September and December. Business and editorial offices: 1600 John F. Kennedy Boulevard, Suite 1800, Philadelphia, PA 19103-2899. Accounting and circulation offices: 6277 Sea Harbor Drive, Orlando, FL 32887-4800. Periodicals postage paid at New York, and additional mailing offices. Subscription prices are $139.00 per year (US individuals), $70.00 (US students), $303.00 (US institutions), $149.00 (Canadian individuals), $85.00 (Canadian students), $279.00 (Canadian institutions), $161.00 (foreign individuals), $92.00 (foreign students), and $326.00 (foreign institutions). Foreign air speed delivery is included in all *Clinics* subscription prices. All prices are subject to change without notice. POSTMASTER: Send address changes to *Sleep Medicine Clinics*, Elsevier Journals Customer Service, 6277 Sea Harbor Drive, FL 32887-4800. Customer Service: 1-800-654-2452 (US). From outside the United States, call 1-407-563-6020. Fax: 1-407-363-9661. E-mail: JournalsCustomerService-usa@elsevier.com.

Reprints: For copies of 100 or more, of articles in this publication, please contact the Commercial Reprints Department, Elsevier Inc., 360 Park Avenue South, New York, New York 10010-1710. Tel.: (212) 633-3813, Fax: (212) 462-1935, e-mail: reprints@elsevier.com.

Printed in the United States of America.

SLEEP AND DISORDERS OF SLEEP IN WOMEN

CONSULTING EDITOR

TEOFILO LEE-CHIONG, JR., MD
Head, Section of Sleep Medicine, National Jewish
Medical and Research Center; Associate Professor
of Medicine, University of Colorado Health
Sciences Center, Denver, Colorado

GUEST EDITOR

HELEN S. DRIVER, PhD, RPSGT, DABSM
Sleep Disorders Laboratory, Kingston General
Hospital, Kingston, Ontario, Canada; Brain
Function Research Group, School of Physiology,
University of Witwatersrand, Johannesburg,
South Africa

CONTRIBUTORS

SONIA ANCOLI-ISRAEL, PhD
Professor, Department of Psychiatry, University
of California, San Diego; Director, Patient and
Family Support Services; Co-Director, Doris Howell
Palliative Care Service, Moores University of
California, San Diego, Cancer Center, La Jolla;
Veterans Affairs San Diego Healthcare System,
San Diego, California

FIONA C. BAKER, PhD
Human Sleep Research Program, SRI International,
Menlo Park, California; Brain Function Research
Group, School of Physiology, University of the
Witwatersrand, Johannesburg, South Africa

KATSUHISA BANNO, MD
Sleep Disorders Center, Kitatsushima Hospital,
Inazawa-city, Aichi, Japan

WAYNE A. BARDWELL, PhD, MBA
Assistant Professor, Department of Psychiatry,
University of California, San Diego, San Diego;
Director, Patient and Family Support Services;
Co-Director, Doris Howell Palliative Care Service,
Moores University of California, San Diego,
Cancer Center, La Jolla, California

DIANE B. BOIVIN, MD, PhD
Centre for Study and Treatment of Circadian
Rhythms, Douglas Mental Health University

Institute; Department of Psychiatry, McGill
University, Montreal, Quebec, Canada

ALEXANDER A. BORBÉLY, MD
Institute of Pharmacology and Toxicology,
University of Zürich, Zürich, Switzerland

IAN M. COLRAIN, PhD
Human Sleep Research Program, SRI International,
Menlo Park, California; Department of Psychology,
University of Melbourne, Parkville, Victoria,
Australia

JUDITH R. DAVIDSON, PhD
Assistant Professor (Adjunct), Department
of Psychology; Assistant Professor, Department
of Oncology, Queen's University; Psychologist,
Kingston Family Health Team, Kingston, Ontario,
Canada

DERK-JAN DIJK, PhD
Sleep Research Center, University of Surrey,
Guildford, Surrey, United Kingdom

HELEN S. DRIVER, PhD, RPSGT, DABSM
Sleep Disorders Laboratory, Kingston General
Hospital, Kingston, Ontario, Canada; Brain
Function Research Group, School of Physiology,
University of Witwatersrand, Johannesburg,
South Africa

NATALIE EDWARDS, PhD
Senior Research Fellow, David Read Laboratory,
Department of Medicine, The University of Sydney,
New South Wales, Australia

DAVID A. EHRMANN, MD
Professor of Medicine, Section of Endocrinology,
Diabetes, and Metabolism, Department of
Medicine, University of Chicago, Chicago, Illinois

STELLA IACOVIDES, BS
Brain Function Research Group, School of
Physiology, University of the Witwatersrand,
Johannesburg, South Africa

FRANCINE O. JAMES, PhD
Centre for Study and Treatment of Circadian
Rhythms, Douglas Mental Health University
Institute; Department of Psychiatry, McGill
University, Montreal, Quebec, Canada

MEIR H. KRYGER, MD, FRCPC
Sleep Research and Education, Gaylord Hospital,
Wallingford, Connecticut

LYNNE J. LAMARCHE, PhD
School of Psychology, University of Ottawa,
Whitby, Ontario, Canada

JUDITH A. OWENS, MD, MPH
Director, Learning, Attention, and Behavior
Program; Director, Pediatric Sleep Disorders Clinic,
Division of Pediatric Ambulatory Medicine, Rhode
Island Hospital; Associate Professor of Pediatrics,
Warren Alpert School of Medicine at Brown
University, Providence, Rhode Island

PÄIVI POLO-KANTOLA, MD, PhD
Department of Obstetrics and Gynecology,
University Central Hospital of Turku; Sleep

Research Center Dentalia, University of Turku,
Turku, Finland

JOAN L.F. SHAVER, PhD, RN, FAAN
Professor and Dean, University of Illinois at
Chicago, College of Nursing, Chicago, Illinois

ARI SHECHTER, BSc
Centre for Study and Treatment of Circadian
Rhythms, Douglas Mental Health University
Institute; Department of Neurology and
Neurosurgery, McGill University, Montreal,
Quebec, Canada

EILEEN P. SLOAN, MD, PhD, FRCPC
Staff Psychiatrist, Maternal/Infant Mental Health
Program, Mount Sinai Hospital; Assistant Professor,
Department of Psychiatry, University of Toronto,
Toronto, Ontario, Canada

COLIN E. SULLIVAN, MD, PhD
Professor of Medicine, David Read Laboratory,
Department of Medicine, The University of Sydney,
New South Wales, Australia

ESRA TASALI, MD
Assistant Professor of Medicine, Section of
Pulmonary and Critical Care Medicine, Department
of Medicine, University of Chicago, Chicago,
Illinois

EVE VAN CAUTER, PhD
Professor of Medicine, Section of Endocrinology,
Diabetes, and Metabolism, Department of
Medicine, University of Chicago, Chicago, Illinois

ESTHER WERTH, PhD
Center of Sleep/Wake Disturbances, Department of
Neurology, University Hospital Zürich, Zürich,
Switzerland

SLEEP AND DISORDERS OF SLEEP IN WOMEN

Volume 3 • Number 1 • March 2008

Contents

The Menstrual Cycle Effects on Sleep

Helen S. Driver, Esther Werth, Derk-Jan Dijk, and Alexander A. Borbély

Women with ovulatory cycles have a biphasic change in body temperature, reduced subjective sleep quality premenstrually and at menstruation, while sleep homeostatic mechanisms, as reflected by slow wave sleep (SWS), are unaltered. The mid-luteal phase increase in body temperature is associated with more stage 2 sleep, higher spindle frequency activity, reduced REM sleep, and elevated heart rates during sleep when compared to the mid-follicular phase. Based on a few studies the effects of oral contraceptives (OC) appear small: women taking OCs have more stage 2 compared to naturally cycling women but less SWS than naturally cycling women in the luteal phase.

Circadian Rhythms and Shift Working Women

Ari Shechter, Francine O. James, and Diane B. Boivin

Approximately a quarter of the female workforce in Canada works shifts. Shift workers experience a misalignment between their endogenous circadian rhythms and their sleep/wake cycle, which can result in various health and psychosocial problems, including sleep disruptions, cardiovascular and gastrointestinal disorders, and effects on relationships and mood. Shift-working women also have several gender-specific health concerns and may be especially at risk for developing menstrual cycle irregularities, problems with reproductive health, and breast cancer. This article includes a theoretical background on circadian rhythms and clock genes, presents general problems of circadian misalignment, and discusses the specific issues associated with shift work as they pertain to women.

There are few studies of sleep in menstrual-related disorders. Preliminary evidence indicates subtle differences in sleep and circadian regulation in women with severe premenstrual syndrome, and increased subjective sleepiness in the premenstrual phase. Symptoms may be relieved in some sufferers with partial sleep deprivation. Primary dysmenorrhea occurs in approximately 25% of women who self-report sleep disturbance, a finding confirmed by laboratory-based study of sleep in these women. Menstrual cycle-related sleep disturbance appears to be highly prevalent; more research is needed to investigate the role of sleep in the etiology of menstrual disorders and the role of sleep manipulation in their treatment.

Polycystic ovary syndrome (PCOS), the most common endocrine disorder of premenopausal women, is characterized by chronic hyperandrogenism, oligo- or anovulation, obesity, and insulin resistance. Women who have PCOS are at increased risk for glucose intolerance, type 2 diabetes mellitus, and cardiovascular disorders. Recent reports indicate an unexpectedly high prevalence of obstructive sleep apnea (OSA) in women who have PCOS. Alterations in sex steroids and increased visceral adiposity could potentially contribute to the increased prevalence of OSA in this disorder, and there may be strong associations between the presence and severity of OSA and the metabolic disturbances that characterize PCOS. Causal mechanisms in the link between PCOS and OSA remain to be elucidated. Clinicians who manage PCOS patients should be aware of the high prevalence of OSA and should systematically evaluate these women for sleep disturbances.

In this article evidence is discussed related to the reciprocal features of sleep and pain across three chronic multisymptom conditions, referred to as functional somatic syndromes, that are disproportionately found in women. Light and fragmented polysomnography sleep patterns, although often of lesser severity, match subjective reports of nonrestorative sleep quality and excess risk for sleep-related disorders. Health ecology factors (personal and environmental) contributing to women's vulnerability to these stress-embedded conditions and potential mechanisms related to emotional arousal and inflammatory/immune activation are discussed as linked to pain processing and poor sleep.

Fatigue is a common and disabling symptom in patients who have breast cancer and in breast cancer survivors. A rather nebulous concept, fatigue overlaps with sleepiness and depressed mood. This article addresses methods for assessing fatigue; describes the occurrence of fatigue before, during, and after initial treatment; presents possible underlying mechanisms of fatigue; and enumerates approaches to its treatment.

Pregnancy and the postpartum period are associated with significant changes in sleep architecture and the subjective quality of sleep. These changes are caused by the many physiologic changes that occur during pregnancy (eg, altered hormone levels, increased urination at night, changes in body size) and post partum, especially with a newborn to tend. Although most women negotiate the disruption to their sleep very well, others may experience such severe disruption to sleep that it compromises their physical well-being and mental health. Physicians providing care for pregnant women must inquire about sleep patterns; if a woman is reporting significant difficulty coping with the disruption, a thorough history should be taken. Primary sleep disorders are common in pregnancy and further investigation and treatment may be warranted.

The prevalence of sleep-disordered breathing (SDB) in late pregnancy is as high as 15%, a result of normal physiologic processes occurring during pregnancy, and its prevalence in pre-eclampsia is even higher. The cardiovascular risks associated with SDB have an even stronger association in pregnancy: with SDB in pregnancy there is an eightfold relative risk of developing systemic hypertension, primarily because the vascular inflammatory processes leading to endothelial dysfunction that occur in SDB are increased during pregnancy. The fetal effects of maternal cardiovascular compromise arising from SDB include growth restriction and impaired movement.

In addition to biologic mechanisms, cultural factors are important determinants of sleep practices and behaviors in infants, children, and adolescents and influence both the type and frequency of sleep problems found in the pediatric population. This article discusses some of the key sleep practices most influenced by cultural practices and beliefs: cosleeping, bedtime rituals, the sleeping environment, napping, and parental expectations regarding sleep in children. The importance of clinical and educational cross-cultural collaboration and the need for future research that uses culturally sensitive and comparable methodologies to explore cultural differences and similarities are emphasized.

This article describes the circumstances under which women may develop insomnia and the various treatment options, including hypnotic medication and nonpharmacologic approaches. The efficacy and safety of these treatments are reviewed. The choice of treatment depends on the nature of the insomnia, the stage of a woman's life, the presence of medical or mental-health conditions, the availability of treatments, and personal preference. For immediate, short-term relief of acute insomnia, hypnotic medication, especially the nonbenzodiazepines (zolpidem, zopiclone, eszopiclone) are options. For chronic insomnia, insomnia-specific cognitive and behavioral therapies are generally the interventions of choice.

During the climacterium, which covers the menopausal transition through to postmenopause, women experience vasomotor symptoms (hot flashes and sweating) and sleep disturbances. Hormone therapy is generally acknowledged as the most effective therapy for reducing climacteric vasomotor symptoms and related secondary insomnia. This review describes the effects on sleep of the gradual cessation of hormonal secretion, specifically estrogen and progesterone, by the ovaries and evaluates different treatment options. Aging is briefly discussed with a focus on menopausal transition and related changes in biological functions.

Some sleep disorders are common in women, but gender differences in the clinical presentation of the sleep disorders and lack of awareness of sleep disorders by medical practitioners may lead to a delayed diagnosis. Underlying medical or psychiatric diseases may cause sleep problems; conversely primary sleep disorders could lead to the development of medical and mental conditions. Untreated sleep disorders lead to increased resource utilization of health care systems with reductions in health care utilization following compliance with therapy. Earlier diagnosis and treatment of the sleep disorders may reduce health care utilization in women.

SLEEP
MEDICINE
CLINICS

Sleep Med Clin 3 (2008) xi–xii

Foreword

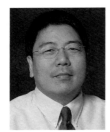

Teofilo Lee-Chiong, Jr., MD
Consulting Editor

Teofilo Lee-Chiong, Jr., MD
Section of Sleep Medicine
National Jewish Medical and Research Center
University of Colorado Health Sciences Center
1400 Jackson Street
Room J232
Denver, CO 80206, USA

E-mail address:
lee-chiongt@njc.org

Across the lifespan of women, reproductive cycles can significantly affect sleep. In general, women appear to describe more subjective complaints of unsatisfactory sleep quality, as well as non-restorative sleep, but also tend to report a greater need for sleep compared to men.

During the menstrual cycle, sleep quality is commonly poorer immediately before and during the initial part of menstruation. Duration of nighttime sleep is also longer prior to menses. Many factors potentially contribute to sleep disturbance during this time, including mood changes and physical complaints (eg, breast tenderness, abdominal bloating, cramping, and headaches). The luteal phase of the menstrual cycle is associated with increased subjective sleepiness, as well as decreased sleep efficiency and more prolonged sleep latency. There is also commonly an increase in non-rapid eye movement (NREM) stage 2 sleep, increase in frequency of sleep spindles, and decrease in rapid eye movement (REM) sleep during the luteal phase as compared to the follicular phase. Menstruation itself can be accompanied by an increase in latency to slow-wave sleep.

Specific sleep disturbances can also develop during the menstrual cycle, secondary to dysmenorrhea (painful uterine cramping), endometriosis (presence of endometrial tissue in the pelvis or abdomen), premenstrual syndrome, and premenstrual dysphoric disorder. Dysmenorrhea can result in diminished sleep quality and duration of REM sleep. Sleep can be disturbed by pain from endometriosis. Premenstrual syndrome (PMS) is characterized by bloating, irritability, and fatigue that develop prior to menses during the late luteal phase. PMS can be associated with poor sleep, frequent awakenings, unpleasant dreams, and complaints of insomnia or excessive sleepiness. Considered a more severe form of PMS, premenstrual dysphoric disorder can also be complicated by complaints of insomnia or excessive sleepiness, along with functional impairment and mood changes. Finally, parasomnias, including sleepwalking and sleep terrors, occurring repeatedly during the luteal phase of menstruation have been described.

The use of oral contraceptives can also produce significant changes in NREM stage 2 sleep and decreases in REM sleep latency; however, no

doi:10.1016/j.jsmc.2008.01.008

changes in daytime alertness have been noted with oral contraceptive use.

Sleep quality and duration are profoundly affected by pregnancy. Increase in frequency of awakenings and wake time after sleep onset, as well as decrease in nighttime sleep duration and increase in daytime napping, can occur as early as the first trimester of pregnancy. Sleep tends to improve during the second trimester, only to significantly deteriorate again during the final months of pregnancy. Causes of sleep disturbance during pregnancy vary from one individual to the next but may be due to a combination of any of the following factors: breast tenderness, dyspnea, nausea, urinary frequency, fetal movements, leg cramps, or anxiety. Sleep-related breathing disorders, including snoring and obstructive sleep apnea, and restless legs syndrome may be precipitated or aggravated by pregnancy. Excessive sleepiness may extend into the postpartum period, and mothers may experience significant sleep loss, changes in mood, and frequent napping.

Finally, peri-menopausal and post-menopausal phases with their declining levels of estrogen and progesterone, and irregular menstrual cycles can lead to the development of hot flashes, night sweats, headaches, and urinary frequency; these, in turn, can give rise to excessive sleepiness, sleep fragmentation, and insomnia. In addition to insomnia, obstructive sleep apnea also has a higher prevalence during this period compared to the pre-menopausal period.

SLEEP
MEDICINE
CLINICS

Sleep Med Clin 3 (2008) xiii–xiv

Preface

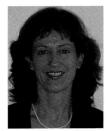

Helen S. Driver, PhD, RPSGT, DABSM
Guest Editor

Helen S. Driver, PhD, RPSGT, DABSM
Sleep Disorders Laboratory
Kingston General Hospital
Departments of Medicine and Psychology
Queen's University
Kingston, Ontario K7L 2V6, Canada

Brain Function Research Group
School of Physiology
University of the Witwatersrand
Johannesburg, South Africa

E-mail address: driverh@kgh.kari.net

This issue of *Sleep Medicine Clinics* highlights the emerging scientific consensus on the importance of female-specific sleep changes through a diverse and high-level set of articles. The authors' unique voices and distinct scientific and clinical perspectives ensure that this issue on sleep and sleep disorders in women fully encompasses a woman's reproductive lifespan, with topics related to menstrual cycles, pregnancy, childrearing, and menopause. Its clinical components cover medical conditions that are either specific to or more prevalent in women, such as insomnia, or that demonstrate sex-based differences, such as obstructive sleep apnea (OSA). Data-driven articles from well-known research groups and reviews by clinical specialists from across the world link the pure science to clinical practice.

The first three articles cover a series of discussions on menstrual cycle. Sleep homeostasis is relatively unaffected by menstrual cycle changes, but many women experience subjectively poorer sleep around menstruation. Driver, Werth, Dijk and Borbély describe their findings that changes in the post-ovulation sleep EEG coincide with a progesterone-mediated increase in nocturnal body temperature

and elevated heart rates during sleep. Shechter, James, and Boivin review reproductive and health issues for the approximately 25% of Canadian women in the work force who are shift workers. Shift work causes a misalignment of circadian rhythms resulting in menstrual cycle irregularities, weight gain, increased risk of cardiovascular disease, functional bowel disorders, and breast cancer. Baker, Lamarche, Iacovides and Colrain describe menstrual-related disturbances. They review the influence of dysmenorrhea (pain at menstruation), and the impact of premenstrual syndrome and premenstrual dysphoric disorder on sleep.

A series of papers examines disturbed sleep caused by pain, fatigue, and depression. Women experience pain acutely in predictable recurring cycles, such as dysmenorrhoea, and they also are disproportionately prone to manifest chronically widespread and regional painful, multi-symptom syndromes including fibromyalgia, irritable bowel syndrome, and chronic pelvic pain. Sleep disturbance, with complaints of poor and unrefreshing sleep, in relation to menstrual-related disorders in women who have functional somatic syndromes, as

doi:10.1016/j.jsmc.2007.11.002

outlined by Shaver, appears to be highly prevalent. In addition to the menstrual-related disorders and functional somatic syndromes, breast cancer survivor's fatigue, reviewed by Bardwell and Ancoli-Israel, is linked to pain and sleep disturbance, worse physical health, less physical activity, and depressive symptoms.

Two articles examine the altered hormone profiles of pregnancy and menopause and their effect on sleep. In her article, Sloan summarizes sleep changes during pregnancy and postpartum, emphasizing sleep disruption, insomnia, depression, and restless legs syndrome and their response to various treatment strategies. The gradual withdrawal of estrogen and progesterone around menopause results in an increase in sleep problems. Polo-Kantola considers these changes and therapies, including hormone replacement.

Women are at increased risk for developing insomnia in pivotal periods such as pregnancy, childbirth, and especially menopause. These periods are associated with changing hormone profiles and changes in lifestyle and/or environment. For example, sleep behaviors and practices often are radically altered with the arrival of an infant in the home. Owens discusses how biological determinants of sleep, cultural influences, and lifestyles contribute to sleep practices, particularly during the formative years. Davidson outlines insomnia predisposing, precipitating, and perpetuating factors and therapeutic options. Since persistent insomnia correlates with increased use of healthcare services and the risk of developing depression (as highlighted by Banno and Kryger and by Davidson), appropriate pharmacologic and nonpharmacologic interventions described in this issue should be given serious consideration.

Another set of articles highlight women's unique challenges from sleep disorders. Women with sleep disordered breathing are more likely to present with depression, and complain of fatigue and unrefreshing sleep rather than the more traditionally accepted symptom of excessive daytime sleepiness, as summarized by Banno and Kryger. Women are more likely to have increased upper airway resistance syndrome rather than frank apneas. Edwards and Sullivan review these sex-differences in their discussion of unique changes during pregnancy and the impact on sleep disordered breathing, while Polo-Katola examines the increased incidence of OSA in postmenopausal women. The influence of hormones is particularly relevant during pregnancy when women traditionally have been thought to be "protected" from developing breathing disorders during sleep. However, there is growing concern regarding increased risk for OSA in this population, particularly in women who have preeclampsia and in those who are obese. Tasali, Van Cauter, and Ehrmann conclude that not only do women who have polycystic ovary syndrome have higher levels of androgens, lower levels of progesterone and estrogen, menstrual irregularity, and obesity, but also they are at increased risk for insulin resistance, hypertension, and OSA. The multi-faceted influence of hormones, weight gain, and the possible role of proinflammatory cytokines in developing OSA is also described in the articles on polycystic ovaray syndrome, pregnancy and menopause.

With this issue of *Sleep Medicine Clinics* the reader is provided with the background to be able to identify and consider treatment options for women who are at high risk for sleep disorders. I thank the authors who have contributed to this issue on women's sleep matters from childbirth to menopause, and I thank the editors and publishers who helped bring it to publication.

SLEEP
MEDICINE
CLINICS

Sleep Med Clin 3 (2008) 1–11

The Menstrual Cycle Effects on Sleep

Helen S. Driver, PhD, RPSGT, DABSM[a,b],*, Esther Werth, PhD[c],
Derk-Jan Dijk, PhD[d], Alexander A. Borbély, MD[e]

The physiology of menstrual cycles provides inherent challenges for research, given the variability in cycle length, the presence or absence of ovulation, individual and cycle-to-cycle differences, changes with age, and the interaction with mood, discomfort, and pain around menstruation. Research on young women has been complicated by concerns around the need to select discrete times in the cycle during which to study women, the frequency of data sampling required, and the use of oral contraceptives (OCs). To control for potential confounds across the menstrual cycle, many researchers opt to study women in the follicular phase. With ovulatory cycles, and with the associated changes in estrogen and progesterone in particular, there are changes in body temperature and effects on subjective and objective measures of sleep that have been described in recent reviews [1–4] and are summarized in this article.

The most remarkable effects on the sleep electroencephalograph (EEG) occur in the luteal phase when progesterone predominates compared with the follicular phase when estrogen predominates. The authors have conducted an analysis of changes

[a] Sleep Disorders Laboratory, Kingston General Hospital and Department of Medicine, Room 20-303 Richardson House, Queen's University, 102 Stuart Street, Kingston, Ontario, Canada
[b] Brain Function Research Group, School of Physiology, University of the Witwatersrand, Johannesburg, South Africa
[c] Center of Sleep/Wake Disturbances, Department of Neurology, University Hospital Zürich, Frauenklinikstrasse 26, 8091 Zürich, Switzerland
[d] Sleep Research Center, University of Surrey, Egerton Road, Guildford, Surrey GU2 7XP, UK
[e] Institute of Pharmacology and Toxicology, Winterthurerstrasse 190, University of Zürich, CH-8057 Zürich, Switzerland
* Corresponding author. Department of Medicine, Room 20-303 Richardson House, Queen's University, 102 Stuart Street, Kingston, Ontario K7L 2V6, Canada
E-mail address: driverh@kgh.kari.net (H.S. Driver).

doi:10.1016/j.jsmc.2007.10.003

in sleep, the sleep EEG, body temperature, and heart rate across 1 night at the midpoints of the follicular and luteal phases. These data extend the discussion of the influence of progesterone and temperature on sleep and include the changes in temperature and heart rate in rapid-eye-movement (REM) and non-REM sleep during the first four sleep cycles.

Although about 100 million women worldwide use OCs, there has been very little research on their effects on sleep and temperature. These influences may be small, but the relatively undocumented effects have contributed to the exclusion of women taking OC therapy from studies. This article concludes with a summary and suggestions for future research.

Ovulatory menstrual cycles

In an ovulatory menstrual cycle there are cyclical changes in four reproductive hormones, namely the pituitary gonadotropins—luteinizing hormone and follicle-stimulating hormone—and estrogen and progesterone that occur in conjunction with a bi-phasic change in body temperature [5]. The common identification, based on the days of the cycle, starts with the first day of menstruation as day 1 and continues until the start of the next bleeding period. Menstrual cycle length decreases from an average of 28 days for women in their twenties to 26 days for women in their forties [6]; an average cycle lasts 28 days but may range from 25 to 35 days.

On the day menstruation begins, all four key reproductive hormones are low. As follicle-stimulating hormone and estrogen rise, ovarian follicles develop and mature during this follicular or proliferative phase. The follicular phase, which precedes ovulation, may vary in length. Luteinizing hormone peaks about 16 hours before ovulation, and the appearance of luteinizing hormone in urine is a reliable marker of ovulation. At ovulation an oocyte is released from the follicle. Thereafter, the corpus luteum evolves from the ruptured follicle and secretes progesterone and estrogen in the luteal phase (also called the "secretory phase"). If ovulation has occurred, body temperature, when measured at the same time every morning, increases by about 0.4°C [1,7,8]. About 10 days after ovulation, and if fertilization does not occur, the corpus luteum begins to degenerate, and hormone production begins to decline, leading to shedding of the endometrium and the start of a new cycle. The luteal phase usually is constant, lasting 14 days. Most negative menstrual symptoms are experienced during the last 4 to 8 days of the cycle (as estrogen and progesterone concentrations decline) and the first few days of menstruation (when ovarian hormones are low).

Subjective effects of the menstrual cycle on sleep

Subjective sleep quality is reduced both premenstrually and at menstruation [1,9–11]. In a telephone survey of 514 women, approximately 70% reported that their sleep is affected adversely by menstrual symptoms such as bloating, tender breasts, headaches, and cramps, on average 2.5 days every month [12]. Earlier retrospective surveys found that 16% to 32% of women report increased fatigue, difficulty in concentrating, or lethargy in the premenstrual period ([13–14]; for reviews see Refs. [2–4]).

Prospective studies also show that sleep disturbance increases around menstruation [9–11]. A study of 32 women who kept daily diaries across two menstrual cycles found no change in sleep duration, but sleep disturbances increased, with poorer sleep quality, in the late luteal phase as compared with the mid-follicular phase [11]. There was a delay in sleep onset and an increased number of awakenings premenstrually. Laessle and colleagues [10] however, found no change in sleep quality or sleep duration in young women (n = 30) who had normal menstrual cycles. A more recent study by Baker and Driver [9], in which ovulatory cycles were confirmed, found that young women (n = 26) without significant menstrual-associated complaints reported poorer sleep quality 3 to 6 days premenstrually and during the first 4 days of menstruation.

In general, women across a wide age range (18–50 years) report more sleep disturbances, including time to sleep onset and number of awakenings [11,13] and decreased sleep efficiency or quality [9] during the premenstrual week than at other times. As discussed in more detail in the article by Baker and colleagues in this issue, the experience of pain at menstruation and the severity of premenstrual symptoms should be considered. Women who have more severe symptoms have reported more unpleasant dreams and a lower quality of sleep in the luteal phase [14] and increased sleepiness [15] than women who have minimal symptoms. Similarly, women who have dysmenorrhea, who experience extremely painful cramps during menstruation, and women who have endometriosis, who suffer extreme menstrual pain caused by misplaced uterine (endometrial) tissue in the abdominal and pelvic area, report poorer sleep quality and higher anxiety during menstruation than symptom-free women. Baker and colleagues [16] found that dysmenorrheic women had more disturbed sleep and subjective sleepiness than controls.

Given the cyclical, although modest, reduction in sleep quality around menstruation in women who do not have sleep complaints, investigation of insomnia in women who have ovulatory cycles should consider the temporal relationship of sleep complaints and the phase of the menstrual cycle.

Objective polysomnographic findings across the menstrual cycle

Early gender-specific laboratory studies yielded limited information on sleep changes across normal ovulatory cycles. These studies were based on small sample sizes, usually in young women (< 30 years of age) with heterogeneous groups including those who had affective symptoms and those taking OCs, often without verification that ovulation had occurred [1,2,4]. Two controlled studies addressed this issue [7,17]. These studies conducted more frequent recordings across the cycle—3 nights/week [17] and every other night [7], respectively—in nonsymptomatic, good sleepers who had verified ovulatory cycles and included temperature measurements and spectral analysis of the sleep EEG.

Slow-wave sleep (SWS) [7,17,18] or slow-wave activity (SWA) in the power spectrum [7] was not different across the cycle, suggesting that sleep homeostatic mechanisms are not altered by menstrual phase.

REM sleep seems to be influenced slightly by menstrual phase. Some studies have found that REM sleep has an earlier onset in the luteal phase [18]. The percentage of REM sleep tends to be decreased [8,16,19,20] in association with raised body temperature in the luteal phase compared with the follicular phase. The authors found that REM sleep tended to decrease from the early follicular phase (27.4%) to the late luteal phase (22.9%) [7].

A consistent finding was a menstrual cycle–associated variation in stage 2 sleep, which was higher in the luteal phase than in the follicular phase. In the study by Driver and colleagues [7], stage 2 sleep increased from (50%) in the late follicular phase to (55.3%) in the early luteal phase. Selected sleep parameters for a full night during the mid-follicular and mid-luteal phases are provided in Table 1. The only significant difference in visually scored sleep was in the proportion of stage 2 sleep.

Specific effects on the sleep EEG was a prominent variation in sleep spindles in the upper frequency range (14.25–15 Hz), which were lowest in the mid-follicular phase and maximal in the mid-luteal phase [7]. Because the menstrual effect on the spindle frequency region in non-REM sleep coincided with the progesterone-mediated increase in rectal temperature [21], it was proposed that the variation could be a temperature-dependent response [22].

Table 1: Mean over the whole night for selected sleep measures based on visual scoring body temperature, and heart rate during the first four episodes of non-REM and REM sleep from nine women who had ovulatory menstrual cycles for 1 night in the mid-follicular phase and 1 night in the mid-luteal phase (Age 20–30 years)

Parameter	Follicular phase (SD)	Luteal phase (SD)
TST (mins)	449.5 (30.6)	455.1 (30.2)
SOL (mins)	14.9 (7.0)	14.3 (10.5)
ROL (mins)	66.1 (10.2)	64.0 (8.8)
Stage 1 (% of TST)	4.8 (1.9)	4.2 (1.5)
Stage 2 (% of TST)[a]	49.6 (3.2)	53.7 (3.2)
Stage 3 (% of TST)	5.3 (2.5)	5.5 (2.4)
Stage 4 (% of TST)	14.5 (3.3)	12.0 (3.4)
SWS (% of TST)	19.8 (4.9)	17.5 (4.2)
REM (% of TST)	25.8 (2.7)	24.6 (3.5)
WASO (% of TST)	3.3 (4.8)	2.5 (3.3)
MT (% of TST)	2.6 (1.2)	2.3 (0.7)
SE (% of TST)	91.7 (3.8)	92.8 (3.6)
$Temp_{sleep}$ (°C)[a]	36.7 (0.2)	37.1 (0.2)
HR_{SO}(bpm)	63.9 (10.1)	65.7 (10.9)
HR_{sleep}(bpm)[a]	59.8 (5.5)	63.5 (7.0)

Abbreviations: TST, total sleep time; SOL, sleep onset latency; ROL, REM sleep onset latency; SWS, slow wave sleep; WASO, wakefulness after sleep onset; MT, movement time; SE, sleep efficiency (TST as percentage of time in bed); % as a percentage of TST; $Temp_{sleep}$, rectal temperature during the first four nonREM and REM sleep episodes; HR_{SO}, heart rate (beats per min (bpm)) during wake preceding sleep onset; HR_{sleep}, overnight heart rate during the first four nonREM and REM sleep episodes.
[a] $P < .05$, paired *t*-test.
Data from Driver HS, Dijk DJ, Werth E, et al. Menstrual cycle effects on sleep EEG in young healthy women. J Clin Endocrinol Metab 1996;81:728–35.

Alternatively, it might be induced by progesterone and other agonistic modulators of γ-aminobutyric acid$_A$ ($GABA_A$) receptors, such as benzodiazepines and non-benzodiazepines [23] and neuroactive metabolites of progesterone, that facilitate $GABA_A$ receptor functioning independent of the temperature response ([24–26]; for review see Ref. [27]).

Menstrual, diurnal, and sleep-associated changes in body temperature

In addition to the menstrual cycle–associated changes in body temperature, there are also diurnal fluctuations. Circadian disruption, such as occurs with shift work or increased nocturnal exposure to light, may lead to an increased risk for breast cancer in women [28], as discussed in more detail in the article by Shechter and colleagues in this issue. The largest difference in body temperature between the follicular and luteal phase occurs during the early hours of the morning [29–31]. Studies that have reported thermoregulatory effects of the menstrual cycle are those that have taken cognizance of the circadian profile influencing the thermogenic effect of progesterone [32,33]. There is a rapid increase in body temperature in response to progesterone administration [34], and body temperature in women increases about 24 hours after a detectable increase in progesterone plasma concentration [21]. Estrogen, on the other hand, lowers body temperature [35]. Considering that body temperature in women who have ovulatory menstrual cycles has both a menstrual and a circadian profile (for review, see Ref. [28]), compensatory responses to the temperature changes (eg, on the cardiovascular system) may be more evident at night than during the day [36].

Sleep-related electroencephalographic spectra, temperature, and heart rate during the mid-follicular and mid-luteal phases

The most remarkable changes in polysomnographically recorded sleep seem to be from the mid-follicular phase, when nocturnal body temperature is low and estrogen predominates, to the mid-luteal phase, when progesterone and temperature are elevated. This finding is in contrast to a subjective increase in sleep disturbances and reduced sleep quality around menstruation, when endogenous levels of these steroid hormones are low.

Methods for investigating the temporal evolution of sleep, temperature, and heart rate

To investigate the temporal evolution of the changes during sleep through one night in the mid-follicular and mid-luteal phase, the authors examined the sleep EEG, nocturnal body temperature, and heart rate during the first four sleep cycles. These data were from nine healthy young women aged 20 to 30 years, with normal body mass indices (mean ± SD 22.1 ± 2.4 kg/m^2) and documented ovulatory cycles, as previously reported [7]. Recordings of sleep, rectal temperature, and heart rate were made every alternate night over 32 to 36 days for the duration of one menstrual cycle. Estradiol, progesterone, and prolactin hormone concentrations measured 6 to 8 days after ovulation were in the normal range for the luteal phase [7]. Progesterone levels ranged from 22.5 to 44.1 nmol/L (normal luteal-phase levels, 20–90 nmol/L), the estradiol concentrations ranged from 190 to 470 pmol/L (normal luteal-phase levels, 180–1100 pmol/L), and prolactin levels ranged from 7.9 to 21.1 µg/L. For the present analysis, one night in the mid-follicular and one night in the mid-luteal phase were selected for each woman relative to her temperature, ovulation, and the onset of menstruation.

For the temporal evolution of changes through the night, sleep cycles of non-REM and REM sleep were defined according to modified criteria described by Aeschbach and Borbély [37]. A cycle that comprised non-REM and REM sleep began with stage 2 sleep, contained at least 15 minutes of stages 2, 3, and 4 sleep, and ended with an REM sleep episode of at least 5 minutes. For the first cycle no minimum duration of REM sleep was required.

The power spectra were calculated over the first 7.5 hours for non-REM sleep (stages 2, 3, and 4) and for REM sleep. Individual power density values in the 0.625 to 4.625 Hz band, defined as SWA, and EEG power in the 12.125 to 15.125 Hz region, defined as spindle frequency activity (SFA), were computed. The time course of the changes in sleep power spectra for each woman was analyzed for the wake period between lights-out and sleep onset and for the first four non-REM and REM sleep episodes (sleep cycles). For the period before sleep onset the individual means were calculated for one time bin. In each of the four sleep cycles, individual non-REM sleep episodes were subdivided into 20 equal parts (percentiles), and REM sleep was divided into four equal parts. For each subdivision in the four cycles, the means for SWA and SFA were calculated then averaged over subjects and plotted with respect to the mean duration of each non-REM and REM sleep episode in Fig. 1.

Rectal temperatures were recorded continuously while the women were sleeping in the sleep laboratory (ambient temperature, 19°C–22°C). The data were digitized and stored at 60-second intervals on an ambulatory monitoring system. Heart rate (beats per minute) was calculated based on beat-to-beat intervals, determined as the time between successive R-waves and stored for 20-second epochs as described previously [38]. R-waves were detected by a level-crossing algorithm. Twenty-second intervals containing RR intervals of 20 milliseconds or less were considered as artifact and removed from further analysis.

For the cycle analysis, the relative heart rates and temperatures were calculated in parts of consecutive non-REM and REM sleep episodes for each woman. To align the 60-second temperature data with the 20-second sleep epochs, the same temperature value was taken for three consecutive epochs. As in the analysis of sleep and EEG power density, individual heart rates and temperatures were calculated for one time bin before sleep onset. For non-REM sleep and REM sleep episodes heart rate and temperature data were subdivided into 20 equal parts for non-REM sleep and into four equal parts for REM sleep for each woman. Thereafter the

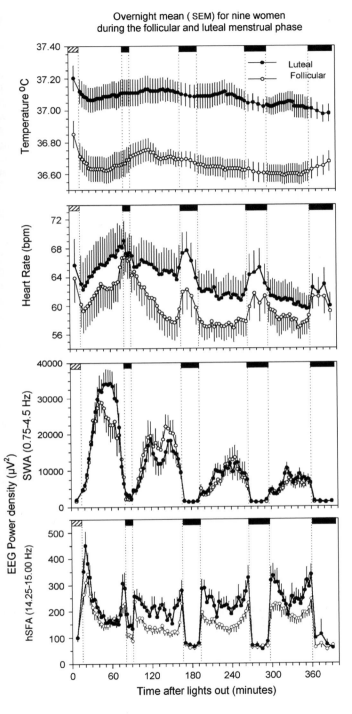

Overnight mean (SEM) for nine women
during the follicular and luteal menstrual phase

Fig. 1. Overnight mean values (± 1 SEM) for rectal temperature, heart rate, and slow-wave activity power (SWA) in the frequency range from 0.625 to 4.625 Hz and high spindle frequency activity (hSFA: 14.125–15.125 Hz) from nine young women during the mid-follicular (*open symbols*) and mid-luteal (*closed symbols*) menstrual phases. Data were aligned with respect to lights-out at time zero, sleep onset as the first occurrence of stage 2 sleep, and the mean timing of the first four complete non-REM–REM sleep cycles for all nights (n = 18). The first dotted vertical line denotes sleep onset. Dotted lines thereafter mark episodes of REM sleep (indicated by the black bars at the top of the panels). One time bin was allocated to the wake period before the onset of sleep (*hashed bar*). Individual non-REM sleep episodes were subdivided into 20 equal time bins, and REM sleep episodes were divided into four equal timebins. Rectal temperature was significantly higher at all time points in the luteal phase than the follicular phase. (Paired *t*-test based on means per non-REM and REM sleep episode, *P* ≤ .0125, for heart rate: non-REM cycles 1–4, REM cycles 2 and 3; SWA: non-REM cycles 1, 2, and 4; hSFA: non-REM cycles 1–4).

means in sleep cycles 1 to 4 were computed for non-REM (20 percentiles) and REM sleep (four percentiles) and averaged across subjects.

Initial comparisons were for the 7.5-hour all-night data, then by cycles 1 through 4, and over the mean for cycles 1 to 4 (390 minutes). Absolute values for the EEG power spectra were log-transformed before statistical analysis. Statistical differences based on repeated measures of ANOVA were followed by paired *t*-test comparisons using a software statistical package (SAS Institute Inc., Cary, North Carolina). Missing values in non-REM sleep were replaced with the mean for the two parts adjacent to the missing value for that subject, and missing REM sleep values were replaced with the subject mean from that REM period. For two women in the follicular phase, heart rate data were missing from non-REM cycle 2, through to REM cycle 3 for one woman and to the end of the recording for the other woman. Statistical analysis of the heart rate data was performed without replacing data after cycle 1 for these two women. Missing values for temperature and heart rate before sleep onset were replaced with the group mean of the menstrual phase for which data were missing. Significant differences for all-night data were Huynh-Feldt adjusted and set at $P \leq .05$ and at $P \leq .0125$ for the cycle data because of repeated comparisons over the four sleep episodes.

Changes in temperature and heart rate across the first four sleep cycles

Luteal phase overnight body temperature was increased by about 0.4°C compared with the follicular phase (see Table 1 and Fig. 1, top panel). This temperature difference ($F_{1,95}1949.73; P = .0001$) was present from before lights-out and over all four non-REM (20 parts per episode) and REM sleep episodes (four parts per episode).

Changes in temperature were correlated with heart rate. Combining the two study nights, the Pearson correlation coefficient for the means of temperature and heart rate during wake preceding sleep onset and during the first four episodes of non-REM and REM sleep was 0.522 ($P = .026$). During the wake period before sleep onset, there was no difference in mean heart rate, as shown in Table 1 (HR_{so}) and Fig. 1 (second graph from the top, first data point). The mean non-REM– and REM sleep–associated heart rate (HR_{sleep}) during the first four sleep cycles differed between the two phases, however. The mean heart rate during the four sleep cycles was higher in the luteal phase ($F_{1,95}75.44; P = .0001$) than during the follicular phase. This difference was significant for all non-REM sleep episodes and in the second and third REM sleep episodes. Heart rate initially decreased on going to sleep, then increased gradually during the first non-REM sleep episode, decreased again in the second non-REM sleep episode, and remained low during the third sleep cycle (see Fig. 1). Cyclical changes in heart rate were evident, with lower rates during non-REM sleep and increases during REM sleep episodes.

Changes in sleep across the first four sleep cycles

The length of the sleep cycle and the length of the REM sleep episode were affected by menstrual phase (Table 2). The first sleep cycle and the first REM sleep episode were shorter in the luteal phase than in the follicular phase. In addition, REM sleep episodes showed a significant interaction (see Table 2), indicating a different evolution in the course of the night during the two phases of the menstrual cycle. During the follicular phase, REM sleep episodes increased progressively in duration across the first four episodes, whereas in the luteal phase the duration of the REM sleep episode increased from the first to the second episode and then remained on a similar level for the second, third, and fourth cycles. Thus, over the first four non-REM–REM sleep cycles, there was a menstrual-phase effect on the time spent in REM sleep ($F_{1,71}5.18; P = .026$) that was not evident over the whole night (see Table 1). In the luteal phase compared with the follicular phase, there was less REM sleep in the first and fourth sleep cycles whereas during the second sleep cycle there was more stage 2 sleep (menstrual phase× sleep cycle: $F_{3,71}2.89; P = .042$), and less SWS (menstrual phase×sleep cycle: $F_{3,71}4.00; P = .011$; stage 4 sleep $F_{3,71}3.83; P = .014$).

Relative power density in the luteal phase expressed relative to the follicular phase revealed a significant effect of frequency ($F_{99,792} = 5.59; P < .0001$; 1-way rANOVA on log-transformed relative values; factor 'frequency') for the all-night non-REM sleep spectrum and no effect for the REM sleep spectrum. In the first non-REM sleep cycle, menstrual-phase differences were noted in the lower frequency range corresponding to SWA (0.75–4.5 Hz) that were less evident in the second cycle and absent in the third cycle. The menstrual-phase effect on frequency in non-REM sleep was in the range of sleep spindles, from 14 to 16 Hz. The luteal-phase increase in power in the frequency region of sleep spindles was evident in the high range of spindle frequency activity (hSFA) at 14.25 to 15.00 Hz in all non-REM sleep episodes and was particularly noticeable after the first episode.

The temporal evolution of the two frequency ranges with a menstrual-phase effect is illustrated in Fig. 1. The bottom two graphs depict SWA and hSFA. Significant menstrual differences in SWA were present in non-REM sleep episodes 1, 2, and 4—higher in the luteal-phase first cycle and lower in the second cycle than in the mid-follicular phase ($F_{1,95}10.3; P = .0015$). EEG activity in the hSFA range ($F_{1,95}162.87; P = .0001$) also was higher in the luteal phase than in the follicular phase (see Fig. 1, bottom panel).

Are progesterone and/or temperature associated with sleep and heart rate changes?

The relative absence of progesterone in the follicular phase suggest that it plays a major role in orchestrating the changes in the sleep EEG noted in the

Table 2: Mean duration of non-REM–REM sleep cycles (CYC-1 to CYC-4) and non-REM (non-REM-1 to non-REM-4) and REM sleep (REM-1 to REM-4) episodes for nine young women during 1 night in the follicular phase and 1 night in the luteal phase

Cycle or episode	Follicular phase in minutes (SD)	Luteal phase in minutes (SD)	Statistics[a]		
CYC-1	82.0 (11.5)	70.7 (7.3)	Menstrual phase	Cycle or episode	Interaction
Non-REM-1	66.1 (10.2)	64.0 (8.8)	P $(F_{1,8})$	P $(F_{3,24})$	P $(F_{3,24})$
REM-1[a]	15.2 (9.2)	6.5 (4.1)			
CYC-2	103.3 (15.2)	100.4 (20.4)		Cycle duration	
Non-REM-2	77.1 (13.0)	72.6 (13.9)	0.032 (6.68)	0.0004 (10.71)	Not significant
REM-2	25.5 (9.0)	27.6 (9.4)			
CYC-3	107.9 (22.6)	101.6 (25.4)		Non-REM episodes	
Non-REM-3	73.7 (14.0)	72.6 (13.2)	Not significant	0.071 (2.66)	Not significant
REM-3	32.9 (15.0)	28.1 (14.6)			
CYC-4	106.9 (13.1)	96.4 (16.4)		REM episodes	
Non-REM-4	65.8 (12.8)	61.1 (5.8)	0.007 (12.92)	0.0004 (14.47)	0.035 (3.61)
REM-4	39.8 (12.2)	30.6 (10.8)			

Statistical details: P (F value) based on a two-way ANOVA for repeated measures on log-transformed values (factors: menstrual phase, cycle or episode, and their interaction).
[a] P < .05, paired t-test (performed if ANOVA revealed significant effect of 'menstrual phase' or a significant interaction).

luteal phase, and its effect may be in addition to, or in association with, other effects such as elevating body temperature. From the mid-follicular to the mid-luteal menstrual phase an increase in body temperature was associated with more stage 2 sleep, higher SFA, and elevated heart rates during sleep. The trend for a reduction in REM sleep when body temperature was higher that the authors have reported [7] is small and has not has been a consistent finding in other studies (reviewed in [1,28]). In the present analysis, the difference in REM sleep proportion was found over the first four sleep cycles but not for the whole night, suggesting an effect of sleep duration.

Although the higher luteal temperatures were sustained during the night, the SWA effect was transient (see Fig. 1), being elevated in the first cycle of the luteal phase and reduced in the second cycle when differences in SFA with the follicular phase became more pronounced. The time course of the overall decline in SWA during the first four sleep cycles with a decrease in temperature from sleep onset showed the overall monotonic slope as for a normal night [37] rather than the modification seen with sleep deprivation [39] or napping [40]. The suggestion that the higher luteal-phase temperatures during sleep may be caused by poorer sleep [30] is not supported by the present and other recent studies [1,28]. Rather, sleep in the early part of the night may be improved in the mid-luteal phase. Mid-luteal sleep did not seem to be disturbed, and reported detriments in subjective sleep occur from the late luteal phase, when the levels of the steroid hormones estrogen and progesterone are

decreasing, and during menstruation [11,12]. The higher SWA in the first cycle of the luteal phase may be attributed to the higher temperature, because studies in the rat have shown SWA to be increased with elevated body temperature [41].

The difference in temperature also could explain the SFA effects, in part [22]. Studies have shown that administration of progesterone raises body temperature in rats [42] and in human males [43] and females [21]. Compared with single doses of exogenous steroids, secretory hormone profiles during the menstrual cycle and the additional priming or interactions of progesterone with estrogen influencing the central nervous system need to be considered also. Thus, the effects may not be entirely temperature dependent, because progesterone administration induced changes in sleep in male rats without affecting body temperature [25].

There may be an interplay between progesterone and its metabolites and their effects on the sleep EEG. Progesterone has been found to induce changes in sleep in young men and in rats [24,25]. In young men, administration of progesterone at 21:30 resulted in marked increases in plasma levels of progesterone and the metabolites, allopregnanolone and pregnanolone, and led to increased stage 2 sleep and a tendency to reduced REM and stage 4 sleep [24]. There was a slight reduction in SWA and enhanced activity in the higher spindle frequency range (> 15 Hz), particularly in the first hours after progesterone administration. In contrast, elevated SWS and depressed EEG sigma power (10.26–14.1 Hz) has been reported with pregnanolone in young men [44]. Elevated SWA has been found in rats given pregnanolone [45] and with a selective $GABA_A$ agonist [46].

Sleep spindles, reflected by SFA, have been considered to indicate inhibitory activity in the central nervous system and are modulated by the circadian pacemaker [47] and the menstrual rhythm [7]. The hormonal milieu with progesterone and its metabolites, as well as estrogen, which has been shown to decrease binding to $GABA_A$ receptors [1,27], influences the balance between neural excitation and inhibition across the menstrual cycle. Even though inhibitory processes with higher SFA may be amplified in the mid-luteal phase, an increase in sleep intensity (SWA) was accommodated early in the night during normal menstrual cycles.

With the elevated body temperature in the luteal phase, the authors found that nocturnal heart rates were higher (by 3%–5%) than during the follicular phase. This finding is in contrast with studies of the effects of menstrual cycle on autonomic activity, measuring heart rate variability during the daytime, which found that heart rate was not different between the two phases [48,49]. These studies, however, did find an influence of the menstrual cycle on heart rate variability, with increased sympathetic activity at rest in the luteal versus the follicular phase, [48,49]. The largest progesterone-induced temperature effects are timed to occur during sleep, even though they seem to be independent of this state [50], possibly explaining why these studies found that the menstrual cycle had no effect on heart rate, whereas the authors' study did.

During sleep itself there are variations in heart rate as well as in blood pressure and cardiac output [51]. As reported in studies on men [51], there was a graded decrease in heart rate during non-REM sleep, followed by increases during REM sleep and wake periods. These effects result from central sympathetic nervous system activation, with depression of this system in non-REM sleep [38,52]. A gender difference in heart rate has been reported, tending to be lower in healthy men between 20 and 69 years of age than in women [53]. Along with the elevated temperature and metabolic rate in the luteal phase, heart rate and arm blood flow have been found to increased by 5% at thermoneutral conditions [32]. Possibly, with the relative lowering of the heart rate during sleep, any potential stress on the cardiovascular system with hormone- and/or temperature-associated elevations in heart rates would be reduced. Because young, healthy women have the lowest cardiovascular risk among adults [36], the small but predictable changes in heart rate may contribute to affording them more cardiovascular plasticity and protection from cardiovascular disease than men. Whether this effect on heart rate, nocturnal temperature and sleep is present with OCs, which carry a concern for cardiovascular risk, should be investigated.

Oral contraceptives

Remarkably few studies have examined the effects of OCs on sleep. Studies are also complicated by the different levels of synthetic estrogen and progestin within the various monophasic and triphasic pills. OCs contain synthetic estrogen and/or progestin, with 21 days of active hormone and the last 7 days inactive. Monophasic pills provide the same dosage of hormones through the entire active cycle; triphasic pills give different dosage levels during each week of the month, more closely duplicating the natural hormonal pattern. These "combined" pills contain estrogen and progesterone, whereas "minipills" contain only progestin. Oral contraceptives prevent ovulation by suppressing endogenous reproductive hormones so that women taking these preparations do not have normal cycles. The progestin is responsible for the contraceptive effects, and the estrogen component is included for cycle control; ethinyl estradiol (EE) is a potent suppressor of pituitary gonadotropins.

During the 40-plus years since the introduction of OCs in the 1960s, there has been a trend to lowering the dose of EE and, more recently, extending the use of EE over 84 days and 7 days of placebo. This trend developed because of a concern about the cardiovascular risks, particularly venous thromboembolism, and the side effects commonly associated with OCs, such as weight gain, nausea, breast tenderness, and bleeding, as well as greater acceptance and understanding of the OCs [54,55]. Effects of OCs on sleep may vary, depending on hormonal concentrations and combinations. Although disturbed sleep is not one of the reported symptoms in studies investigating side effects and contraceptive tolerance [56], OCs have been found to alter temperature and sleep architecture.

Oral contraceptives and body temperature

Progestins contained in the contraceptive pill seem to have the same thermogenic effect as endogenous progesterone, in that the 24-hour body temperature profiles in women taking OCs are similar to those of women in the luteal phase of ovulatory cycles. The temperature nadir occurs at a similar time [30,57] or slightly later [58]. In contrast to the rapid decrease in body temperature with the withdrawal of endogenous progesterone before menstruation [59], body temperatures in women taking OCs remain elevated at least 3 days after they have taken the final active contraceptive pill [58]. Thus synthetic steroid hormones have a more prolonged

Table 3: Changes in temperature and sleep as a function of menstrual cycle phase and oral contraceptive use and the main effects of shift-work on reproductive function in women

Condition and parameter	Effect/consequence
Women who have normal menstrual cycles	
Body temperature	LP versus FP: ↑ mean temperature, ↓ amplitude
Sleep	LP versus FP: ↑ SFA (high frequency 14.25–15.00 Hz), ↓ REM sleep (first four sleep cycles), No change in night-time SWS/SWA, ↑ daytime SWS (naps)
Heart rate during sleep	LP versus FP: ↑
Women taking oral contraceptives	
Body temperature	OC versus FP: ↑ mean temperature, ↓ amplitude
	OC versus LP: Similar temperature rhythm
Sleep	OC versus LP: ↓ SWS
	OC versus FP, LP, and placebo: ↑ Stage 2 sleep
Shift-work	
Menstrual cycle	↑ irregularities and painful menses
	↑ fertility problems
Breast cancer	↑ incidence in shift-workers

Abbreviations: FP, follicular phase; LP, luteal phase; OC, oral contraceptive; SFA, spindle frequency activity; SWA, slow wave activity; SWS, slow wave sleep.
Data from Baker F, Driver HS. Circadian rhythms, sleep and the menstrual cycle. Sleep Medicine 2007;8:613–22.

effect on body temperature rhythms than does the endogenous hormone.

Effects of oral contraceptives on sleep

In an archival analysis that compared women diagnosed as having major depressive disorder and healthy controls, but in which menstrual phase or type of contraceptive was not controlled [60], a reduction in SWS was found to be associated with OC use. OC use, however, does not seem to affect sleep efficiency [58,60] or subjective sleep quality. Reduced REM latency has been reported in healthy women taking OCs [60].

In the active phase of the OC, the proportion of stage 2 sleep was increased compared with placebo [58]. Women taking OCs also had more stage 2 sleep than the naturally cycling women in both menstrual cycle phases but had less SWS than naturally cycling women in the luteal phase. On balance, because the effects of OCs on sleep seem modest, the use of OCs to attenuate pain and mood symptoms may improve sleep in women who have premenstrual and menstrual symptoms.

Summary

In the presence of progesterone, the mid-luteal phase has an increase in body temperature that is associated with more stage 2 sleep, higher SFA, reduced REM sleep, higher SWA in the first cycle, and elevated heart rates during sleep than occur in the mid-follicular phase. A summary of changes in sleep, body temperature, and heart rate is provided in Table 3. The relative stability in all-night sleep processes may be an important factor in affording women the flexibility to adapt to the thermoregulatory and cardiovascular challenges of the menstrual cycle. Most of the studies have been conducted in young women in their early twenties. For women in their forties, waning ovarian function leads to decreased ovulation and increased cycle irregularity, which in turn may negatively influence their sleep. Changes in sleep with OCs seem small (ie, increasing stage 2 sleep), but the effects of OCs and fertility treatments on the sleep EEG and nocturnal heart rate have not been investigated.

References

[1] Driver HS, Baker FC. Menstrual factors in sleep. Sleep Med Rev 1998;2:213–29.

[2] Dzaja A, Arber S, Hislop J, et al. Women's sleep in health and disease. J Psychiatr Res 2005;39: 55–76.

[3] Manber R, Armitage R. Sex, steroids, and sleep; a review. Sleep 1999;22:540–55.

[4] Moline ML, Broch L, Zak R, et al. Sleep in women across the life cycle from adulthood through menopause. Sleep Med Rev 2003;7: 155–78.

[5] Mishell JDR. Reproductive endocrinology. In: Stenchever MA, Droegemueller W, Herbst AL, editors. Comprehensive gynecology. 4th edition. St. Louis (MO): Mosby Inc.; 2001. p. 71–124.

[6] Rousseau ME. Women's midlife health. Reframing menopause. J Nurse Midwifery 1998;43: 208–23.

[7] Driver HS, Dijk DJ, Werth E, et al. Menstrual cycle effects on sleep EEG in young healthy women. J Clin Endocrinol Metab 1996;81: 728–35.

[8] Baker FC, Waner JI, Vieira EF, et al. Sleep and 24-hour body temperatures: a comparison in young men, naturally-cycling women, and in women taking hormonal contraceptives. J Physiol 2001; 530:565–74.

[9] Baker FC, Driver HS. Self-reported sleep across the menstrual cycle in young, healthy women. J Psychosom Res 2004;56:239–43.

[10] Laessle RG, Tuschl R, Schweiger U, et al. Mood changes and physical complaints during the normal menstrual cycle in healthy young women. Psychoneuroendocrinology 1990;15:131–8.

[11] Manber R, RR Bootzin. Sleep and the menstrual cycle. Health Psychol 1997;16:209–14.

[12] National Sleep Foundation (NSF) 1998. Women and sleep poll. Available at: www.sleepfoundation. org. Accessed March 13, 2006.

[13] Patkai P, Johannson G, Post B. Mood, alertness and sympathetic-adrenal medullary activity during the menstrual cycle. Psychosom Med 1974; 36:503–12.

[14] Mauri M, Reid RL, MacLean AW. Sleep in the premenstrual phase: a self-report study of PMS patients and normal controls. Acta Psychiatr Scand 1988;78:82–6.

[15] Lamarche LJ, Driver HS, Wiebe S, et al. Nocturnal sleep, daytime sleepiness, and napping among women with significant emotional/behavioral premenstrual symptoms. J Sleep Res 2007;16(3):262–8.

[16] Baker FC, Driver HS, Rogers G, et al. High nocturnal body temperatures and disturbed sleep in women with primary dysmenorrhea. Am J Physiol 1999;277:E1013–21.

[17] Ishizuka Y, Pollak CP, Shirakawa S, et al. Sleep spindle frequency changes across the menstrual cycle. J Sleep Res 1994;3:26–9.

[18] Lee KA, Shaver JF, Giblin EC, et al. Sleep patterns related to menstrual cycle phase and premenstrual affective symptoms. Sleep 1990;13: 403–9.

[19] Baker FC, Driver HS, Paiker J, et al. Acetaminophen does not affect 24-h body temperature or sleep in the luteal phase of the menstrual cycle. J Appl Physiol 2002;92:1684–91.

[20] Parry BL, Mostofi N, LeVeau B, et al. Sleep EEG studies during early and late partial sleep deprivation in premenstrual dysphoric disorder and normal control subjects. Psychiatry Res 1999; 85:127–43.

[21] Israel SL, Schneller O. The thermogenic property of progesterone. Fertil Steril 1950;1:53–65.

[22] Deboer T. Brain temperature dependent changes in the electroencephalogram power spectrum of humans and animals. J Sleep Res 1998;7: 254–62.

[23] Trachsel L, Dijk DJ, Brunner DP, et al. Effect of zopiclone and midazolam on sleep and EEG spectra in a phase-advanced sleep schedule. Neuropsychopharmacology 1990;3:11–8.

[24] Friess E, Tagaya H, Trachsel L, et al. Progesterone-induced changes in sleep in male subjects. Am J Physiol 1997;35:E885–91.

[25] Lancel M, Faulhaber J, Holsboer F, et al. Progesterone induces changes in sleep comparable to those of agonistic GABA$_A$ receptor modulators. Am J Physiol 1996;271:E763–72.

[26] Lancel M, Faulhaber J, Schiffelholz T, et al. Allopregnanolone affects sleep in a benzodiazepine-like fashion. J Pharmacol Exp Ther 1997;282: 1213–8.

[27] Smith SS, Shen H, Gong QH, et al. Neurosteroid regulation of GABAA receptors: focus on the α4 and δ subunits. Pharmacol Ther 2007;116(1): 58–76.

[28] Baker SS, Driver HS. Circadian rhythms, sleep and the menstrual cycle. Sleep Med [special issue on circadian rhythms disorders] 2007;8(6): 613–22.

[29] Cagnacci A, Soldani R, Laughlin GA, et al. Modification of circadian body temperature rhythm during the luteal menstrual phase: role of melatonin. J Appl Physiol 1996;80:25–9.

[30] Kattapong KR, Fogg LF, Eastman C. Effect of sex, menstrual cycle phase and oral contraceptive use on circadian temperature rhythms. Chronobiol Int 1995;12:257–66.

[31] Lee KA. Circadian temperature rhythms in relation to menstrual cycle phase. J Biol Rhythms 1988;8:348–50.

[32] Hessemer V, Brück K. Influence of menstrual cycle on shivering, skin blood flow, and sweating responses measured at night. J Appl Physiol 1985;59:1902–10.

[33] Meijer GAL, Westerterp KR, Saris WHM, et al. Sleeping metabolic rate in relation to body composition and the menstrual cycle. Am J Clin Nutr 1992;55:637–40.

[34] Nakayama T, Suzuki M, Ishizuka N. Action of progesterone on preoptic thermosensitive neurones. Nature 1975;258:80.

[35] Brooks EM, Morgan AL, Pierzga JM, et al. Chronic hormone replacement therapy alters thermoregulatory and vasomotor function in postmenopausal women. J Appl Physiol 1997; 83:477–84.

[36] Larsen JA, Kadish AH. Effects of gender on cardiac arrhythmias. J Cardiovasc Electrophysiol 1998;9:655–64.

[37] Aeschbach D, Borbély AA. All-night dynamics of the human sleep EEG. J Sleep Res 1993;2:70–81.

[38] Cajochen C, Pischke J, Aeschbach D, et al. Heart rate dynamics during human sleep. Physiol Behav 1994;55:769–74.

[39] Dijk DJ, Hayes B, Czeisler CA. Dynamics of electroencephalographic sleep spindles and slow wave activity: effect of sleep deprivation. Brain Res 1993;626:190–9.

[40] Werth E, Dijk DJ, Achermann P, et al. Dynamics of the sleep EEG after an early evening nap:

experimental data and simulations. Am J Physiol 1996;271:R501–10.

[41] Gao B, Franken P, Tobler I, et al. Effect of elevated ambient temperature on sleep EEG spectra, and brain temperature in the rat. Am J Phyiol 1995;37:R1365–73.

[42] Marrone BL, Gentry RT, Wade GN. Gonadal hormones and body temperature in rats: effects of estrous cycles, castration and steroid replacement. Physiol Behav 1976;17:419–25.

[43] Rothchild I, Barnes AC. The effects of dosage, and of estrogen, androgen or salicylate administration on the degree of body temperature elevation induced by progesterone. Endocrinology 1952;50:485–96.

[44] Steiger A, Trachsel L, Guldner J, et al. Neurosteroid pregnenolone induces sleep-EEG changes in man compatible with inverse agonistic GABA$_A$-receptor modulation. Brain Res 1993;615:267–74.

[45] Lancel M, Crönlein TAM, Müller-Preuss, et al. Pregnenolone enhances EEG delta activity during non-rapid eye movement sleep in the rat, in contrast to midazolam. Brain Res 1994;646:85–94.

[46] Lancel M. The GABA$_A$ agonist THIP increases non-REM sleep and enhances non-REM sleep-specific delta activity in the rat during the dark period. Sleep 1997;20:1099–104.

[47] Dijk D-J, Shanahan TL, Duffy JF, et al. Variation of electroencephalographic activity during non-rapid eye movement and rapid eye movement sleep with phase of circadian melatonin rhythm in humans. J Physiol 1997;505:851–8.

[48] Sato N, Miyake S, Akatsu J, et al. Power spectral analysis of heart rate variability in healthy young women during the normal menstrual cycle. Psychosom Med 1995;57:331–5.

[49] Yildirir A, Kabakci G, Akgul E, et al. Effects of menstrual cycle on cardiac autonomic

innervation as assessed by heart rate variability. Ann Noninvasive Electrocardiol 2002;7:60–3.

[50] Rogacz S, Duffy JF, Ronda JM, et al. The increase in body temperature during the luteal phase of the menstrual cycle is only observed during the subjective night and is independent of sleep. Sleep Res 1988;17:395.

[51] George CF, Kryger MH. Sleep and control of heart rate. Clin Chest Med 1985;6:595–601.

[52] Bonnet MH, Arand DL. Heart rate variability: sleep stage, time of night, and arousal influences. Electroencephogr Clin Neurophysiol 1997;102:390–6.

[53] Jensen-Urstad K, Storck N, Bouvier F, et al. Heart rate variability in healthy subjects is related to age and gender. Acta Physiol Scand 1997;160:235–41.

[54] Poindexter A. The emerging use of the 20-µg oral contraceptive. Fertil Steril 2001;75:457–65.

[55] Zurawin RK, Ayensu-Coker L. Innovations in contraception: a review. Clin Obstet Gynecol 2007;50:425–39.

[56] Moreau C, Trussel J, Gilbert F, et al. Oral contraceptive tolerance. Obstet Gynecol 2007;109:1277–85.

[57] Wright KP Jr, Badia P. Effects of menstrual cycle phase and oral contraceptives on alertness, cognitive performance, and circadian rhythms during sleep deprivation. Behav Brain Res 1999;103:185–94.

[58] Baker FC, Mitchell D, Driver HS. Oral contraceptives alter sleep and raise body temperature in young women. Pflugers Arch 2001;442:729–37.

[59] Coyne MD, Kesick CM, Doherty TJ, et al. Circadian rhythm changes in core temperature over the menstrual cycle: method for noninvasive monitoring. Am J Physiol Regul Integr Comp Physiol 2000;279:R1316–20.

[60] Burdick RS, Hoffmann R, Armitage RA. Short note: oral contraceptives and sleep in depressed and healthy women. Sleep 2002;25:347–9.

SLEEP
MEDICINE
CLINICS

Sleep Med Clin 3 (2008) 13–24

Circadian Rhythms and Shift Working Women

Ari Shechter, BSc[a,b], Francine O. James, PhD[c,d],
Diane B. Boivin, MD, PhD[c,e,*]

- The central circadian clock
- Circadian and sleep/wake disorganization in shift work
- Health effects of shift work in women: menstrual cycle, fertility/reproduction, and breast cancer
  Menstrual cycle effects
  Fertility, pregnancy, and fetal development
  Breast cancer, light at night, and melatonin
- Clock genes, peripheral circadian clocks, cancer development, and shift work
- More health effects of shift work in women: nutrition, cardiovascular, and gastrointestinal disorders
  Nutrition, eating, and weight
  Cardiovascular disease and smoking
  Gastrointestinal disease
- Psychosocial and behavioral
  Domestic and family life
  Psychological effects
- Countermeasures
- Summary
- References

Shift work, defined as working on schedules that are outside of the typical nine-to-five workday, is a necessity in and a product of the 24/7, "around-the-clock" society. As recently as 2001, 30% of employed Canadian men between ages 18 and 54 years worked on nonstandard shifts [1]. Over the past few decades, the number of employed women has increased, with many working shifts. Almost 75% of women who have children younger than 16 years participate in the workforce [2], and in Canada 26% of employed women between ages 18 and 54 years are involved in shift work [1]. Shift work can result in a severe disruption of the temporal harmony between various physiologic and

This work was supported by a grant from the *Institut de recherche Robert-Sauvé en santé et en sécurité du travail* (IRSST), the Canadian Institutes of Health Research (CIHR), and the Fonds de la Recherche en Santé du Québec (FRSQ). Dr. James was supported by a fellowship from the IRSST. Dr. Boivin was supported by a career award from the CIHR.

a Centre for Study and Treatment of Circadian Rhythms, Douglas Mental Health University Institute, 6875 LaSalle Boulevard, F-1115, Montreal, Quebec, Canada H4H 1R3
b Department of Neurology and Neurosurgery, McGill University, Montreal, Quebec, Canada
c Department of Psychiatry, McGill University, Montreal, Quebec, Canada
d Centre for Study and Treatment of Circadian Rhythms, Douglas Mental Health University Institute, 6875 LaSalle Boulevard, F-1126, Montreal, Quebec, Canada H4H 1R3
e Centre for Study and Treatment of Circadian Rhythms, Douglas Mental Health University Institute, 6875 LaSalle Boulevard, F-1127, Montreal, Quebec, Canada H4H 1R3
* Corresponding author. Centre for Study and Treatment of Circadian Rhythms, Douglas Mental Health University Institute, 6875 LaSalle Boulevard, F-1127, Montreal, Quebec, Canada H4H 1R3.
E-mail address: diane.boivin@douglas.mcgill.ca (D.B. Boivin).

doi:10.1016/j.jsmc.2007.10.008

psychological rhythms, contributing to several medical and psychosocial health problems.

Women have more difficulty adapting to shift work than men [3]; they are especially at risk for several female-specific disorders, including menstrual cycle disruption, problems with fertility and reproduction, and breast cancer. The recent identification of functional clocks in tissues outside the brain suggests that circadian desynchronization experienced by shift workers is complex [4]. For women, the finding that neurons in the central 24-hour or circadian clock, the suprachiasmatic nucleus (SCN), contain receptors for estrogen and progesterone [5] indicates a functional interaction between the circadian system and the menstrual cycle that adds another level of complexity to perturbations in their circadian rhythm and sleep/wake schedule. This article explores concerns for the female shift worker, from physiologic to personal and family life, and addresses the relationship between an altered sleep/wake cycle and the circadian system as a consequence of shift work, and various associated health and psychosocial disorders.

The central circadian clock

Twenty four–hour rhythmicity is observed in many aspects of human physiology and behavior, including levels of hormone secretion [6], sleep propensity and architecture [7,8], and subjective and electroencephalographic-estimated alertness [9,10] throughout the day. Experiments identifying an intrinsic 24-hour mean activity in the neurons of the SCN together with studies showing that ablation of the SCN abrogates rhythmic behavior confirm that the SCN is the location of the central circadian clock [11]. Lesion of the SCN in nocturnal and diurnal mammals results in a loss of sleep/wake rhythmicity [12].

In humans, just as in many other organisms, the most powerful synchronizer of the central circadian clock is light [13,14]. Nonphotic synchronizers, such as exercise and melatonin, also have demonstrable effects on circadian phase, although the efficacy of these measures is less well characterized than light stimuli [15,16]. The synchronizing effect of light permits the central circadian clock to predictably coordinate internal physiology with the external environment.

The pattern of light exposure can be planned to rapidly reset the central circadian pacemaker to earlier or later phases [14]. The central circadian clock is especially sensitive to light in the 440 to 480 nm range [17,18], and therefore shorter wavelength light (eg, in the blue visible light range) can more efficiently induce significantly larger phase shifts in the temperature and melatonin rhythms than light of longer wavelengths [19,20]. The central

circadian clock is also sensitive to low intensities of light, including ordinary indoor room light [14,21], and integrates light information so that the effect of light exposure is sustained even when light is intermittently interrupted by darkness [22].

The consolidation of human sleep is the result of a complex interaction, including homeostatic and circadian components [7,8]. The circadian phase at which sleep is initiated and the time passed since a previous sleep episode interact to regulate the length of sleep [7,13]. Sleep parameters measurable with polysomnography, such as sleep propensity, sleep latency, sleep efficiency, the proportion of rapid eye movement (REM) sleep, REM sleep latency, and the fraction of sigma activity (12–15 Hz) (ie, sleep spindles) in non-REM sleep, co-vary with circadian rhythms of core body temperature (CBT) and plasma melatonin concentration [7,13,23]. Under normally entrained conditions, sleep is initiated on the falling limb of the CBT rhythm, approximately 6 hours before the temperature minimum, resulting in sleep durations approximating 8 hours [24].

Circadian and sleep/wake disorganization in shift work

A misalignment between the endogenous circadian system and the timing of sleep contributes to sleep disruption and impaired vigilance. Initiating sleep close to the temperature nadir, as is the case for many shift workers, results in abbreviated sleep length with an increase in the amount of wakefulness in the later part of the displaced sleep episode [7,13,25]. Night shift work in particular is associated with the most sleep disruption. In one study, almost one third of night shift workers reported symptoms of insomnia or excessive sleepiness, whereas these symptoms were reported in only 18% of day workers from the same sample population [26]. Data from actigraphy [27], sleep diary [26,28], and polysomnography-based studies [10,29,30] indicate a disruption in sleep associated with the night shift in particular, so that the duration of daytime sleep in night shift workers typically ranges from 4 to 7 hours.

The central circadian pacemaker does not adapt to rapid reorientations in the shift worker's sleep/wake schedule. In most individuals, circadian adjustment of cortisol and melatonin rhythms to the shifted sleep/wake schedule remains incomplete and may persist despite consecutive shifts worked [31]. Slow-rotating shift arrangements could favor some circadian realignment to the work schedule, because consecutive sleep episodes on the same schedule may lead to larger phase shifts of temperature, melatonin, and cortisol rhythms [32,33].

sleep duration is also influenced by the length and timing of shifts (eg, longer periods between shifts may foster longer sleep times) [34].

Shift work sleep disorder, as described by the International Classification of Sleep Disorders, is characterized by excessive sleepiness or insomnia [35]. Shift work–related sleep disruptions, sleep deprivation, and especially working during night hours can result in lapses in vigilance and attention, decrement in performance, and reduced cognitive throughput [10]. Recent work has used waking electroencephalographic and imaging techniques (positron emission tomography and functional MRI) to more objectively explore the effects of sleep loss on neurocognitive function [36]. In addition to the effects on workplace productivity and the safety of others, decreased vigilance and attention after a night or extended shift was shown to be associated with increased risk for motor vehicle crashes and accidents [10,37].

Health effects of shift work in women: menstrual cycle, fertility/reproduction, and breast cancer

In women who work shifts, the disruption of the circadian clock and its immediate effect on hormonal production, sleep, and clock gene expression form the background on which sex-specific issues may present themselves.

Menstrual cycle effects

Circadian rhythms, most notably the circadian curve of CBT, vary as a function of the changing hormone profile across the menstrual cycle [38], which may have implications on sleep quality [39–41]. Recently, neurons in the SCN were found to contain receptors for both estrogen and progesterone, the two main steroid hormones associated with the menstrual cycle [5], which further suggests a functional interaction between the circadian system and the menstrual cycle.

Female shift workers, who experience atypical sleep/wake schedules and a desynchronization of their daily rhythms, experience several menstrual cycle irregularities. An early study by Tasto and colleagues [42] investigated, among other health consequences, the effects of shift-working on menstrual function in a large group of nurses. The results showed that nurses on a rotating schedule experience the most disruption. Compared with all other fixed schedules (including night only), rotating nurses reported lengthened menstrual cycles, visited the clinic more often with menstrual-associated complaints, and experienced more "tension, nervousness, weakness, and sickness at menstruation." Another survey of 2264 shift-working women

found an increased occurrence of menstrual irregularity and dysmenorrhea (painful menstruation) in night-shift workers [43]. Although some investigators have found no evidence of altered menstrual cycle length or other irregularities in shift workers [44], a recent report showed that 60% of night-shift nurses who had regularly occurring cycles experienced cycles of fewer than 25 days [45]. In another study, 53% of shift-working nurses experienced altered menstrual function, with symptoms including dysmenorrhea, changes in menstrual flow and length, and duration of bleeding [46].

Hormonal changes (specifically, increased amounts of circulating progesterone) associated with the luteal, or postovulatory, phase of the menstrual cycle influence mood, circadian rhythms, and sleep, and the possibility exists that these factors may contribute to and influence shift-work maladaptation. An interaction between shift work and menstrual phase has been observed, with decreased subjective sleep quality in evening shift workers and increased irritability and decreased alertness in night-shift workers during the premenstrual (late luteal) phase compared with the follicular phase [47]. Therefore, in addition to social and familial conditions that are unique to women, the physiology of the menstrual cycle should be considered when discussing problems with shift work.

Fertility, pregnancy, and fetal development

As a consequence of alterations in their menstrual cycle, a decline in the reproductive health of night and rotating shift workers is likely. A series of studies, although not unequivocal [48], indicate that exposure to shift work [44,49], rotating shifts [50], and evening/night shifts [51] resulted in subfecundity (longer time to pregnancy). However, a meta-analysis of the literature published between 1966 and 2005 investigating the occurrence of preterm delivery, low–birth weight, and preeclampsia as a result of various unusual working conditions concluded that shift work poses only a minimal risk to the reproductive system [52]. Nevertheless, evidence suggests that shift work during pregnancy has consequences for fetal development. Fixed night work was associated with increased incidence of fetal loss [53–55], especially during the first trimester, which resulted in a 60% increased risk for miscarriage compared with workers on a day schedule [56]. Compared with day workers, young women working rotating shifts showed significant reductions in gestational age and birth weight in live births [57], although no increased risk for fetal loss was seen [54–56].

Breast cancer, light at night, and melatonin

Breast cancer, a sex hormone–dependent malignancy with a possible estrogen-related origin, is the second leading cause of death and the most frequently reported cancer in women [58]. Several epidemiologic studies, although not all [59], have found a disproportionate incidence of breast cancer in shift-working women, including those on rotating shifts [60–62] and fixed-night schedules [63–65], and in radio/telegraph operators at sea [66] and flight attendants [67]. Exposure to artificial light at night and subsequent melatonin suppression may increase the risk for breast cancer [68].

The melatonin hypothesis proposed by Stevens [69] suggests that factors (eg, magnetic fields, light at night) that decrease nocturnal melatonin levels can influence breast cancer development. Melatonin secretion is suppressed by light [70] of intensities as low as 200 lux [71]. This hypothesis is supported by evidence of melatonin's oncostatic properties. Ablation of the pineal gland (eliminating all melatonin secretion) in 20-day-old rats [72], and "functionally pinealectomizing" rats by keeping them in constant light from birth [73], significantly increased the incidence of 7,12-dimethylbenz(α)anthracene (DMBA)–induced mammary tumors. Cancer development was reduced from 95% (in DMBA + vehicle treated rats) to 25% (in DMBA + melatonin treated rats) after a 500 µg/d melatonin administration [73]. Furthermore, addition of 10^{-9} to 10^{-11} M concentrations of melatonin (ie, physiological nocturnal concentrations) significantly reduced tumor proliferation in human breast cancer cells in vitro, with a loss of this inhibition with melatonin-free medium [74]. These results were recently reinforced by Blask and colleagues [75], who first implanted human breast cancer xenografts or rat hepatomas in rats, and then perfused them with blood samples from premenopausal women. Increased cell proliferation was found in tumors perfused with melatonin-deficient blood (collected either during the day or at night after suppression by bright white light) compared with those perfused with melatonin-rich blood (collected during night time in darkness). Finally, blind women, who are less sensitive to light and therefore melatonin suppression from light exposure at night, show a reduced risk for developing breast cancer [76–78].

In shift workers, exposure to light at night was proposed as the means through which nocturnal levels of melatonin are blunted, which in turn reduces melatonin's oncostatic function in night-shift workers [79]. In a nested case-control study, almost twice as many cases of breast cancer were identified in nurses who provided a morning urine sample within the lower quartile of urinary 6-sulfatoxymelatonin concentrations compared with nurses who provided samples within the highest quartile of urinary 6-sulfatoxymelatonin concentration [80]. However, this particular study included no control for the light intensities at sampling, the number of night shifts worked before the sample, or the shape of the melatonin rhythm. A separate investigation could identify no association between 24-hour urinary 6-sulfatoxymelatonin concentration and breast cancer risk [81].

Clock genes, peripheral circadian clocks, cancer development, and shift work

Recent studies elucidating the mechanisms that underlie circadian rhythmicity bring an added dimension to our understanding of the physiological consequences of shift work. The intrinsic function of SCN neurons depends on a regulated loop of clock genes that includes *Clock* and *Bmal1*, three Period genes (*Per 1, 2, 3*), and two cryptochrome genes (*Cry 1, 2*) [4,82]. The autoregulatory loops are organized so that protein complexes of transcription factors CLOCK and BMAL1, or alternatively NPAS2 and BMAL1, promote the expression of the *Per* and *Cry* genes and clock-controlled genes that are the output of the pacemaker [82]. The PER and CRY proteins in turn heterodimerize in the cytoplasm and repress their own transcription in the nucleus. The CLOCK:BMAL1 protein dimer is also believed to promote the transcription of orphan nuclear receptors *Rev-erb* (α and β) and *Ror* (α and β) which in turn promote or repress *Bmal1* transcription [83]. The result of this organization is that a circadian rhythm in the levels of clock gene RNA and protein products can be discerned within the SCN. Rhythmicity in the expression of a modified clock protein also exists outside the SCN [84]. *Per* and *Bmal1* RNA levels peak in antiphase to each other in peripheral tissues just as in the SCN, suggesting that the molecular organization of these clocks is similar [4]. The central circadian clock of the SCN is considered dominant because it is required for coordination of clock gene expression [85,86].

Peripheral clocks have also been sampled in humans in vivo under entrainment [87–89] and constant conditions [89–91]. In human peripheral blood mononuclear cells (PBMCs) and polymorphonuclear white blood cells, *HPER1* expression peaks near the habitual time of awakening and after the peak of plasma melatonin concentration [89–91]. *HPER2* levels are also higher in the morning, near the time of habitual awakening [89,91,92]. In humans, as in animals, clock gene expression can become aligned to a shifted light/dark schedule; patterns of *HPER1* and *HPER2* expression in PBMCs are in their habitual alignment with a shifted sleep/wake schedule after 11 days of simulated night shift work in the presence of light intervention that produced shifts in the circadian rhythms of melatonin and cortisol [93]. However, shifts in the light/dark cycle resynchronize peripheral oscillators more slowly than the SCN; phase shifts in peripheral tissues may follow shifts observed in the SCN by several days [84]. As a result, a desynchronization may exist among tissues or the SCN and peripheral clocks after a shift in the light/dark schedule. Early evidence suggests that peripheral clocks are directly related to the function of their tissue [94–96]. Thus, deregulation of the local clock in addition to the relationship between central and peripheral clocks may significantly impact shift work maladjustment.

Recent evidence found a link between disrupted circadian rhythms and cancer development. Bilateral lesions of the SCN in mice caused an acceleration of tumor growth [97]. Furthermore, recent research also explored the association between clock genes and cancer development [98–101].

Mutant mice deficient in *Per2*, which is involved in the p53 apoptosis pathway, have a higher incidence of inducible cancer development from deregulation of the tumor suppressors *Cyclin D1*, *Cyclin A*, *Mdm-2*, and *Gadd45α* [98]. Three recent studies found an association between clock genes and breast cancer development in humans [99–101]. Analysis of cancerous tissue taken from women who had breast cancer showed differences in the expression of *Per1*, *Per2*, and *Per3* compared with tissue from controls [99]. An increased risk for breast cancer was detected in young (premenopausal) women who had either the homozygous or heterozygous five-repeat allele of *Per3* [100]. Finally, genotyping of women who had breast cancer and controls showed that the Ala394Thr polymorphism of the *NPAS2* gene was associated with breast cancer risk in both pre- and postmenopausal women [101]. These data suggest that a desynchronized rhythm of clock gene expression in peripheral tissue could contribute to an increased risk for cancer development.

The accumulation of information on the function of peripheral clocks will likely add to the discussion on the association between shift work and cancer. In light of the interaction between clock genes and the apoptotic pathway [98], the fact that implanted tumors grow more quickly in animals experiencing chronic disruptions of the light/darkness cycle is of particular interest to researchers [102,103]. Therefore a persistent misalignment between central and peripheral clocks, or between the central clock and the environment, may contribute to cancer risks associated with shift work.

More health effects of shift work in women: nutrition, cardiovascular, and gastrointestinal disorders

An unavoidable consequence of shift work is altered mealtimes. Changes in eating habits and other behavioral risk factors, such as smoking, in shift-working women may be related to several health outcomes, including weight gain, increased incidence of cardiovascular disease, and various gastrointestinal disorders.

Nutrition, eating, and weight

As a function of their unusual working hours and altered sleep/wake cycles, shift workers must also change their eating habits in terms of when and how they eat. Compared with day nurses, night-working nurses reported having fewer meals per day [42,104], which were replaced by more frequent snacking [42]. Night nurses often willingly eat unhealthy foods as a "means of staying awake" (eg, candy or sweets, and caffeinated beverages and energy drinks with a high sugar content) and frequently resort to eating fast food during shifts [105]. Some of these qualitative differences were quantified through comparing the nutrient adequacy rate (NAR) in female shift workers [106]. Compared with day workers, nutritional status was worse in shift workers, as illustrated with a lower and inadequate NAR for energy intake (a possible result of reduced meal frequency) [106]. These different habits may contribute to the increased weight gain [104,107] and higher body mass index (BMI) [56,106,108] reported in female shift workers. Increased BMI was also associated with longer duration of shift work [109,110]. Finally, lack of time, motivation, or energy to participate in exercise and physical fitness may also be an important contributor [105,111].

Cardiovascular disease and smoking

Cardiovascular disease is one of the leading causes of death in women, and the prognosis for women who have coronary heart disease is worse than men [112]. Although a circadian or sleep/wake cycle–dependent cause of cardiovascular disease has not been fully established, shift workers have an increased risk for cardiovascular disease [113], and atypical work schedules have been linked to increased incidence of ischemic heart disease [114], serum triglyceride levels [114,115], circulatory disease [116], and weight gain. Studies conducted specifically on female shift workers have reported an increased risk for myocardial infarction [113] and coronary heart disease [109], and also found associations between the length of shift work ($\geq$ 10 years) and high cholesterol [117], hypertension, and diabetes mellitus [109].

Results from several studies [44,51,54–56,109,110], although not all [104,118], indicate a strong association between shift-working women and smoking, contributing to the increased prevalence of cardiovascular disease. A recent proposal is that, rather than being considered a confounding factor to be corrected for in analyses, smoking should be viewed as a "factor in the causative pathway" from shift work to cardiovascular disease [119]. A reasonable assumption is that nicotine, a stimulant of the central nervous system, is used in many night and shift workers to counteract increased sleepiness and decreased vigilance [120]. Moreover, a recent study shows the negative impact of smoking on polysomnography parameters, including increased sleep-onset latency and stage 1 sleep, with decreased total sleep time and slow-wave sleep [121]. Therefore, nicotine (and also caffeine [122]) may be an arm in a feedback loop that continually perturbs sleep in shift-working individuals.

Gastrointestinal disease

Gastrointestinal diseases are a serious medical problem for women, and some, such as irritable bowel syndrome (IBS), occur more frequently in women than men (see the article by Shaver elsewhere in this issue). Furthermore, various gastrointestinal complaints have been disproportionately reported in shift workers [113], with diet and eating habits possibly contributing. Female shift workers reported an increased incidence of gastrointestinal symptoms (eg, peptic ulcer, gastritis, and gastroduodenitis) [123], functional bowel disorders (eg, IBS, abdominal bloating, constipation, dyspepsia, and diarrhea), and increased risk for colorectal cancer [124], with rotating nurses often experiencing more of these symptoms than their day-working counterparts [42,118,125]. Evidence from the past decade indicates a positive correlation [125] or causal relationship [126] between sleep disturbances and gastrointestinal symptoms, an association that is important for shift workers' health.

A proposed but controversial [127] theory is that gastrointestinal symptoms are influenced by the menstrual cycle [128], which is also a consideration for shift-working women. Two recent studies, one with all female participants [129], advocate melatonin as a therapeutic agent for the treatment of gastrointestinal symptoms [129,130]. Each study reported that, compared with placebo, melatonin was successful in alleviating IBS symptom scores without affecting nocturnal subjective [129,130] or objective [130] sleep parameters. Melatonin

treatment as a sleep aid and countermeasure used by shift workers is discussed later.

Psychosocial and behavioral

An unfortunate but inevitable consequence of shift work is a disruption of social, familial, and psychological well-being. This effect is often particularly deleterious in women shift workers who, because of societal expectations or personal preference, continue to be responsible for various domestic duties.

Domestic and family life

In addition to a full-time work schedule of approximately 35 to 40 hours per week, female health care shift workers reported spending an additional 30 hours per week on domestic responsibilities and housework [117]. Shift-working women living with their spouse and/or children are especially vulnerable to sleep disturbances. A comparison of daytime sleep episodes in unmarried night shift nurses and night nurses who were married with two children showed that the latter had a reduced sleep duration of approximately 1.5 hours [131]. These workers, because of various maternal obligations, were found to postpone their bedtime to later in the day after the end of their night shifts (eg, to 10:00 AM) [131]. This delay can lead to further reduction of sleep duration and increased sleep-onset latency [24]. Additionally, a shorter and often interrupted daytime sleep episode (eg, because of preparing or participating in the midday meal [131]) has been reported to be another factor contributing to disturbed sleep in shift-working mothers [131,132].

Qualitative assessments show that family relationships are also affected by shift work. Female night workers complain of a lack of time for children [117] and, compared with day/afternoon workers, rotating and night nurses reported most complaints from their spouses, a lower level of satisfying time spent with spouses, and more interference with sexual activities [42]. An innovative line of investigation explored the relationship between parental work schedules and sleep in adolescent children, and concluded that shift work had a negative impact on sleep patterns in these children, although polysomnography recordings were not conducted [133]. Along these lines, maternal shift work during the first few years of a child's life has been associated with negative childhood cognitive development [134].

Psychological effects

A nonadditive interaction between circadian and sleep/wake processes influences subjective mood fluctuations across the 24-hour day [135]. Circadian processes indicate that subjective mood is lowest at times surrounding the nadir of the CBT curve, and the precise timing of this mood rhythm is modulated by the duration of prior wakefulness [135]. Because shift workers, especially those with night shifts who are working during the declining limb and trough of the endogenous CBT curve, typically experience a misalignment between their sleep/wake and circadian systems and also report increased sleep disruption, they are at risk for developing mood and psychological disorders. Mood also fluctuates across the menstrual cycle, with complaints associated with the late luteal phase in women who experience the broadly defined premenstrual syndrome, and surely those who have the more severe premenstrual dysphoric disorder characterized by the *Diagnostic and Statistical Manual of Mental Disorders, Fourth Edition* [136] (see the article by Baker and colleagues elsewhere in this issue). Therefore, physiologic and hormonal variations across the menstrual cycle in female shift workers may further modulate the interaction known to exist between sleep/wake and circadian processes to significantly influence mood in these women.

Surveys of nurses determined that night and rotating shift workers scored higher on measures of tension–anxiety [42,137] and that night nurses had significantly higher scores of depression, anger-hostility, fatigue, and confusion than those working other shifts [137]. Assessing quality of life scores through questionnaire, Kaliterna and colleagues [111] suggest that, despite nonsignificant differences in overall happiness and life satisfaction between shift and non–shift workers, night work is an important factor influencing various quality of life indices. For example, compared with day-shift workers, night workers reported fewer opportunities to improve their psychological "being" (ie, psychological health, cognitions, feelings, and personal evaluations) and personal growth, and gave a lower rating on community belonging. Compared with non–shift workers, these night workers also reported lower scores on the spiritual "being" subdomain (eg, personal values, standards, spiritual beliefs) and fewer opportunities to improve their practical "becoming" (eg, domestic activities, school, volunteer work) [111].

Countermeasures

Strategies are available to promote circadian adaptation to the work schedule, increase total sleep time, or increase alertness and performance levels at work. Improving the alignment of the central circadian clock, such as with light or taking naps, can result in an extension of the sleep period and better reported daytime sleep quality [138,139].

Enlightened scheduling practices that anticipate the effects of circadian physiology and extended work hours can promote an increase in sleep time and reduce the number of serious work-related errors [140]. Shaping the pattern of light exposure with combinations of phototherapy and light avoidance (eg, bright light at work, wearing dark glasses on the commute home, sleeping in a darkened room) can shift the circadian pacemaker to a more appropriate phase [31,32] and may counteract the potential effects of chronic circadian misalignment on central and peripheral clock function. Attempts to reduce the likelihood of sleep debt may be a healthy and beneficial approach to coping with shift work. Supplementing abbreviated sleep episodes with nap opportunities can counteract decreases in vigilance during work periods [141,142] and may have long-term benefits, because chronically abbreviated sleep augments the likelihood of obesity [143,144], hypertension [145], and endocrine deregulation [144]. Under medical supervision, prescribed hypnotics may be a short-term solution to increase the total duration of sleep per workday [139,146]. The hypnotic effect of melatonin has been effectively used to increase sleepiness levels and total sleep time [139,147].

Shift workers may also use the direct effect of light, including blue light in the 440 to 480 nm range, to increase objective and subjective measures of alertness and performance during shifts [148,149]. Various stimulants, including caffeine and modafinil, may also increase a worker's alertness during shifts [139,146,150].

Summary

Shift-working women, who compose a significant portion of the shift-working population, experience an acute circadian disruption that can have several effects on their health and well-being, including but probably not limited to disturbed sleep, increased gastrointestinal disorders and cardiovascular disease, nutritional deficit or weight gain, deteriorations in interpersonal and domestic life, and changes in mood and quality of life indices. Emerging evidence points to a functional interaction between the circadian system and the menstrual cycle, and therefore shift-working women are also at risk for developing menstrual cycle irregularities and problems with reproductive health. Additionally, exposure to light at night and subsequent melatonin suppression, and disrupted clock gene expression, may contribute to the increased incidence of breast cancer seen in shift-working women. Various tools have been developed to help shift workers become better adapted to their altered sleep/wake cycles, although strategies specifically for women are rare. Unfortunately, a relative dearth exists of studies investigating sleep in women, because researchers often exclude menstruating women from their experiments as a result of the "confounding" effects of the menstrual cycle [151]. To form a more complete picture, research must explore the influence of and interactions among the menstrual cycle, sleep, and circadian rhythms. Along these lines, new research conducted on shift-working women, and ultimately workforce administrative decisions, scheduling, and policy-making, should take into account the specific issues of female shift workers.

References

[1] Shields M. Shift work and health. Health Reports (Statistics Canada report 82-003) 2002; 13(4):11–33.

[2] Almey M. Women in the workplace. Women in Canada: Work Chapter Updates (Statistics Canada, Catalogue 89F0133) 2006;1–23.

[3] Tepas DI, Duchon JC, Gersten AH. Shiftwork and the older worker. Exp Aging Res 1993; 19(4):295–320.

[4] Lamont EW, James FO, Boivin DB, et al. From circadian clock gene expression to pathologies. Sleep Med 2007;8(6):547–56.

[5] Kruijver FP, Swaab DF. Sex hormone receptors are present in the human suprachiasmatic nucleus. Neuroendocrinology 2002;75(5): 296–305.

[6] Boivin DB. Disturbances of hormonal circadian rhythms in shift workers. In: Cardinali DP, Pandi-Perumal SR, editors. Neuroendocrine correlates of sleep/wakefulness. New York: Springer; 2005. p. 325–54.

[7] Dijk DJ, Franken P. Interaction of sleep homeostasis and circadian rhythmicity: dependent or independent systems?. In: Kryger MH, Roth T, Dement WC, editors. Principles and practice of sleep medicine. Philadelphia: Elsevier; 2005. p. 418–34.

[8] Borbely AA, Achermann P. Sleep homeostasis and models of sleep regulation. J Biol Rhythms 1999;14(6):557–68.

[9] Van Dongen HPA, Dinges DF. Circadian rhythms in sleepiness, alertness, and performance. In: Kryger MH, Roth T, Dement WC, editors. Principles and practice of sleep medicine. Philadelphia: Elsevier; 2005. p. 435–43.

[10] Akerstedt T. Altered sleep/wake patterns and mental performance. Physiol Behav 2007; 90(2–3):209–18.

[11] Silver R, Schwartz WJ. The Suprachiasmatic nucleus is a functionally heterogeneous timekeeping organ. Methods Enzymol 2005;393:451–65.

[12] Mistlberger RE. Circadian regulation of sleep in mammals: role of the suprachiasmatic nucleus. Brain Res Brain Res Rev 2005;49(3):429–54.

[13] Czeisler CA, Buxton OM, Khalsa SB. The human circadian timing system and sleep-wake regulation. In: Kryger M, Roth T, Dement WC, editors. Principles and practice of sleep medicine. Philadelphia: Elsevier; 2005.

[14] Duffy JF, Wright KP Jr. Entrainment of the human circadian system by light. J Biol Rhythms 2005;20(4):326–38.

[15] Arendt J, Skene DJ. Melatonin as a chronobiotic. Sleep Med Rev 2005;9(1):25–39.

[16] Mistlberger RE, Skene DJ. Nonphotic entrainment in humans? J Biol Rhythms 2005;20(4): 339–52.

[17] Thapan K, Arendt J, Skene DJ. An action spectrum for melatonin suppression: evidence for a novel non-rod, non-cone photoreceptor system in humans. J Physiol 2001;535(Pt 1): 261–7.

[18] Brainard GC, Hanifin JP, Greeson JM, et al. Action spectrum for melatonin regulation in humans: evidence for a novel circadian photoreceptor. J Neurosci 2001;21(16): 6405–12.

[19] Lockley SW, Brainard GC, Czeisler CA. High sensitivity of the human circadian melatonin rhythm to resetting by short wavelength light. J Clin Endocrinol Metab 2003;88(9):4502–5.

[20] Revell VL, Arendt J, Terman M, et al. Short-wavelength sensitivity of the human circadian system to phase-advancing light. J Biol Rhythms 2005;20(3):270–2.

[21] Boivin DB, James FO. Circadian adaptation to night-shift work by judicious light and darkness exposure. J Biol Rhythms 2002;17(6):556–67.

[22] Gronfier C, Wright KP Jr, Kronauer RE, et al. Efficacy of a single sequence of intermittent bright light pulses for delaying circadian phase in humans. Am J Physiol Endocrinol Metab 2004; 287(1):E174–81.

[23] Wyatt JK, Ritz-De Cecco A, Czeisler CA, et al. Circadian temperature and melatonin rhythms, sleep, and neurobehavioral function in humans living on a 20-h day. Am J Physiol 1999;277(4 Pt 2):R1152–63.

[24] Dijk DJ, von Schantz M. Timing and consolidation of human sleep, wakefulness, and performance by a symphony of oscillators. J Biol Rhythms 2005;20(4):279–90.

[25] Akerstedt T, Hume K, Minors D, et al. Regulation of sleep and naps on an irregular schedule. Sleep 1993;16(8):736–43.

[26] Drake CL, Roehrs T, Richardson G, et al. Shift work sleep disorder: prevalence and consequences beyond that of symptomatic day workers. Sleep 2004;27(8):1453–62.

[27] Burch JB, Yost MG, Johnson W, et al. Melatonin, sleep, and shift work adaptation. J Occup Environ Med 2005;47(9):893–901.

[28] Ursin R, Bjorvatn B, Holsten F. Sleep duration, subjective sleep need, and sleep habits of 40- to 45-year-olds in the Hordaland Health Study. Sleep 2005;28(10):1260–9.

[29] Torsvall L, Akerstedt T, Gillander K, et al. Sleep on the night shift: 24-hour EEG monitoring of spontaneous sleep/wake behavior. Psychophysiology 1989;26(3):352–8.

[30] Lockley SW, Cronin JW, Evans EE, et al. Effect of reducing interns' weekly work hours on sleep and attentional failures. N Engl J Med 2004; 351(18):1829–37.

[31] Boivin DB, James FO. Light treatment and circadian adaptation to shift work. Ind Health 2005; 43(1):34–48.

[32] Horowitz TS, Cade BE, Wolfe JM, et al. Efficacy of bright light and sleep/darkness scheduling in alleviating circadian maladaptation to night work. Am J Physiol Endocrinol Metab 2001; 281(2):E384–91.

[33] Hennig J, Kieferdorf P, Moritz C, et al. Changes in cortisol secretion during shiftwork: implications for tolerance to shiftwork? Ergonomics 1998;41(5):610–21.

[34] Kurumatani N, Koda S, Nakagiri S, et al. The effects of frequently rotating shiftwork on sleep and the family life of hospital nurses. Ergonomics 1994;37(6):995–1007.

[35] American Academy of Sleep Medicine. International classification of sleep disorders, revised: diagnostic and coding manual. Chicago: American Academy of Sleep Medicine; 2001.

[36] Boonstra TW, Stins JF, Daffertshofer A, et al. Effects of sleep deprivation on neural functioning: an integrative review. Cell Mol Life Sci 2007;64(7–8):934–46.

[37] Sigurdson K, Ayas NT. The public health and safety consequences of sleep disorders. Can J Physiol Pharmacol 2007;85(1):179–83.

[38] Baker FC, Driver HS. Circadian rhythms, sleep, and the menstrual cycle. Sleep Med 2007;8(6): 613–22.

[39] Shechter A, Boivin DB. Thermoregulatory changes across the menstrual cycle: implications for sleep quality. Presented at the 21st Annual Meeting of the Associated Professional Sleep Societies 2007. Minneapolis, June 9–14, 2007.

[40] Baker FC, Driver HS, Rogers GG, et al. High nocturnal body temperatures and disturbed sleep in women with primary dysmenorrhea. Am J Physiol 1999;277(6 Pt 1):E1013–21.

[41] Shibui K, Uchiyama M, Okawa M, et al. Diurnal fluctuation of sleep propensity and hormonal secretion across the menstrual cycle. Biol Psychiatry 2000;48(11):1062–8.

[42] Tasto DL, Colligan MJ, Skjei EW, et al. Health consequences of shift work. In: DHEW (NIOSH) Publication No. 78-154. Cincinnati (OH): US Dept of Health, Education, and Welfare; 1978.

[43] Uehata T, Sasakawa N. The fatigue and maternity disturbances of night workwomen. J Hum Ergol (Tokyo) 1982;11(Suppl 4):65–74.

[44] Bisanti L, Olsen J, Basso O, et al. Shift work and subfecundity: a European multicenter study. European Study Group on Infertility and Subfecundity. J Occup Environ Med 1996;38(4): 352–8.

[45] Chung FF, Yao CC, Wan GH. The associations between menstrual function and life style/ working conditions among nurses in Taiwan. J Occup Health 2005;47(2):149–56.

[46] Labyak S, Lava S, Turek F, et al. Effects of shift-work on sleep and menstrual function in nurses. Health Care Women Int 2002;23(6–7): 703–14.

[47] Totterdell P, Spelten E, Pokorski J. The effects of nightwork on psychological changes during the menstrual cycle. J Adv Nurs 1995;21(5): 996–1005.

[48] Tuntiseranee P, Olsen J, Geater A, et al. Are long working hours and shiftwork risk factors for subfecundity? A study among couples from southern Thailand. Occup Environ Med 1998; 55(2):99–105.

[49] Spinelli A, Figa-Talamanca I, Osborn J. Time to pregnancy and occupation in a group of Italian women. Int J Epidemiol 1997;26(3):601–9.

[50] Ahlborg G Jr, Axelsson G, Bodin L. Shift work, nitrous oxide exposure and subfertility among Swedish midwives. Int J Epidemiol 1996; 25(4):783–90.

[51] Zhu JL, Hjollund NH, Boggild H, et al. Shift work and subfecundity: a causal link or an artefact? Occup Environ Med 2003;60(9):E12.

[52] Bonzini M, Coggon D, Palmer KT. Risk of prematurity, low birthweight and pre-eclampsia in relation to working hours and physical activities: a systematic review. Occup Environ Med 2007;64(4):228–43.

[53] Infante-Rivard C, David M, Gauthier R, et al. Pregnancy loss and work schedule during pregnancy. Epidemiology 1993;4(1):73–5.

[54] Zhu JL, Hjollund NH, Andersen AM, et al. Shift work, job stress, and late fetal loss: the National Birth Cohort in Denmark. J Occup Environ Med 2004;46(11):1144–9.

[55] Zhu JL, Hjollund NH, Olsen J. Shift work, duration of pregnancy, and birth weight: the National Birth Cohort in Denmark. Am J Obstet Gynecol 2004;191(1):285–91.

[56] Whelan EA, Lawson CC, Grajewski B, et al. Work schedule during pregnancy and spontaneous abortion. Epidemiology 2007;18(3):350–5.

[57] Xu X, Ding M, Li B, et al. Association of rotating shiftwork with preterm births and low birth weight among never smoking women textile workers in China. Occup Environ Med 1994; 51(7):470–4.

[58] Cos S, Gonzalez A, Martinez-Campa C, et al. Estrogen-signaling pathway: a link between breast cancer and melatonin oncostatic actions. Cancer Detect Prev 2006;30(2):118–28.

[59] O'Leary ES, Schoenfeld ER, Stevens RG, et al. Shift work, light at night, and breast cancer on Long Island, New York. Am J Epidemiol 2006;164(4):358–66.

[60] Schernhammer ES, Kroenke CH, Dowsett M, et al. Urinary 6-sulfatoxymelatonin levels and their correlations with lifestyle factors and steroid hormone levels. J Pineal Res 2006;40(2):116–24.

[61] Schernhammer ES, Kroenke CH, Laden F, et al. Night work and risk of breast cancer. Epidemiology 2006;17(1):108–11.

[62] Schernhammer ES, Laden F, Speizer FE, et al. Rotating night shifts and risk of breast cancer in women participating in the nurses' health study. J Natl Cancer Inst 2001;93(20):1563–8.

[63] Lie JA, Roessink J, Kjaerheim K. Breast cancer and night work among Norwegian nurses. Cancer Causes Control 2006;17(1):39–44.

[64] Davis S, Mirick DK, Stevens RG. Night shift work, light at night, and risk of breast cancer. J Natl Cancer Inst 2001;93(20):1557–62.

[65] Hansen J. Increased breast cancer risk among women who work predominantly at night. Epidemiology 2001;12(1):74–7.

[66] Tynes T, Hannevik M, Andersen A, et al. Incidence of breast cancer in Norwegian female radio and telegraph operators. Cancer Causes Control 1996;7(2):197–204.

[67] Rafnsson V, Tulinius H, Jonasson JG, et al. Risk of breast cancer in female flight attendants: a population-based study (Iceland). Cancer Causes Control 2001;12(2):95–101.

[68] Stevens RG, Davis S, Thomas DB, et al. Electric power, pineal function, and the risk of breast cancer. FASEB J 1992;6(3):853–60.

[69] Stevens RG. Electric power use and breast cancer: a hypothesis. Am J Epidemiol 1987;125(4):556–61.

[70] Lewy AJ, Wehr TA, Goodwin FK, et al. Light suppresses melatonin secretion in humans. Science 1980;210(4475):1267–9.

[71] Brainard GC, Rollag MD, Hanifin JP. Photic regulation of melatonin in humans: ocular and neural signal transduction. J Biol Rhythms 1997;12(6):537–46.

[72] Tamarkin L, Cohen M, Roselle D, et al. Melatonin inhibition and pinealectomy enhancement of 7,12-dimethylbenz(a)anthracene-induced mammary tumors in the rat. Cancer Res 1981;41(11 Pt 1):4432–6.

[73] Shah PN, Mhatre MC, Kothari LS. Effect of melatonin on mammary carcinogenesis in intact and pinealectomized rats in varying photoperiods. Cancer Res 1984;44(8):3403–7.

[74] Hill SM, Blask DE. Effects of the pineal hormone melatonin on the proliferation and morphological characteristics of human breast cancer cells (MCF-7) in culture. Cancer Res 1988;48(21):6121–6.

[75] Blask DE, Brainard GC, Dauchy RT, et al. Melatonin-depleted blood from premenopausal women exposed to light at night stimulates growth of human breast cancer xenografts in nude rats. Cancer Res 2005;65(23):11174–84.

[76] Verkasalo PK, Pukkala E, Stevens RG, et al. Inverse association between breast cancer incidence and degree of visual impairment in Finland. Br J Cancer 1999;80(9):1459–60.

[77] Hahn RA. Profound bilateral blindness and the incidence of breast cancer. Epidemiology 1991;2(3):208–10.

[78] Kliukiene J, Tynes T, Andersen A. Risk of breast cancer among Norwegian women with visual impairment. Br J Cancer 2001;84(3):397–9.

[79] Schernhammer ES, Rosner B, Willett WC, et al. Epidemiology of urinary melatonin in women and its relation to other hormones and night work. Cancer Epidemiol Biomarkers Prev 2004;13(6):936–43.

[80] Schernhammer ES, Hankinson SE. Urinary melatonin levels and breast cancer risk. J Natl Cancer Inst 2005;97(14):1084–7.

[81] Travis RC, Allen DS, Fentiman IS, et al. Melatonin and breast cancer: a prospective study. Natl Cancer Inst 2004;96(6):475–82.

[82] Levi F, Schibler U. Circadian rhythms: mechanisms and therapeutic implications. Annu Rev Pharmacol Toxicol 2007;47:593–628.

[83] Guillaumond F, Dardente H, Giguere V, et al. Differential control of Bmal1 circadian transcription by REV-ERB and ROR nuclear receptors. J Biol Rhythms 2005;20(5):391–403.

[84] Yamazaki S, Numano R, Abe M, et al. Resetting central and peripheral circadian oscillators in transgenic rats. Science 2000;288(5466):682–5.

[85] Yoo SH, Yamazaki S, Lowrey PL, et al. PERIOD2: LUCIFERASE real-time reporting of circadian dynamics reveals persistent circadian oscillations in mouse peripheral tissues. Proc Natl Acad Sci U S A 2004;101(15):5339–46.

[86] Pando MP, Morse D, Cermakian N, et al. Phenotypic rescue of a peripheral clock genetic defect via SCN hierarchical dominance. Cell 2002;110(1):107–17.

[87] Teboul M, Barrat-Petit MA, Li XM, et al. Atypical patterns of circadian clock gene expression in human peripheral blood mononuclear cells. Mol Med 2005;83(9):693–9.

[88] Bjarnason GA, Jordan RC, Wood PA, et al. Circadian expression of clock genes in human oral mucosa and skin: association with specific cell-cycle phases. Am J Pathol 2001;158(5):1793–801.

[89] James FO, Boivin DB, Charbonneau S, et al. Expression of clock genes in human peripheral blood mononuclear cells throughout the circadian and sleep/wake cycles. Chronobiol Int in press.

[90] Kusanagi H, Mishima K, Satoh K, et al. Similar profiles in human period1 gene expression in peripheral mononuclear and polymorphonuclear cells. Neurosci Lett 2004;365(2):124–7.

[91] Boivin DB, James FO, Wu A, et al. Circadian clock genes oscillate in human peripheral blood mononuclear cells. Blood 2003;102(12):4143–5.

[92] Takata M, Burioka N, Ohdo S, et al. Daily expression of mRNAs for the mammalian Clock genes Per2 and clock in mouse suprachiasmatic nuclei and liver and human peripheral blood mononuclear cells. Jpn J Pharmacol 2002; 90(3):263–9.

[93] James FO, Cermakian N, Boivin DB. Circadian rhythms of melatonin, cortisol and clock gene expression during simulated night shift work. Sleep 2007;30(11):1427–36.

[94] Zvonic S, Ptitsyn AA, Conrad SA, et al. Characterization of peripheral circadian clocks in adipose tissues. Diabetes 2006;55(4):962–70.

[95] Durgan DJ, Trexler NA, Egbejimi O, et al. The circadian clock within the cardiomyocyte is essential for responsiveness of the heart to fatty acids. J Biol Chem 2006;281(34):24254–69.

[96] Sun Y, Yang Z, Niu Z, et al. MOP3, a component of the molecular clock, regulates the development of B cells. Immunology 2006;119(4): 451–60.

[97] Filipski E, King VM, Li X, et al. Host circadian clock as a control point in tumor progression. J Natl Cancer Inst 2002;94(9):690–7.

[98] Fu L, Pelicano H, Liu J, et al. The circadian gene Period2 plays an important role in tumor suppression and DNA damage response in vivo. Cell 2002;111(1):41–50.

[99] Chen ST, Choo KB, Hou MF, et al. Deregulated expression of the PER1, PER2 and PER3 genes in breast cancers. Carcinogenesis 2005;26(7): 1241–6.

[100] Zhu Y, Brown HN, Zhang Y, et al. Period3 structural variation: a circadian biomarker associated with breast cancer in young women. Cancer Epidemiol Biomarkers Prev 2005; 14(1):268–70.

[101] Zhu Y, Stevens RG, Leaderer D, et al. Non-synonymous polymorphisms in the circadian gene NPAS2 and breast cancer risk. Breast Cancer Res Treat, in press

[102] Filipski E, Delaunay F, King VM, et al. Effects of chronic jet lag on tumor progression in mice. Cancer Res 2004;64(21):7879–85.

[103] Filipski E, Li XM, Levi F. Disruption of circadian coordination and malignant growth. Cancer Causes Control 2006;17(4):509–14.

[104] Geliebter A, Gluck ME, Tanowitz M, et al. Work-shift period and weight change. Nutrition 2000; 16(1):27–9.

[105] Persson M, Martensson J. Situations influencing habits in diet and exercise among nurses working night shift. J Nurs Manag 2006;14(5): 414–23.

[106] Sudo N, Ohtsuka R. Nutrient intake among female shift workers in a computer factory in Japan. Int J Food Sci Nutr 2001;52(4): 367–78.

[107] Niedhammer I, Lert F, Marne MJ. Prevalence of overweight and weight gain in relation to night work in a nurses' cohort. Int J Obes Relat Metab Disord 1996;20(7):625–33.

[108] Ha M, Park J. Shiftwork and metabolic risk factors of cardiovascular disease. J Occup Health 2005;47(2):89–95.

[109] Kawachi I, Colditz GA, Stampfer MJ, et al. Prospective study of shift work and risk of coronary heart disease in women. Circulation 1995; 92(11):3178–82.

[110] Chen H, Schernhammer E, Schwarzschild MA, et al. A prospective study of night shift work, sleep duration, and risk of Parkinson's disease. Am J Epidemiol 2006;163(8):726–30.

[111] Kaliterna LL, Prizmic LZ, Zganec N. Quality of life, life satisfaction and happiness in shift- and non-shiftworkers. Rev Sauda Publica 2004; 38(Suppl):3–10.

[112] Mosca L, Manson JE, Sutherland SE, et al. Cardiovascular disease in women: a statement for healthcare professionals from the American Heart Association. Writing Group. Circulation 1997;96(7):2468–82.

[113] Knutsson A. Health disorders of shift workers. Occup Med (Lond) 2003;53(2):103–8.

[114] Knutsson A, Akerstedt T, Jonsson BG. Prevalence of risk factors for coronary artery disease among day and shift workers. Scand J Work Environ Health 1988;14(5):317–21.

[115] Romon M, Nuttens MC, Fievet C, et al. Increased triglyceride levels in shift workers. Am J Med 1992;93(3):259–62.

[116] Tuchsen F, Hannerz H, Burr H. A 12 year prospective study of circulatory disease among Danish shift workers. Occup Environ Med 2006;63(7):451–5.

[117] Portela LF, Rotenberg L, Waissmann W. Self-reported health and sleep complaints among nursing personnel working under 12 h night and day shifts. Chronobiol Int 2004;21(6): 859–70.

[118] Sveinsdottir H. Self-assessed quality of sleep, occupational health, working environment, illness experience and job satisfaction of female nurses working different combination of shifts. Scand J Caring Sci 2006;20(2):229–37.

[119] van Amelsvoort LG, Jansen NW, Kant I. Smoking among shift workers: more than a confounding factor. Chronobiol Int 2006;23(6):1105–13.

[120] Kageyama T, Kobayashi T, Nishikido N, et al. Associations of sleep problems and recent life events with smoking behaviors among female staff nurses in Japanese hospitals. Ind Health 2005;43(1):133–41.

[121] Zhang L, Samet J, Caffo B, et al. Cigarette smoking and nocturnal sleep architecture. Am J Epidemiol 2006;164(6):529–37.

[122] Carrier J, Fernandez-Bolanos M, Robillard R, et al. Effects of caffeine are more marked on daytime recovery sleep than on nocturnal sleep. Neuropsychopharmacology 2007;32:964–72.

[123] Costa G. The impact of shift and night work on health. Appl Ergon 1996;27(1):9–16.

[124] Schernhammer ES, Laden F, Speizer FE, et al. Night-shift work and risk of colorectal cancer

in the nurses' health study. J Natl Cancer Inst 2003;95(11):825–8.

[125] Lu WZ, Gwee KA, Ho KY. Functional bowel disorders in rotating shift nurses may be related to sleep disturbances. Eur J Gastroenterol Hepatol 2006;18(6):623–7.

[126] Jarrett M, Heitkemper M, Cain KC, et al. Sleep disturbance influences gastrointestinal symptoms in women with irritable bowel syndrome. Dig Dis Sci 2000;45(5):952–9.

[127] Degen LP, Phillips SF. Variability of gastrointestinal transit in healthy women and men. Gut 1996;39(2):299–305.

[128] Heitkemper MM, Cain KC, Jarrett ME, et al. Symptoms across the menstrual cycle in women with irritable bowel syndrome. Am J Gastroenterol 2003;98(2):420–30.

[129] Lu WZ, Gwee KA, Moochhalla S, et al. Melatonin improves bowel symptoms in female patients with irritable bowel syndrome: a double-blind placebo-controlled study. Aliment Pharmacol Ther 2005;22(10):927–34.

[130] Song GH, Leng PH, Gwee KA, et al. Melatonin improves abdominal pain in irritable bowel syndrome patients who have sleep disturbances: a randomised, double blind, placebo controlled study. Gut 2005;54(10):1402–7.

[131] Gadbois C, Reinberg A, Vieux N, et al. Women on night shift: interdependence of sleep and Off-The-Job activities. In: Reinberg A, Vieux N, Andlauer P, editors. Night and shift work biological and social aspects. Toronto: Pergamon Press; 1980. p. 223–7.

[132] Rotenberg L, Moreno C, Portela LF, et al. The amount of diurnal sleep, and complaints of fatigue and poor sleep, in Night-Working women: the effects of having children. Biol Rhythm Res 2000;31(4):515–22.

[133] Radosevic-Vidacek B, Koscec A. Shiftworking families: parents' working schedule and sleep patterns of adolescents attending school in two shifts. Rev Saude Publica 2004;38(Suppl): 38–46.

[134] Han WJ. Maternal nonstandard work schedules and child cognitive outcomes. Child Dev 2005; 76(1):137–54.

[135] Boivin DB, Czeisler CA, Dijk DJ, et al. Complex interaction of the sleep-wake cycle and circadian phase modulates mood in healthy subjects. Arch Gen Psychiatry 1997;54(2): 145–52.

[136] Di Giulio G, Reissing ED. Premenstrual dysphoric disorder: prevalence, diagnostic considerations, and controversies. J Psychosom Obstet Gynaecol 2006;27(4):201–10.

[137] Munakata M, Ichi S, Nunokawa T, et al. Influence of night shift work on psychologic state and cardiovascular and neuroendocrine responses in healthy nurses. Hypertens Res 2001;24(1):25–31.

[138] Crowley SJ, Lee C, Tseng CY, et al. Complete or partial circadian re-entrainment improves performance, alertness, and mood during night-shift work. Sleep 2004;27(6):1077–87.

[139] Boivin DB, Tremblay GM, James FO. Working on atypical schedules. Sleep Med 2007;8(6):578–89.

[140] Lockley SW, Landrigan CP, Barger LK, et al. When policy meets physiology: the challenge of reducing resident work hours. Clin Orthop Relat Res 2006;449:116–27.

[141] Schweitzer PK, Randazzo AC, Stone K, et al. Laboratory and field studies of naps and caffeine as practical countermeasures for sleep-wake problems associated with night work. Sleep 2006;29(1):39–50.

[142] Sallinen M, Harma M, Akerstedt T, et al. Promoting alertness with a short nap during a night shift. J Sleep Res 1998;7(4):240–7.

[143] Gangwisch JE, Malaspina D, Boden-Albala B, et al. Inadequate sleep as a risk factor for obesity: analyses of the NHANES I. Sleep 2005; 28(10):1289–96.

[144] Knutson KL, Spiegel K, Penev P, et al. The metabolic consequences of sleep deprivation. Sleep Med Rev 2007;11(3):163–78.

[145] Gottlieb DJ, Redline S, Nieto FJ, et al. Association of usual sleep duration with hypertension: the Sleep Heart Health Study. Sleep 2006; 29(8):1009–14.

[146] Schwartz JR, Roth T. Shift work sleep disorder: burden of illness and approaches to management. Drugs 2006;66(18):2357–70.

[147] Rajaratnam SM, Middleton B, Stone BM, et al. Melatonin advances the circadian timing of EEG sleep and directly facilitates sleep without altering its duration in extended sleep opportunities in humans. J Physiol 2004;561(Pt 1): 339–51.

[148] Phipps-Nelson J, Redman JR, Dijk DJ, et al. Daytime exposure to bright light, as compared to dim light, decreases sleepiness and improves psychomotor vigilance performance. Sleep 2003;26(6):695–700.

[149] Cajochen C, Munch M, Kobialka S, et al. High sensitivity of human melatonin, alertness, thermoregulation, and heart rate to short wavelength light. J Clin Endocrinol Metab 2005; 90(3):1311–6.

[150] Czeisler CA, Walsh JK, Roth T, et al. Modafinil for excessive sleepiness associated with shift-work sleep disorder. N Engl J Med 2005; 353(5):476–86.

[151] Driver HS, Baker FC. Menstrual factors in sleep. Sleep Med Rev 1998;2(4):213–29.

SLEEP
MEDICINE
CLINICS

Sleep Med Clin 3 (2008) 25–35

Sleep and Menstrual-Related Disorders

Fiona C. Baker, PhD[a,b,*], Lynne J. Lamarche, PhD[c],
Stella Iacovides, BS[b], Ian M. Colrain, PhD[a,d]

Many women of reproductive age have recurrent emotional and physical symptoms in association with the menstrual cycle, particularly during the late luteal (premenstrual) and menstruation phases. These symptoms may interfere with social and occupational functioning, as well as with sleep; women who have menstrual-related problems are between two and three times more likely than other women to report insomnia and excessive sleepiness during the day [1]. This article reviews studies that have investigated sleep in women who suffer from significant menstrual-related disturbances, particularly premenstrual syndrome (PMS) and physical pain that occurs in association with menstruation (primary dysmenorrhea). It also discusses specific sleep disorders that are related to the menstrual cycle: premenstrual insomnia and premenstrual hypersomnia.

An important issue when investigating conditions characterized by recurring bouts of symptoms is whether group differences in measured variables between patients and controls occur only in association with symptom occurrence or whether they also are present when the patients are asymptomatic. In the present context, the persistence of group differences across all phases of the menstrual cycle would argue for the existence of an underlying trait difference, perhaps associated with some subclinical symptom presentation, which manifests clinically when an additional stressor such as menstruation (or the hormonal changes associated with menstruation) is present. Group differences that occur only in conjunction with symptoms are more likely to reflect state-related phenomena. The determination of trait versus state differences may provide insight into the underlying mechanisms of

[a] Human Sleep Research Program, SRI International, 333 Ravenswood Avenue, Menlo Park, CA 94025, USA
[b] Brain Function Research Group, School of Physiology, University of the Witwatersrand, 7 York Road, Parktown, 2193, Johannesburg, South Africa
[c] School of Psychology, University of Ottawa, 405 Powell Road, Whitby, Ontario, Canada, L1N 2H5
[d] Department of Psychology, University of Melbourne, Parkville, Victoria, Australia
* Corresponding author. Human Sleep Research Program, SRI International, 333 Ravenswood Avenue, Menlo Park, CA 94043.
E-mail address: fiona.baker@sri.com (F.C. Baker).

doi:10.1016/j.jsmc.2007.10.001

the pathology and guide the nature and timing of appropriate treatment.

Premenstrual syndrome and premenstrual dysphoric disorder

Definitions and etiology

The definition of PMS varies in the literature [2] but generally is characterized by "emotional, behavioral, and physical symptoms that occur in the premenstrual phase of the menstrual cycle, with resolution after menses" [3]. PMS is classified in the International Classification of Diseases under "pain and other conditions associated with female genital organs and menstrual cycle" [4]. Many women of reproductive age experience some physical or emotional symptoms premenstrually, but approximately 22% of women have moderate to severe premenstrual symptoms that they perceive as distressing and that impact their work and/or social relationships [5]. Premenstrual dysphoric disorder (PMDD, previously known as "late luteal phase dysphoric disorder") is a severe form of PMS that occurs in 3% to 8% of women [6]. PMDD is classified as a "depressive disorder not otherwise specified" in the American Psychiatric Association's *Diagnostic and Statistical Manual of Mental Disorders,* fourth edition (DSM-IV) [7]. A diagnosis of PMDD requires the occurrence of five specified symptoms, of which at least one must be a mood-related symptom, during the late luteal phase, for at least two consecutive cycles (Box 1) [7]. Diagnostic criteria for PMS are not so clearly defined; the difference between PMS and PMDD lies in the minimal number of symptoms required for diagnosis. Both severe PMS and PMDD are associated with significant functional impairment with an impact on quality of life [8].

Several instruments have been developed to assess PMS/PMDD. Ideally, assessment should be made prospectively using daily symptom reports to document accurately an increase in symptom expression and severity during the late luteal phase compared with the early/mid-follicular phase [8]. Confirmation of a PMDD diagnosis requires prospective documentation of symptoms over two menstrual cycles [7]. With prospective evaluation of symptoms, it also is possible to rule out pre-existing, underlying psychiatric disorders, which is of particular importance given the high comorbidity of PMDD and depressive disorders [9]. Women who participate in studies of PMS and PMDD therefore need to go through rigorous and lengthy screening procedures.

Although the cause of PMS and PMDD remains unknown, biologic, psychosocial, and biopsychosocial hypotheses have been proposed. There is

---

Box 1:   Research criteria for premenstrual dysphoric disorder

A. In most menstrual cycles during the past year, five (or more) of the following symptoms were present for most of the time during the last week of the luteal phase, began to remit within a few days after the onset of the follicular phase, and were absent in the week postmenses, with at least one of the symptoms being either (1), (2), (3), or (4):

   (1) markedly depressed mood, feelings of hopelessness, or self-deprecating thoughts
   (2) marked anxiety, tension, feelings of being "keyed up" or "on edge"
   (3) marked affective lability (eg, feeling suddenly sad or tearful or increased sensitivity to rejection)
   (4) persistent and marked anger or irritability or increased interpersonal conflicts
   (5) decreased interest in usual activities (eg, work, school, friends, hobbies)
   (6) subjective sense of difficulty in concentrating
   (7) lethargy, easy fatigability, or marked lack of energy
   (8) marked change in appetite, overeating, or specific food cravings
   (9) hypersomnia or insomnia
   (10) a subjective sense of being overwhelmed or out of control
   (11) other physical symptoms, such as breast tenderness or swelling, headache, joint or muscle pain, a sensation of "bloating," weight gain

B. The disturbance markedly interferes with work or school or with usual social activities and relationships with others (eg, avoidance of social activities, decreased productivity and efficiency at work or school).
C. The disturbance is not merely an exacerbation of the symptoms of another disorder, such as Major Depressive Disorder, Panic Disorder, Dysthymic Disorder, or a Personality Disorder (although it may be superimposed on any of these disorders)
D. Criteria A, B, and C must be confirmed by prospective daily ratings during at least two consecutive symptomatic cycles. (The diagnosis may be made provisionally before this confirmation).

(*From* Diagnostic and statistical manual of mental disorders. 4th edition. Text revision. Washington, DC: American Psychiatric Association, 2000. p. 717–8; with permission.)

evidence suggesting that women who have PMS may be more sensitive to usual changes in gonadal hormones such as estrogen and progesterone [10]. Abnormalities in the serotonin neurotransmitter system [6,11] and in the GABAergic system [12–14] also have been linked with the development of premenstrual symptoms. Some theories related to the cause of premenstrual symptoms are multi-faceted and include the relationship between bio-logic, social, and psychologic factors [15]. For example, it is suggested that some women have a predisposition to the development of premen-strual symptoms and syndromes [6] and that such biologic vulnerabilities interact with environmental factors and stresses that are present during the luteal phase [16], leading to the development of premen-strual symptoms [6].

Sleep disturbances

Among the most common symptoms reported by women who have PMS are problems with sleep [17]. Women who have PMS typically report sleep-related disturbances, such as insomnia and disturbing dreams or nightmares, during the pre-menstrual phase [18]. Further, sleep disturbance (hypersomnia or insomnia) is listed as one of the defining criteria for a diagnosis of PMDD in the DSM-IV (Box 1).

Mauri and colleagues [19] conducted the first de-tailed study of sleep disturbances in women who have PMS. Assessment of sleep quality and premen-strual symptoms was based on retrospective self-reports from 14 patients attending a PMS clinic, which were compared with controls. Women from the PMS clinic group reported having more un-pleasant dreams, tossing and turning, frequent awakenings, and needing a long time to fall back asleep after an awakening during the night when they were experiencing premenstrual symptoms in the late luteal phase. A subsequent small, prospec-tive laboratory study (n = 9) indicated that PMS clinic patients seemed to have more awakenings, body movements, and morning tiredness in the lu-teal and menstruation phases, but details of the study were not provided [18]. Parry and colleagues [20], however, found no differences between the late luteal phase and the follicular phase in sleep time or time spent awake, as recorded in daily sleep logs, in a group of 23 patients who met criteria for a diagnosis of PMDD. Patients reported less sleep than controls, however, in both the asymptomatic follicular and symptomatic luteal phases of the menstrual cycle. A recent study in a small group of nine women who had severe PMS or PMDD based on prospective ratings also found no men-strual-phase difference in self-reported total sleep time [21]. The women, however, rated their sleep

quality, measured on a 100-mm visual analogue scale, as significantly poorer during the late luteal phase (56 ± 15 mm) than during the asymptomatic follicular phase (73 ± 12 mm) [21]. Women who had more severe depression ratings were more likely to rate their sleep quality as poorer (Fig. 1). Other studies have found that even women who do not have significant premenstrual symptoms may rate their sleep quality as poorer in the late lu-teal phase than in the follicular phase [22,23]; how-ever the degree of change seems to be less than that of women who have severe PMS [21].

Taken together, findings suggest that women who have severe PMS or PMDD perceive their sleep to be more disturbed in association with other premen-strual symptoms, although not necessarily in associ-ation with increased perceived time spent awake during the night and not necessarily limited to the time when they are experiencing PMS symptoms. It should be emphasized, however, that only 55 women with PMS have been studied in terms of their subjective experience of sleep, and that variable dis-ease definitions and methodologies were used.

Studies using objective polysomnographic (PSG) recordings have shown little evidence of nocturnal sleep disturbance that is specific to premenstrual symptom expression in the late luteal phase com-pared with other phases of the menstrual cycle [18,21,24–28]. Sleep efficiency (percentage of sleep time relative to time in bed) and wakefulness after sleep onset are similar in women who have PMS or PMDD and women who have minimal symptoms in the late luteal phase [21,24–28]. Although differ-ences in sleep architecture between the late luteal phase and the follicular phase have been found,

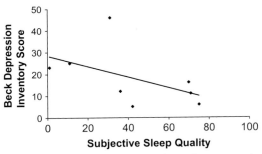

Fig. 1. Scatterplot and regression line of scores on the Beck Depression Inventory versus subjective sleep quality ratings (rated on a visual analogue scale; higher numbers denote better sleep quality) in eight women who had severe PMS during the late luteal phase of the menstrual cycle ($r^2 = 0.5$; $P = .05$). (*From* Baker FC, Kahan TL, Trinder J, et al. Sleep qual-ity and the sleep electroencephalogram in women with severe premenstrual syndrome. Sleep 2007;30(10):1283–91.)

these differences are evident in groups of women who suffer from PMS as well as in those who do not (control groups) [21,25–28] and therefore cannot be attributed solely to PMS.

Some differences in nocturnal sleep architecture have been noted between women who have severe PMS or PMDD and women who have minimal symptoms. These differences, however, occur during both the follicular and luteal phases and are not consistent across studies. Lee [26] studied sleep, based on PSG recordings, in 13 women, 7 of whom met study criteria for PMS. Women were defined as being symptomatic for PMS if they showed at least a 30% increase in scores on the Profile of Mood States or in their 7-day average score on the Woods Women's Health Diary during the luteal phase compared with the follicular phase. Women who had PMS had significantly less slow-wave sleep than women did not have PMS in both the follicular and luteal phases of the menstrual cycle. The symptomatic group also had approximately 7% to 10% more stage 2 sleep than controls, which was statistically significant in the follicular phase [26]. Parry [27] found that eight patients who had severe PMS (based on prospective ratings over 2 months) also had significantly more stage 2 sleep, associated with a significant decrease in REM sleep, than did controls. These effects were evident in the early and late follicular phase as well as in the early and late luteal phase. A subsequent study by the same authors, however, found no differences in sleep architecture between 14 women who had PMDD and 9 controls studied in the follicular and late luteal phases [28]. Both subject groups had quite low sleep efficiencies ($\sim$80%) during recordings, possibly because of experimental conditions, which may have masked any group differences. As part of this study, women underwent a night of partial (early and late) sleep deprivation during their late luteal phase only. During recovery from sleep deprivation, group differences emerged: women who had PMDD had better sleep quality with a shorter sleep-onset latency, less wakefulness after sleep onset, a higher sleep efficiency, and less stage 1 sleep than controls [28]. The authors suggest that sleep deprivation might help restore a healthier circadian regulation of sleep in women who have PMDD [28]. Finally, a recent study found that nine women who had severe PMS or PMDD, determined from prospective ratings, had a longer latency to REM sleep than 12 controls, regardless of menstrual-cycle phase [21].

These inconsistent findings between studies paint a confusing picture as to whether trait-like alterations in sleep architecture are a component of severe PMS and what their relevance might be. Again, it needs to be emphasized that only a small number of patients have been studied in a handful of studies, and variable results may be attributable to differences in methodology, such as instruments used to diagnose PMS and PMDD, time of recordings during the luteal phase, variable (and generally small) sample sizes, and the reliance on Rechtschaffen and Kales [29] criteria for scoring sleep stages, which do not allow the quantification of changes in the microstructure of sleep. The different findings also may be a consequence of variations in the types of symptoms experienced by women who have PMS, with some women experiencing irritability and anxiety as core symptoms and others reporting depression as the core symptom [30].

One study that performed a more detailed analysis of sleep EEG microarchitecture (power spectral analysis and period amplitude analysis) in women who had severe PMS found no differences in the sleep EEG during the late luteal phase compared with the follicular phase that were specific to the PMS group [21]. Women who had PMS, however, showed some trait-like differences across the menstrual cycle with decreased incidence of delta waveforms, increased incidence and amplitude of theta waveforms, and a tendency for increased spectral power in the lower sigma frequency band in non-REM sleep compared with controls [21]. These findings suggest that there may be subtle trait-like differences in sleep architecture and sleep EEG activity in women who have severe PMS that persist in the absence of PMS symptoms. Because this study included only nine women who had severe PMS or PMDD, these findings need to be replicated and confirmed in a larger group.

In summary, women who have severe PMS are likely to report a subjective experience of poorer sleep quality in association with their other premenstrual symptoms. To date, however, studies have not found disturbances in sleep architecture based on PSG recordings or observations of sleep EEG that are specific to premenstrual symptom expression. Possibly, women who have PMS may be more sensitive to subtle changes in sleep architecture that occur in all women during the luteal phase and particularly during the late luteal phase (see [31] for review). For example, some studies have found an increase in intermittent wakefulness [27] or wake time [21] , based on PSG recordings during the late luteal phase, in both women who have significant premenstrual symptoms and those who have minimal symptoms. This increase in sleep fragmentation may affect subjective ratings of sleep quality, particularly in women who have severe PMS. Alternatively, the decline in reported sleep quality in women who have PMS may be a consequence of a negative reporting bias in association with premenstrual symptoms [21]. A similar tendency for negative evaluations of sleep quality has been reported for depressed patients [32] and patients who have irritable bowel syndrome [33].

Age may be a factor that influences the extent of sleep disturbance in association with premenstrual symptoms: preliminary findings indicate that women who have PMS aged 40 years and older report more frequent waking at night as well as more early waking than younger women [34]. Possible differences in sleep structure between women who have severe PMS and women who have minimal symptoms in both the follicular and luteal phases of the menstrual cycle need to be investigated further to determine whether they are linked with specific premenstrual symptoms, such as depressed mood.

Daytime sleepiness and alertness

If sleep disturbance plays a role in the development or exacerbation of PMS symptoms, there should be some measurable impact on daytime sleepiness. As with sleep itself, sleepiness can be assessed both in terms of its subjective experience or more objectively in terms of the propensity to fall asleep (usually measured in minutes) if given the opportunity to do so.

Women who have PMS commonly report sleepiness, fatigue, and an inability to concentrate during the premenstrual phase [18]. Few studies have investigated these symptoms in any detail. Manber and Bootzin [23] analyzed sleep and daytime diaries of 32 women between the ages of 27 and 51 years. At bedtime, the women rated various mood-related variables from which a premenstrual severity index was calculated; three women met criteria for severe PMS. Women also rated their sleepiness levels at bedtime. Sleepiness varied significantly with menstrual phase, being higher in the luteal phase, and the change from the follicular to luteal phase

correlated significantly with the premenstrual index. The authors suggest that women who have more severe symptoms of PMS may need more sleep during the late luteal phase [23]. This interesting possibility has not been tested with laboratory-based studies, because sleep-wake schedules typically are constrained in the laboratory.

Although the complete methodology of the study is not provided, Mauri [18] found that a group of nine PMS clinic patients had greater levels of daytime sleepiness, based on scores on the Stanford Sleepiness Scale [35] in the luteal and menstruation phases of the menstrual cycle. A recent study also used the Stanford Sleepiness Scale in addition to a Subjective Alertness Scale to investigate daytime sleepiness and alertness in women who had significant premenstrual symptoms [25]. Women who had significant symptoms were sleepier and less alert in the late luteal phase than in the follicular phase, whereas no menstrual-phase change in sleepiness was found in a group of women who had minimal symptoms (Fig. 2). In addition, women who had more severe symptoms were significantly sleepier and less alert than women who had minimal symptoms during the late luteal phase but not during the follicular phase of the cycle. Preliminary results from another study showed that women with PMDD had slower reaction times, along with a tendency to feel sleepier, than controls in their late luteal phase [36]. One study has used a nap protocol to investigate daytime sleep characteristics of women in the late luteal phase. Lamarche [25] found no significant differences in sleep architecture during a short mid-afternoon nap between young adult women who had severe and minimal premenstrual symptoms, although two women who had severe symptoms entered REM sleep,

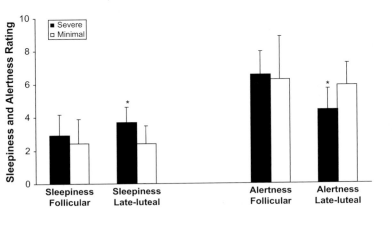

Fig. 2. Levels of sleepiness (rated on the Stanford Sleepiness Scale; higher numbers denote increased sleepiness) and alertness (rated on a Subjective Alertness Scale; lower numbers denote decreased alertness) for 10 women who had severe and 9 women who had minimal premenstrual symptoms during the follicular and late luteal phases of the menstrual cycle. Women who had severe premenstrual symptoms were significantly sleepier and less alert than women who had minimal symptoms in the late luteal phase. *, $P < .05$. (*From* Lamarche L, Driver HS, Wiebe S, et al. Nocturnal sleep, daytime sleepiness, and napping among women with significant emotional/behavioral premenstrual symptoms. J Sleep Res 2007;16(3):262–8.)

whereas none of the women who had minimal symptoms did so. Of note, there were no group differences in sleep-onset latency: the group that had severe premenstrual symptoms fell asleep in 6 minutes, on average, and the group that had minimal symptoms fell asleep in 7 minutes, on average. The short sleep-onset latency found for both groups of women suggests that there was a high sleep need during the late luteal phase regardless of symptom severity, possibly indicating chronic sleep restriction, as may be expected in this age group (mean age 26.7 years) [37].

Although the number of studies is limited, findings indicate that sleepiness is a recognizable component of severe PMS. Because studies show that objective sleep disturbances are minimal in women who have PMS during their late luteal phase, it remains to be determined what factors contribute to the increase in daytime sleepiness.

Circadian rhythm disturbances

Although studies have not been conducted under constant routine conditions, evidence suggests that women who have PMDD may have abnormal regulation of their circadian rhythms. High mean nocturnal temperatures have been reported in women who have severe PMS or PMDD compared with asymptomatic controls, regardless of menstrual-cycle phase [38]. In a larger study, no significant differences were found in temperature amplitude, minimum temperature, or timing of the temperature minimum, although women with PMDD tended to have higher mean nocturnal temperatures than controls [39]. During partial sleep deprivation in the late luteal phase, group differences emerged. Women with PMDD had higher temperature maxima and mesors (rhythm-adjusted mean) than women who had minimal symptoms [39]. Also, women with PMDD had a delayed temperature acrophase (time at which the peak of the rhythm occurs), whereas controls had an advanced acrophase during early sleep deprivation (sleep from 03:00 to 07:00) compared with a baseline recording in the late luteal phase [39]. These timing disturbances in women with PMDD may reflect underlying disturbances in the circadian pacemaker that regulates the temperature rhythm [39].

Disturbances in melatonin rhythms and in the timing of the rhythms of cortisol and thyroid-stimulating hormone also have been reported in women with PMDD [40–43]. Parry and colleagues [40] found that women with PMDD had a phase-delayed melatonin onset in the luteal phase compared with the follicular phase, an effect not found in controls. Also, area under the curve, amplitude, and mean level of melatonin were decreased during the luteal phase compared with the follicular phase

in women with PMDD and compared with controls [40]. A study by Shinohara and colleagues [44] examined the timing of sleep onset during the luteal and follicular phases of the menstrual cycle in one participant who had PMS. Results showed that sleep onset was advanced after menstruation had begun but then was progressively delayed shortly after ovulation until the next menstruation. The follicular phase therefore was characterized by a phase advance, whereas the luteal phase was characterized by a phase delay.

Given these possible disturbances in circadian rhythmicity in women with PMDD, investigators have explored the possibility of treating PMDD by manipulating the timing of sleep with sleep-deprivation protocols (as described later) or with light therapy. Appropriately timed light therapy has shown some promise as a treatment strategy for PMDD, possibly by altering nocturnal melatonin secretion [45,46]. Bright light therapy significantly reduced depression, irritability, and physical premenstrual symptoms compared with a placebo condition, and these improvements were maintained at 12 months [47]. Similarly, Lam and colleagues [48] found that 30 minutes of light therapy in the evening for 2 weeks during the luteal phase resulted in a significant improvement in premenstrual symptoms in women who had PMS compared with baseline levels. These initial findings are promising; however, a meta-analysis of clinical trials of bright light therapy concluded that larger trials are needed to define the role bright light therapy might have in the treatment of PMDD [49].

Sleep deprivation studies

Sleep deprivation has been shown to be effective in reducing depressive symptoms in patients who have major depressive disorder [50]. Given the similarities between PMDD and other mood disorders, such as depression [51], it is of interest to investigate whether sleep deprivation has a similar efficacy in this population. Parry and colleagues have conducted studies to determine the effects of various sleep-deprivation protocols on mood variables in women who have severe PMS or PMDD [20,52]. Parry and Wehr [52] examined the effects of total sleep deprivation (40 hours) during the late luteal phase on the symptoms of women who had premenstrual depression. Eight of 10 women experienced an improvement in premenstrual mood, based on Hamilton ratings, with total sleep deprivation, and the improvement was maintained after a recovery night's sleep. Two consecutive nights of late-night sleep deprivation (sleeping from 20:00 to 02:00) were found to be more effective than early sleep deprivation (sleeping from 02:00 to 08:00) and were as effective as total sleep deprivation [52].

In a subsequent larger study of 22 women who had PMDD and 17 controls, no differences were found between the effectiveness of 1 night of early (sleep from 03:00 to −07:00) versus 1 night of late (sleep from 21:00 to 01:00) sleep deprivation [20]. Both types of partial sleep deprivation had similar positive effects on mood in 60% to 67% of patients, but these effects were significant only after recovery sleep [20]. Predictors of responsiveness to sleep deprivation were sadness and depression, duration and severity of symptoms, history of depression, and personal and family history of suicide. Of interest, changes in REM latency and REM density in the first REM sleep period from baseline to recovery nights were significantly correlated with improvement in mood in responders to sleep deprivation [28].

The effect of sleep deprivation on mood in women with PMDD differs from that found in patients with major depressive disorder, who have improved mood the day following total sleep deprivation but tend to relapse after recovery sleep [50]. The lack of relapse after recovery sleep in women with PMDD makes partial sleep deprivation a potential treatment option for PMDD [20]. Indeed, a follow-up study of seven patients who continued with the treatment of 1 night of partial sleep deprivation at home when they were symptomatic in their luteal phase showed that the deprivation protocol continued to be effective in improving mood in these women [20]. Although these studies show promise, several unanswered questions need to be addressed before sleep deprivation can be considered as a potential treatment strategy for PMDD. For example, it still remains to be determined whether the positive response to sleep deprivation is more than just a placebo effect; if there is a critical window when the sleep-deprivation protocol should be applied to be effective; and if the positive effects of a single night of sleep deprivation can be maintained throughout the late-luteal phase.

In summary, there is evidence that disturbances in sleep and circadian regulation are components of severe PMS and PMDD and that correcting these disturbances with bright light therapy or sleep deprivation may have positive effects on mood. Many findings are preliminary, and there is a need for further study. Future studies need to be more consistent in their assessment measures as well as in their inclusion/exclusion criteria for study participants.

Primary dysmenorrhea

Definition and etiology

Dysmenorrhea, defined as painful menstrual cramps of uterine origin, is the most common gynecologic condition among women of reproductive age [53] and is very severe in approximately 10% to 25% of women [54,55]. Despite its common occurrence, it is underdiagnosed and undertreated. Based on pathophysiology, dysmenorrhea can be classified as either primary or secondary [56]. Primary dysmenorrhea is defined as painful, spasmodic cramping in the lower abdomen, just before and/or during menstruation, in the absence of any discernable macroscopic pelvic pathology [54]. The onset of primary dysmenorrhea usually occurs in adolescence, at or shortly after (6–24 months) menarche [55]. Primary dysmenorrheic pain is most severe during the first or second day of menstruation and typically lasts for 8 to 72 hours [57]. The pain may radiate to the back and thighs and is frequently accompanied by systemic symptoms including nausea, vomiting, diarrhea, fatigue, and insomnia [55,58]. Secondary dysmenorrheic pain, in contrast, may originate from a number of identifiable pathologic conditions including endometriosis, adenomyosis, fibroids (myomas), and pelvic inflammatory disease.

The etiology of primary dysmenorrhea is not entirely understood, but prostaglandins have been implicated as the primary mediators of the pain [54]. Prostaglandins are thought to produce the ischemic pain experienced by women who have dysmenorrhea by causing contraction of the uterine muscle or constriction of uterine blood vessels; both of which ultimately reduce the blood supply to the uterus. Alternatively, prostaglandins may reduce the nerve ending's threshold for pain perception [55,53]. Given the prostaglandin-based origin of primary dysmenorrhea, the most common pharmacologic treatment for dysmenorrhea is nonsteroidal anti-inflammatory drugs (NSAIDs) [59].

Primary dysmenorrhea has characteristics of both chronic and acute pain syndromes: the pain recurs monthly, and, although the pain is severe, it is of short duration with a predictable onset and offset. The painful menstrual cramps experienced by these women every month significantly impact productivity and quality of life [60].

Sleep disturbances

Based on survey data, menstrual cramps are a major disruptor to sleep in women of reproductive age [61]. As far as the authors are aware, only one published study has systematically investigated the impact of dysmenorrheic pain on sleep [62]. The study included 10 women who had primary dysmenorrhea and 8 women who did not have dysmenorrhea (controls) who were studied in the sleep laboratory on the first night of menstruation as well as during the mid-follicular and mid-luteal phases of the menstrual cycle. Although not prospectively documented, none of the women reported significant symptoms of PMS. The women who had primary dysmenorrhea rated their menstrual pain as severe in the evening before going to bed on the first day of menstruation. As shown in Fig. 3, in association with their pain, the dysmenorrheic women (48 ± 24 mm) rated their sleep quality as significantly worse than controls (65 ± 21 mm) during menstruation and compared with their own pain-free follicular and luteal phases [62]. PSG recordings also indicated significant sleep disturbance in the women who had dysmenorrhea. They had a lower sleep efficiency, increased combined time spent awake, moving, and in stage 1 light sleep, and less REM sleep compared with pain-free phases of the menstrual cycle and compared with women who did not suffer from menstrual pain [62]. Four of the women who had dysmenorrhea required pain-relieving medication (mefenamic acid) before their overnight recordings; these women may have experienced even greater sleep disruption in the absence of medication.

Given that NSAIDs are an effective treatment for dysmenorrhea [56], it is likely that treatment of nocturnal pain with NSAIDs would alleviate painful cramps and consequently improve sleep quality in women who have dysmenorrhea. Indeed, Iacovides and colleagues have preliminary evidence that women who have primary dysmenorrhea have a better sleep efficiency and subjective sleep quality when their pain is treated with a NSAID compared with placebo (Stella Iacovides, BSc (Hons), Johannesburg, South Africa, unpublished findings, June 2007).

There is some evidence that women who have dysmenorrhea may have altered sleep architecture even before the onset of pain. Dysmenorrheic women were found to have significantly less REM sleep (in association with higher nocturnal rectal temperatures) compared with controls, during the follicular, luteal, and menstruation phases of the menstrual cycle [62]. A subsequent study that investigated sleep and body temperatures in the follicular and luteal phases of the menstrual cycle in women who had dysmenorrhea and controls (eight women in each group) did not support this finding: there were no differences in the 24-hour temperature rhythms or in REM sleep between women who had dysmenorrhea and controls [63]. Sample sizes were small in both these studies, and it remains to be confirmed whether there are any significant differences in sleep and body temperature in women who have primary dysmenorrhea outside of the painful menstruation phase.

Menstrual-associated sleep disorder

Two sleep disorders that are temporally related to menstruation, premenstrual insomnia and

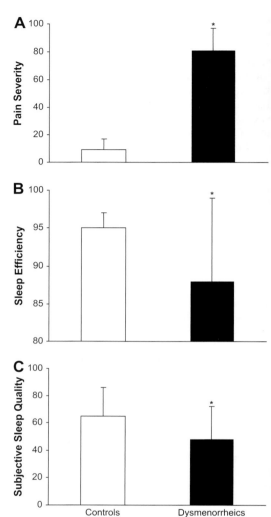

Fig. 3. (*A*) Pain severity (rated on a visual analogue scale; higher numbers denote greater pain), (*B*) PSG-defined sleep efficiency, and (*C*) subjective sleep quality (rated on a visual analogue scale; higher numbers denote better sleep quality) in 10 women who had primary dysmenorrhea and in 8 women who had minimal symptoms on the first night of menstruation. *, $P < .05$. (*Data from* Baker FC, Driver HS, Rogers GG, et al. High nocturnal body temperatures and disturbed sleep in women with primary dysmenorrhea. Am J Physiol 1999;277(6 Pt 1):E1013–21.)

premenstrual hypersomnia, have been proposed in the International Classification of Sleep Disorders [64]. Both of these disorders are rare and have been characterized based on case studies. Importantly, a diagnosis of menstrual-associated sleep disorder is given only if the patient does not meet the criteria for a diagnosis of PMDD.

Premenstrual insomnia is characterized by difficulty in falling asleep or remaining asleep in emporal association with the menstrual cycle. This form of insomnia occurs in the week before the onset of menses and must be present for at least three consecutive months for a diagnosis to be given. The cause of premenstrual insomnia is unknown, but there is some evidence from a case study suggesting that desynchronization of temperature and sleep-wake rhythms in the luteal phase could be a contributing factor [65].

Premenstrual hypersomnia is characterized by sleepiness occurring in the week before the onset of menses. The patient has no complaints of persistent, excessive sleepiness at other times in the menstrual cycle [64]. Some case studies of women who have premenstrual hypersomnia have been published [66–68]. Polygraphic recordings in one patient (13 years old) indicated a 44% increase in total sleep time in a 24-hour period, with a decrease in the percentage of slow-wave sleep and increases in stage 1 and stage 2 sleep but no change in the organization of night-time sleep stages when the patient was symptomatic compared with asymptomatic intervals [67]. Patients who have premenstrual hypersomnia have been treated successfully with estrogen [67] or oral contraceptives [68].

Summary

Menstrual cycle–related pathology has a high prevalence and at least putative links to sleep disturbance and/or daytime sleepiness. Nonetheless, the relationship between sleep and these disorders has been studied in only a very few patients and studies. This paucity is not unsurprising, because such studies have to overcome three major obstacles to research funding. First, although they are debilitating and even potentially personally devastating in terms of their impact on the sufferers, menstrual-related disorders are not life-threatening conditions; second, it often is difficult to convince funding agencies of the importance of sleep as a factor in problems that manifest as daytime symptoms; and third, these problems are "women's issues."

PMS/PMDD demonstrates a trait-like pattern of subtle alterations in sleep architecture and sleep EEG that persists across symptomatic and asymptomatic phases of the menstrual cycle. There is, however, a clear increase in daytime sleepiness in the symptomatic late luteal phase. This dissociation of objective sleep quality from sleepiness is a salutary indicator to sleep researchers that sleepiness is not necessarily linked to poor sleep quality, as it is traditionally measured in the laboratory. Given the preliminary evidence presented in this article that PMS/PMDD may be associated with some form of circadian dysregulation, the sleepiness may be a function of desynchronization of circadian rhythms. Put in terms of Borbely's two-process model of sleep regulation [69], PMS/PMDD could be conceived as being a "Process C" problem rather than a "Process S" problem. This view is supported by the evidence of partial sleep deprivation being a possible treatment of PMS/PMDD symptoms.

It should be self-evident from the material presented that more research is warranted, with continuous routine studies to unmask underlying circadian rhythms effectively and studies to identify subject characteristics that predict treatment efficacy of sleep deprivation as well as determination of the optimal sleep-deprivation protocol for women to use to obtain symptom relief.

It is important to consider the presence of menstrual-associated disorders when evaluating women who have sleep complaints to determine whether there is an association between their sleep disturbance and the menstrual cycle. It also is important for future research studies to assess sleep-related interventions as preventative measures for PMS symptoms and sleep disruptions and to determine that analgesic treatment regimens for menstrual pain do not negatively impact sleep quality.

It is rare to find such a mismatch between the small number of studies investigating a problem and the high prevalence of that problem in society. In this case, the overused and sometimes trite conclusion that "clearly more work needs to be done" is not only warranted but self-evident.

References

[1] Strine TW, Chapman DP, Ahluwalia IB. Menstrual-related problems and psychological distress among women in the United States. J Womens Health (Larchmt) 2005;14(4):316–23.

[2] Graham C, Bancroft J. Women, mood and the menstrual cycle. In: Niven C, Carroll D, editors. The health psychology of women. Langhorne (PA): Harwood Academic Publishers/Gordon; 1993. p. 13–25.

[3] Pearlstein T, Stone AB. Premenstrual syndrome. Psychiatr Clin North Am 1998;21:577–90.

[4] Kahn LS, Halbreich U. Oral contraceptives and mood. Expert Opin Pharmacother 2001;2: 1367–82.

[5] Angst J, Sellaro R, Merikangas KR, et al. The epidemiology of perimenstrual psychological symptoms. Acta Psychiatr Scand 2001;104(2):110–6.

[6] Halbreich U. The etiology, biology, and evolving pathology of premenstrual syndromes. Psychoneuroendocrinology 2003;28(Suppl 3):55–99.

[7] American Psychiatric Association A. Diagnostic and statistical manual of mental disorders. 4th edition. Washington, DC: American Psychiatric Press Inc., American Psychiatric Association; 1994.

[8] Freeman EW. Premenstrual syndrome and premenstrual dysphoric disorder: definitions and diagnosis. Psychoneuroendocrinology 2003; 28(Suppl 3):25–37.

[9] Kim DR, Gyulai L, Freeman EW, et al. Premenstrual dysphoric disorder and psychiatric co-morbidity. Arch Womens Ment Health 2004;7(1): 37–47.

[10] Halbreich U, Endicott J, Goldstein S, et al. Premenstrual changes and changes in gonadal hormones. Acta Psychiatr Scand 1986;74:576–86.

[11] Condon JT. Premenstrual syndrome in primary care: an update. Primary Care Psychiatry 2001; 71:85–90.

[12] Epperson CN, Haga K, Mason GF, et al. Cortical gamma-aminobutyric acid levels across the menstrual cycle in healthy women and those with premenstrual dysphoric disorder: a proton magnetic resonance spectroscopy study. Arch Gen Psychiatry 2002;59(9):851–8.

[13] Halbreich U, Petty F, Yonkers K, et al. Low plasma gamma-aminobutyric acid levels during the late luteal phase of women with premenstrual dysphoric disorder. Am J Psychiatry 1996;153(5):718–20.

[14] Sundstrom I, Backstrom T. Patients with premenstrual syndrome have decreased saccadic eye velocity compared to control subjects. Biol Psychiatry 1998;44(8):755–64.

[15] Walker A. Theory and methodology in premenstrual syndrome research. Social Science & Medicine 1995;41:793–800.

[16] Morse CA, Dennerstein L. Cognitive therapy for premenstrual syndrome. In: Brush MG, Goudsmit EM, editors. Functional disorders of the menstrual cycle. Chichester (UK): John Wiley & Sons Ltd.; 1988. p. 177–90.

[17] Hurt SW, Schnurr PPS, Severino SK, et al. Late-luteal phase dysphoric disorder in 670 women evaluated for premenstrual complaints. Am J Psychiatry 1992;149:525–30.

[18] Mauri M. Sleep and the reproductive cycle: a review. Health Care Women Int 1990;11(4): 409–21.

[19] Mauri M, Reid RL, MacLean AW. Sleep in the premenstrual phase: a self-report study of PMS patients and normal controls. Acta Psychiatr Scand 1988;78(1):82–6.

[20] Parry BL, Cover H, Mostofi N, et al. Early versus late partial sleep deprivation in patients with premenstrual dysphoric disorder and normal comparison subjects. Am J Psychiatry 1995; 152(3):404–12.

[21] Baker FC, Kahan TL, Trinder J, et al. Sleep quality and the sleep electroencephalogram in women with severe premenstrual syndrome. Sleep 2007;30(10):1283–91.

[22] Baker FC, Driver HS. Self-reported sleep across the menstrual cycle in young, healthy women. J Psychosom Res 2004;56(2):239–43.

[23] Manber R, Bootzin RR. Sleep and the menstrual cycle. Health Psychol 1997;16(3):209–14.

[24] Chuong CJ, Kim SR, Taskin O, et al. Sleep pattern changes in menstrual cycles of women with premenstrual syndrome: a preliminary study. Am J Obstet Gynecol 1997;177(3):554–8.

[25] Lamarche L, Driver HS, Wiebe S, et al. Nocturnal sleep, daytime sleepiness, and napping among women with significant emotional/behavioral premenstrual symptoms. J Sleep Res 2007 16(3):262–8.

[26] Lee KA, Shaver JF, Giblin EC, et al. Sleep patterns related to menstrual cycle phase and premenstrual affective symptoms. Sleep 1990;13(5) 403–9.

[27] Parry BL, Mendelson WB, Duncan WC, et al. Longitudinal sleep EEG, temperature, and activity measurements across the menstrual cycle in patients with premenstrual depression and in age-matched controls. Psychiatry Res 1989 30(3):285–303.

[28] Parry BL, Mostofi N, LeVeau B, et al. Sleep EEG studies during early and late partial sleep deprivation in premenstrual dysphoric disorder and normal control subjects. Psychiatry Res 1999 85(2):127–43.

[29] Rechtschaffen A, Kales A. A manual of standardized terminology, techniques, and scoring system for sleep stages of human subjects. National Institutes of Health Publication No 204. Washington, DC: National Institutes of Health; 1968.

[30] Abraham GE. Premenstrual tension. Curr Prob Obstet Gynecol 1980;3:1–39.

[31] Moline ML, Broch L, Zak R, et al. Sleep in women across the life cycle from adulthood through menopause. Sleep Med Rev 2003;7(2) 155–77.

[32] Armitage R, Trivedi M, Hoffmann R, et al. Relationship between objective and subjective sleep measures in depressed patients and healthy controls. Depress Anxiety 1997;5(2):97–102.

[33] Elsenbruch S, Thompson JJ, Hamish MJ, et al. Behavioral and physiological sleep characteristics in women with irritable bowel syndrome. Am J Gastroenterol 2002;97(9):2306–14.

[34] Kuan AJ, Carter DM, Ott FJ. Premenstrual complaints before and after 40 years of age [letter] Can J Psychiatry 2004;49(3):215.

[35] Hoddes E, Dement W, Zarcone V. The development and use of the Stanford Sleepiness Scale (SSS). Psychophysiology 1972;9:150.

[36] Baker FC, DeTar L, Rinkevich M, et al. Psychomotor vigilance performance decrements and reduced P300 event-related amplitude in women with premenstrual dysphoric disorder. Sleep 2006;29:A331.

[37] Klerman EB, Dijk DJ. Interindividual variation in sleep duration and its association with sleep debt in young adults. Sleep 2005;28:1253–9.

[38] Severino SK, Wagner DR, Moline ML, et al. High nocturnal body temperature in premenstrual syndrome and late luteal phase dysphoric disorder. Am J Psychiatry 1991;148(10):1329–35.

39] Parry BL, LeVeau B, Mostofi N, et al. Temperature circadian rhythms during the menstrual cycle and sleep deprivation in premenstrual dysphoric disorder and normal comparison subjects. J Biol Rhythms 1997;12(1):34–46.

40] Parry BL, Berga SL, Mostofi N, et al. Plasma melatonin circadian rhythms during the menstrual cycle and after light therapy in premenstrual dysphoric disorder and normal control subjects. J Biol Rhythms 1997;12(1):47–64.

41] Parry BL, Hauger R, LeVeau B, et al. Circadian rhythms of prolactin and thyroid-stimulating hormone during the menstrual cycle and early versus late sleep deprivation in premenstrual dysphoric disorder. Psychiatry Res 1996;62(2): 147–60.

42] Parry BL, Hauger R, Lin E, et al. Neuroendocrine effects of light therapy in late luteal phase dysphoric disorder. Biol Psychiatry 1994;36(6): 356–64.

43] Parry BL, Javeed S, Laughlin GA, et al. Cortisol circadian rhythms during the menstrual cycle and with sleep deprivation in premenstrual dysphoric disorder and normal control subjects. Biol Psychiatry 2000;48(9):920–31.

44] Shinohara K, Uchiyama M, Okawa M, et al. Menstrual changes in sleep, rectal temperature and melatonin rhythms in a subject with premenstrual syndrome. Neurosci Lett 2000;281(2–3): 159–62.

45] Parry BL, Berga SL, Kripke DF, et al. Melatonin and phototherapy in premenstrual depression. Prog Clin Biol Res 1990;341B:35–43.

46] Parry BL, Udell C, Elliott JA, et al. Blunted phase-shift responses to morning bright light in premenstrual dysphoric disorder. J Biol Rhythms 1997;12(5):443–56.

47] Parry BL, Mahan AM, Mostofi N, et al. Light therapy of late luteal phase dysphoric disorder: an extended study. Am J Psychiatry 1993;150(9): 1417–9.

48] Lam RW, Carter D, Misri S, et al. A controlled study of light therapy in women with late-luteal phase dysphoric disorder. Psychiatry Res 1999; 86:185–92.

49] Krasnik C, Montori VM, Guyatt GH, et al. The effect of bright light therapy on depression associated with premenstrual dysphoric disorder. Am J Obstet Gynecol 2005;193(3 Pt 1): 658–61.

50] Wirz-Justice A, Van den Hoofdakker RH. Sleep deprivation in depression: what do we know, where do we go? Biol Psychiatry 1999;46: 445–53.

51] Yonkers KA. The association between premenstrual dysphoric disorder and other mood disorders. J Clin Psychiatry 1997;58(Suppl 15):19–25.

52] Parry BL, Wehr TA. Therapeutic effect of sleep deprivation in patients with premenstrual syndrome. Am J Psychiatry 1987;144(6):808–10.

53] Coco AS. Primary dysmenorrhea. Am Fam Physician 1999;60(2):489–96.

54] Dawood MY. Dysmenorrhea and prostaglandins. In: Gold JJ, Josimovich JB, editors, Gynecologic endocrinology, vol. 4. New York: Plenum Publishing Corportation; 1987. p. 405–21.

55] Hofmeyr GJ. Dysmenorrhoea. In: Bassin J, editor. Topics in obstetrics and gynaecology. Johannesburg: Julmar Communications; 1996. p. 269–74.

56] Proctor M, Farquhar C. Diagnosis and management of dysmenorrhoea. BMJ 2006;332(7550): 1134–8.

57] Proctor ML, Smith CA, Farquhar CM, et al. Transcutaneous electrical nerve stimulation and acupuncture for primary dysmenorrhoea. Cochrane Database of Syst Rev 2002;1: CD002123.

58] Ruoff G, Lema M. Strategies in pain management: new and potential indications for COX-2 specific inhibitors. J Pain Symptom Manage 2003;25(Suppl 2):S21–31.

59] Harel Z. Cyclooxygenase-2 specific inhibitors in the treatment of dysmenorrhea. J Pediatr Adolesc Gynecol 2004;17(2):75–9.

60] Dawood MY. Dysmenorrhea. Clin Obstet Gynecol 1990;33(1):168–78.

61] National Sleep Foundation NSF. Women and sleep poll. Available at: http://web.archive.org/web/20040608054453/www.sleepfoundation.org/publications/1998womenpoll.cfm. Accessed March 13, 2006.

62] Baker FC, Driver HS, Rogers GG, et al. High nocturnal body temperatures and disturbed sleep in women with primary dysmenorrhea. Am J Physiol 1999;277(6 Pt 1):E1013–21.

63] Baker FC, Driver HS, Paiker J, et al. Acetaminophen does not affect 24-h body temperature or sleep in the luteal phase of the menstrual cycle. J Appl Physiol 2002;92(4):1684–91.

64] American Academy of Sleep Medicine. International Classification of Sleep Disorders, Revised: diagnostic and coding manual. Chicago: American Academy of Sleep Medicine; 2001.

65] Suzuki H, Uchiyama M, Shibui K, et al. Long-term rectal temperature measurements in a patient with menstrual-associated sleep disorder. Psychiatry Clin Neurosci 2002; 56(4):475–8.

66] Bamford CR. Menstrual-associated sleep disorder: an unusual hypersomniac variant associated with both menstruation and amenorrhea with a possible link to prolactin and metoclopramide. Sleep 1993;16(5):484–6.

67] Billiard M, Guilleminault C, Dement WC. A menstruation-linked periodic hypersomnia. Kleine-Levin syndrome or new clinical entity? Neurology 1975;25(5):436–43.

68] Sachs C, Persson HE, Hagenfeldt K. Menstruation-related periodic hypersomnia: a case study with successful treatment. Neurology 1982; 32(12):1376–9.

69] Borbely AA. A two process model of sleep regulation. Hum Neurobiol 1982;1(3):195–204.

ELSEVIER
SAUNDERS

SLEEP
MEDICINE
CLINICS

Sleep Med Clin 3 (2008) 37–46

Polycystic Ovary Syndrome and Obstructive Sleep Apnea

Esra Tasali, MD[a], Eve Van Cauter, PhD[b], David A. Ehrmann, MD[b],*

- Polycystic ovary syndrome: definition and pathogenesis
  Hyperandrogenism
  Insulin resistance
  Progesterone and estrogen
- Metabolic and cardiovascular abnormalities in polycystic ovary syndrome
- Prevalence of obstructive sleep apnea in polycystic ovary syndrome

- Polycystic ovary syndrome and obstructive sleep apnea: role of sex steroids and obesity
  Sex steroids
  Obesity
- Polycystic ovary syndrome and obstructive sleep apnea: insulin resistance, glucose intolerance, and type 2 diabetes mellitus
- Summary
- References

Polycystic ovary syndrome (PCOS) affects approximately 5% to 8% of women in the United States, making it the most common endocrine disorder of premenopausal women [1]. Women who have PCOS have a substantial risk for the development of a number of metabolic [2,3] and cardiovascular [4–6] disorders. Specifically, women who have PCOS have among the highest reported rates of early-onset impaired glucose tolerance (IGT) and type 2 diabetes mellitus [7,8] and a substantial increase in risk for hypertension [9], dyslipidemia, coronary [10], and other vascular disorders [11,12]. A recently identified and potentially important addition to this list of health risks is obstructive sleep apnea (OSA), which is present in PCOS women at rates that are considerably higher than in age- and weight-matched normal women [13].

Current evidence suggests that in non-PCOS populations, OSA is independently linked to adverse metabolic and cardiovascular outcome [14–16]. Most studies that have characterized metabolic and cardiovascular abnormalities in PCOS, however, have not considered the high prevalence of OSA in this syndrome or the possible contribution of OSA to the metabolic and cardiovascular disorders in PCOS.

In this article, the authors provide a brief introduction to PCOS and review the current notions regarding the pathogenesis of the metabolic and cardiovascular abnormalities in PCOS. Studies that have examined the prevalence of OSA in PCOS and the evidence for a role of sex steroids in promoting OSA in women who have PCOS are summarized, and the possible role of OSA in the

This work was supported by RO1 HL075079 and P50 HD057796 to D.A.E., Scholars Grants in Sleep Medicine to E.T., and PO1 AG-11412 to E.V.C.

[a] Section of Pulmonary and Critical Care Medicine, Department of Medicine, MC 6026, University of Chicago, 5841 South Maryland Avenue, Chicago, IL 60637, USA

[b] Section of Endocrinology, Diabetes, and Metabolism, Department of Medicine, MC 1027, University of Chicago, 5841 South Maryland Avenue, Chicago, IL 60637, USA

* Corresponding author.

E-mail address: dehrmann@uchicago.edu (D.A. Ehrmann).

doi:10.1016/j.jsmc.2007.11.001

increased risk of insulin resistance and type 2 diabetes mellitus associated with PCOS is discussed.

Polycystic ovary syndrome: definition and pathogenesis

A diagnosis of PCOS requires that at least two of the three following abnormalities are present: (1) absent or irregular menstrual cycles; (2) elevated levels of circulating androgens or clinical manifestations of hyperandrogenism (eg, hirsutism, acne, alopecia); (3) polycystic ovaries on ultrasonography [17]. Thus, polycystic ovaries need not be present in women who have PCOS, and conversely, the presence of polycystic ovaries alone does not establish a diagnosis of PCOS. PCOS typically manifests at the time of puberty with menstrual irregularity, hirsutism, and obesity (particularly central adiposity) [17].

Hyperandrogenism

The cause of hyperandrogenism in PCOS has been elucidated by in vivo and in vitro studies. In response to stimulation by luteinizing hormone released by the pituitary gland, the ovarian theca cell synthesizes androstenedione and testosterone. Androstenedione is converted by 17β-hydroxysteroid dehydrogenase to form testosterone or is aromatized by the aromatase enzyme (cytochrome P-450arom) to form estrone. Theca cells from PCOS ovaries appear to be more efficient at converting androgenic precursors to testosterone than are normal theca cells [18]. Thus, testosterone levels are generally elevated in women who have PCOS.

Insulin resistance

Insulin resistance is frequently present in women who have PCOS and is considered a hallmark of the syndrome. In insulin-resistant individuals, higher concentrations of insulin (hyperinsulinemia) are needed to compensate and maintain normal glucose tolerance. It has been well documented that in PCOS, the compensatory hyperinsulinemia contributes directly and indirectly [19–21] to the increase in plasma androgen concentrations that characterize PCOS. Insulin acts directly by binding to its cognate receptor on the ovarian theca cell to stimulate testosterone synthesis [22]. Insulin can also act indirectly to raise the serum concentration of free testosterone by lowering the serum concentration of sex hormone binding globulin [21].

Progesterone and estrogen

Women who have PCOS not only have higher levels of androgens but also lower levels of progesterone and estrogen. Over time, circulating progesterone levels in PCOS women are lower than those in normally cycling women [23,24]. These low circulating progesterone levels appear related to the chronic oligo- or anovulation and the resulting absence or reduction of the normal postovulatory surge in progesterone production [25]. Progesterone is thought to "protect" against the development of OSA during pregnancy-associated weight gain [26]; however, as reviewed in the article by Edwards and Sullivan found elsewhere in this issue, emerging evidence suggests the onset or an increase in severity of sleep-disordered breathing (especially snoring) in the last trimester of pregnancy. Physiologic and anatomic changes during pregnancy may be conducive to the development of sleep-disordered breathing, particularly in women who have preeclampsia (abrupt hypertension, hyperalbuminuria, and edema in the third trimester). Progesterone is thought to promote its effects through direct stimulation of respiratory drive by way of an increased ventilatory response to hypercapnea and hypoxia [27,28]. Progesterone may also act to enhance upper airway dilator muscle activity [29] and reduce upper airway resistance as has been found post ovulation in the luteal phase compared with the follicular phase of the menstrual cycle [30]. Reduced progesterone levels in PCOS could be implicated in the high prevalence of OSA.

Underproduction of ovarian estrogen results from low intraovarian aromatase expression and a consequent reduction in the production of the estrogens estrone and estradiol from their respective precursor androgens androstenedione and testosterone. Estrone is also synthesized from peripheral aromatization (especially in adipose tissue), and thus the levels of this steroid are normal or even slightly elevated in PCOS. Estrone, however, is a weak estrogen with approximately one tenth the potency of estradiol [31]. In sum, estrogen levels are subnormal in PCOS [32,33]. It is noteworthy that lower estradiol levels have been reported in association with poor sleep quality among non-PCOS women aged 45 to 49 years [34]. Low estradiol levels have also been associated with a higher frequency of apneic events in women across a broad age spectrum (24–72 years) [35]. The high prevalence of OSA and the related poor sleep quality in PCOS could also thus be associated with the low estrogen levels that characterize this condition.

Metabolic and cardiovascular abnormalities in polycystic ovary syndrome

Women who have PCOS are more insulin resistant than weight-matched control women and have an increased risk of hypertension, dyslipidemia, and cardiovascular disorders [17]. Most of the studies that have focused on the metabolic and cardiovascular abnormalities of PCOS have not controlled for the presence of OSA.

There is ample evidence to support a causal link between hyperinsulinemia and the characteristic features of PCOS. For example, reduction of serum insulin levels in women who have PCOS results in a decrease in ovarian androgen biosynthesis, an increased sex hormone binding globulin concentration, and a resultant decrease in free testosterone concentration [2,36]. Insulin also plays a key role in the higher risk of IGT and type 2 diabetes mellitus in PCOS [2,36]. Attenuation of hyperinsulinemia, whether through weight reduction [37] or administration of metformin [38] or a thiazolidinedione [39–41], substantially attenuates the metabolic perturbations of PCOS.

Although obesity is a major factor in the development of insulin resistance in PCOS, it is now established that a component of insulin resistance in PCOS is independent of body weight [36,42]. Lean and obese women who have PCOS are more insulin resistant than their non-PCOS counterparts matched for total and fat-free body mass, as documented by using a variety of well-established techniques to assess insulin sensitivity [36,40,42,43]. The potential role of OSA in the severity of insulin resistance in PCOS remains to be elucidated. Reduced sleep duration and quality have been shown to result in decreased insulin sensitivity in laboratory studies conducted in healthy young nonobese adults, and most individuals who have OSA have reduced sleep duration and quality [44].

In long-term follow-up studies of women who have PCOS, there is an increased prevalence of type 2 diabetes mellitus compared with appropriate control subjects [9]. Two large, prospective studies in PCOS place the prevalence of IGT between 30% and 40% and the prevalence of type 2 diabetes mellitus between 5% to 10% [7,8]. These prevalences approach those in Pima Indians, a population with one of the highest rates of development of type 2 diabetes mellitus [45]. More recently, Ehrmann and colleagues [7] and Legro and colleagues [46] found that the conversion rates from normal glucose tolerance to IGT or to type 2 diabetes mellitus in PCOS are substantially elevated.

Insulin secretory defects also play an important role in the propensity to develop diabetes in PCOS. Initial evidence for β-cell dysfunction in PCOS was derived from analyses of basal and postprandial insulin secretory responses in women who had PCOS relative to weight-matched control subjects who had normal androgen levels [47]. The incremental insulin secretory response to meals was markedly reduced in nondiabetic women who had PCOS and presented striking similarities with the pattern of meal responses typical of individuals who had established type 2 diabetes mellitus [48]. Reduced β-cell responsiveness to glucose may be experimentally produced in normal healthy individuals by recurrent partial sleep deprivation or reduction of sleep quality, suggesting that sleep disturbances in PCOS may contribute to insulin secretory deficits.

Insulin secretion is most appropriately expressed in relation to the magnitude of ambient insulin resistance. When the initial insulin response to intravenous glucose is analyzed in relation to the degree of insulin resistance, women who have PCOS exhibit a significant impairment in β-cell function [39,43]. β-cell function in PCOS was also quantified by examining the insulin secretory response to a graded increase in plasma glucose and the ability of the β cell to adjust and respond to induced oscillations in the plasma glucose level [43]. Results from provocative stimuli were consistent: when expressed in relation to the degree of insulin resistance, insulin secretion was impaired in PCOS subjects.

Women who have PCOS are frequently characterized as having elevated triglyceride (TG) levels, increased levels of very-low-density lipoprotein and low-density lipoprotein, and a lower level of high-density lipoprotein cholesterol [49]—a lipid pattern similar to that seen in patients who have type 2 diabetes mellitus. The mechanisms responsible for the adverse effects of PCOS on plasma TG homeostasis are not known. Insulin resistance has been postulated to play a key role in causing hypertriglyceridemia in PCOS. The author and colleagues [50], however, found that treatment with the insulin-sensitizing agent troglitazone markedly improved insulin sensitivity in women who had PCOS but had little, if any, effect on plasma TG concentration. In addition, lean women who have PCOS are found to have normal plasma TG concentrations despite being hyperinsulinemic [10].

Lipid and nonlipid criteria identify individuals at increased risk for coronary heart disease and type 2 diabetes mellitus [51,52]. Because women who have PCOS have high rates of IGT, type 2 diabetes mellitus [7,8], and a substantial number of risk factors for cardiovascular disease [50], it has been generally assumed that many are also at increased cardiometabolic risk.

Prevalence of obstructive sleep apnea in polycystic ovary syndrome

The most recent estimate of the prevalence of OSA in the general adult population is approximately 17%. In overweight individuals (body mass index [BMI] ≥ 25 kg/m^2), the proportion of mild to moderate OSA is 41% to 58% [53]. As discussed in the articles by the articles by Edwards and Sullivan and Banno and Kryger found elsewhere in this issue, community and clinic-based studies have consistently noted that men have a higher prevalence of OSA than women [54–57]. The prevalence of OSA is particularly low in premenopausal women and increases after menopause [54,58,59] (see the article by Polo-Kantola found elsewhere in this issue). Among women who have PCOS, however, OSA is considerably more common than expected [13,60,61]. Vgontzas and colleagues [60] assessed the prevalence of OSA in 53 premenopausal women who had PCOS compared with 452 control women. The investigators found that PCOS women were 30 times more likely to have OSA than control subjects and that the difference between the two groups remained significant even after controlling for BMI. An independent study published the same year, comparing 18 overweight women who had PCOS with 18 age- and weight-matched control subjects, showed that PCOS women were significantly more likely to suffer from symptomatic OSA (based on an apnea-hypopnea index (AHI) >5 and the presence of excessive daytime sleepiness) than control women (44.4% versus 5.5%) [13]. In another cohort of 23 obese PCOS women, the prevalence of OSA was found to be 70%, and there was no association between obesity (as assessed by BMI) and the severity of OSA [61]. Recently, survey assessments of the prevalence of sleep apnea risk (using the Berlin questionnaire) in a cohort of 40 women who had PCOS, revealed that three of four women were at high risk for sleep apnea [62]. About two thirds of these PCOS women had poor sleep quality as assessed by the Pittsburgh Sleep Quality questionnaire and 45% had chronic daytime sleepiness as defined by the Epworth Sleepiness Scale. Remarkably, less than 8% of this cohort of 40 women who had PCOS were free of sleep complaints (Fig. 1) [62]. Consistent with the findings of frequent daytime somnolence, in two other studies,

women who had PCOS were found to be subjectively sleepier (as defined by the Epworth Sleepiness Scale) [13] and nine times more likely (80.4% versus 27.0%) to report daytime sleepiness [60] than control subjects. Sleep disturbances thus appear to be an important feature of PCOS. Given the high prevalence of OSA among women who have PCOS, it may be warranted to systematically evaluate them for sleep disorders. Findings from a recent survey, however, suggest that more than 90% of physicians who manage PCOS patients rarely (<25% of the time) order a sleep study [63].

Polycystic ovary syndrome and obstructive sleep apnea: role of sex steroids and obesity

Sex steroids

Differences in concentrations of circulating sex steroids (ie, estrogens, progestins, and androgens) are believed to partly account for the gender disparity in normal sleep architecture [64] and in the prevalence and severity of OSA [65]. Androgens are thought to be "harmful," whereas estrogens and progestins have been generally characterized as "protective" against the development of OSA. Several studies have shown that testosterone administration may have adverse effects on breathing during sleep and may predispose to OSA [65–67]. Testosterone appears to influence the neural control of breathing [68] and upper airway mechanics [69]. Zhou and colleagues [67] examined the effect of testosterone on the hypocapnic apneic threshold in women during sleep. Eight normal, healthy, premenopausal women were studied before and after treatment with transdermal testosterone (5 mg/d) administered in the follicular phase of the menstrual cycle. The investigators concluded that testosterone increases the apneic threshold in premenopausal women, facilitating central apneas, thus leading to breathing instability during sleep.

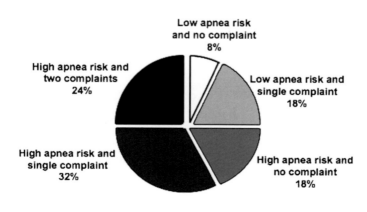

Fig. 1. The frequency distribution of the risk for sleep apnea (derived from responses to the Berlin questionnaire) and sleep complaints (derived from responses to the Pittsburgh Sleep Quality [PSQ] questionnaire and the Epworth Sleepiness Scale [ESS]) in 40 women who have PCOS. A single sleep complaint was defined as a PSQ index greater than 5 or an ESS score of 10 or less. (*From* Tasali E, Van Cauter E, Ehrmann D. Relationships between sleep disordered breathing and glucose metabolism in polycystic ovary syndrome. J Clin Endocrinol Metab 2006;91(1):36–42; with permission. Copyright © 2006, The Endocrine Society.)

Although it is plausible that androgen excess, a defining feature of PCOS, contributes to the higher prevalence of OSA in this disorder, it appears that factors other than the androgen excess may be involved in the increased prevalence of OSA in PCOS. Indeed, two studies found no significant correlations between androgen levels and the severity of OSA [60,62]. In one study of women who had PCOS (N = 53), those taking oral contraceptives (n = 14) were less likely to have OSA [60], consistent with the concept of a "protective role" for estrogens and progesterone in the pathogenesis of OSA [54,58,59]. In contrast, Fogel and colleagues [13] reported that the severity of OSA (as assessed by the AHI) correlated with total and free testosterone levels.

Obesity

The link between obesity and OSA has long been recognized [53]; however, it seems that high prevalence of OSA in PCOS is not simply due to elevated BMI [13,60,61] but may be more closely related to the degree of visceral adiposity. Visceral fat appears to be more metabolically active, and the quantity of visceral fat has been shown to highly correlate with OSA risk [53]. The relative proportion of visceral fat to total body fat is higher in obese men compared with obese women. This difference is thought to contribute to the higher prevalence of OSA in men than in women. Women who have PCOS typically have a high prevalence of visceral adiposity, as assessed, for example, by higher waist-to-hip circumferences than non-PCOS BMI-matched women. Fogel and colleagues [13] reported a significant relationship between waist-to-hip ratio (a measure of central obesity) and severity of OSA in women who have PCOS. The investigators suggested that high androgen levels promote central obesity, which in turn leads to OSA. These findings are consistent with the studies in non-PCOS populations indicating that visceral obesity is closely associated with OSA [53].

In summary, the current evidence suggests that the increased prevalence of OSA in PCOS cannot be fully explained by elevated BMI and high androgen levels. Further well-controlled studies with careful characterization of the levels of sex steroids and assessments of body fat distribution are needed to fully elucidate the complex interactions among obesity, androgen excess, and the presence and severity of OSA in the PCOS population.

Polycystic ovary syndrome and obstructive sleep apnea: insulin resistance, glucose intolerance, and type 2 diabetes mellitus

In non-PCOS populations, there is substantial evidence from cross-sectional studies that supports an independent association between the presence and severity of OSA and alterations in glucose metabolism, including glucose intolerance, insulin resistance, and type 2 diabetes mellitus [14–16]. A number of interventional studies have shown that the treatment of OSA with continuous positive airway pressure improves insulin sensitivity [70] and is associated with a reduction in postprandial glucose and glycohemoglobin levels in individuals who have type 2 diabetes mellitus [71]. So far, only two previous studies have examined the relationships between OSA and alterations in glucose metabolism in women who have PCOS [60,62].

In the first study, Vgontzas and colleagues [60] found that PCOS patients who were recommended treatment for OSA (based on the severity of symptoms) had significantly higher plasma insulin levels and a lower glucose-to-insulin ratio than those who did not have clinically significant OSA, independent of BMI. These findings suggest that in the presence of clinically significant OSA, women who have PCOS may present with a more severe insulin-resistant state. Using a logistic regression model, the investigators also concluded that insulin resistance was the strongest predictor of OSA after controlling for age, BMI, and circulating testosterone concentrations [60].

In the second study, the authors [62] explored the relationships between glucose metabolism and OSA in two cohorts of nondiabetic PCOS women. In the first cohort, sleep apnea risk was determined by the Berlin questionnaire, and glucose metabolism was assessed by the oral glucose tolerance test in 32 women who had PCOS. Fasting insulin levels and the homeostatic model assessment index (defined as the normalized product of fasting glucose by fasting insulin and used as a measure of insulin resistance) were significantly higher in the women who were at high risk for sleep apnea. Furthermore, among the 19 women who had normal glucose tolerance, the insulin response to glucose ingestion was more than twofold higher in women at high risk for sleep apnea compared with those at low risk (Fig. 2). These findings suggest that sleep apnea may contribute to the accelerated conversion rate from normal to IGT in PCOS.

In the second cohort, the authors [62] assessed eight women who had PCOS by overnight polysomnography and the oral glucose tolerance test. The women who had PCOS had reduced sleep efficiency compared with age-matched, healthy nonobese control subjects (mean ± SEM: 80% ± 5% versus 92% ± 1%) and reduced REM (rapid eye movement) sleep time—about half that of the control group (mean ± SEM: 46 ± 10 minutes versus 96 ± 8 minutes). Women who have OSA tend to have a clustering of events during REM sleep [72];

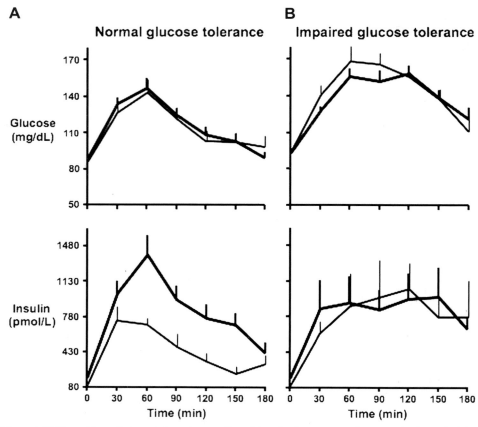

A   **Normal glucose tolerance**   **B**   **Impaired glucose tolerance**

Fig. 2. Mean ± SEM profiles of glucose (*upper panel*) and insulin (*lower panel*) concentrations during the oral glucose tolerance test in women who have PCOS with normal glucose tolerance (n = 19) (*A*) and in women who have PCOS with IGT (n = 13) (*B*). Wide lines represent women who have PCOS at high risk for sleep apnea; narrow lines represent women who have PCOS at low risk for sleep apnea. (*From* Tasali E, Van Cauter E, Ehrmann D. Relationships between sleep disordered breathing and glucose metabolism in polycystic ovary syndrome. J Clin Endocrinol Metab 2006;91(1):36–42; with permission. Copyright © 2006, The Endocrine Society.)

the authors' cohort of women who had PCOS were found to have severe REM-related OSA, with a mean ± SEM AHI of 42 ± 6 per hour of REM sleep. In this small cohort of women who had PCOS, remarkable associations between measures of glucose tolerance and the severity of OSA were detected. Specifically, the markers of the severity of OSA, as quantified by the total AHI of 7 ± 1 per hour of sleep (mean ± SEM), or the number of desaturations, as quantified by at least 3% from baseline in REM sleep (the mean ± SEM of the oxygen desaturation index was 36 ± 4 per hour of REM sleep), were strong predictors of glucose tolerance (Fig. 3).

Several studies have demonstrated that insulin resistance, visceral fat, and higher circulating levels of proinflammatory cytokines are independently and strongly associated with OSA and excessive daytime sleepiness [73,74]. In a recent report [75]

comparing 42 obese PCOS women who did not have OSA, 17 obese women who did not have OSA, and 15 normal-weight control subjects, it was shown that interleukin-6 levels were elevated in obese women who had PCOS independent of obesity or OSA, suggesting that proinflammatory cytokines may be one of the pathways leading to insulin resistance in PCOS.

In summary, limited evidence suggests the existence of strong associations between OSA and abnormalities in glucose metabolism among women who have PCOS. Causal mechanisms underlying these relationships remain to be elucidated. In particular, systematic screening for OSA and carefully designed interventional studies to examine the impact of continuous positive airway pressure treatment of OSA would be important in women who have PCOS and may lead to better treatment options.

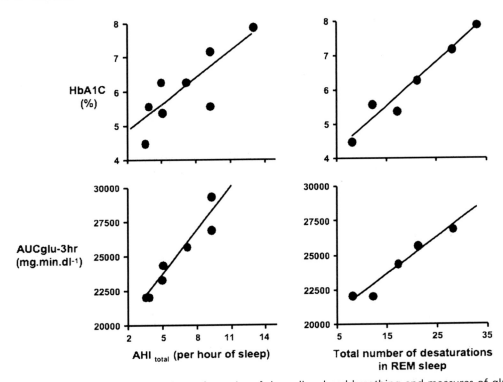

Fig. 3. Relationships between the markers of severity of sleep-disordered breathing and measures of glucose tolerance in eight women who have PCOS. (*Left upper panel*) Relationship between the total AHI (AHI$_{total}$) and glycosylated hemoglobin (HbA1C). (*Left lower panel*) Relationship between AHI$_{total}$ and the area under the glucose curve (AUCglu-3hr). (*Right upper panel*) Relationship between total number of ≥3% desaturations in REM sleep and HbA1C. (*Right lower panel*) Relationship between total number of ≥3% desaturations in REM sleep and AUCglu-3hr. (*From* Tasali E, Van Cauter E, Ehrmann D. Relationships between sleep disordered breathing and glucose metabolism in polycystic ovary syndrome. J Clin Endocrinol Metab 2006;91(1):36–42; with permission. Copyright © 2006, The Endocrine Society.)

Summary

PCOS is one of the most common endocrine disorders affecting women. This syndrome involves a number of reproductive, metabolic, and cardiovascular abnormalities. Affected women are at increased risk for the development of early-onset IGT and type 2 diabetes mellitus. Androgen excess and insulin resistance are the main characteristics in the pathogenesis of PCOS. Recent evidence shows that sleep disturbances appear to be an important feature in PCOS and that OSA is considerably more common than expected in women who have PCOS. The high prevalence of OSA, however, is under-recognized among clinicians who manage PCOS patients. Limited evidence summarized in this review suggests that androgen excess, subnormal estrogen levels, and visceral adiposity could be involved in the increased risk of OSA in PCOS and that there may be a strong association among the severity of OSA and glucose intolerance and insulin resistance. Further research is needed to fully elucidate the causal mechanisms. A better understanding of the link between OSA and PCOS could lead to better treatment options. Systematic screening for OSA in women who have PCOS may be warranted.

References

[1] Knochenhauer E, Key T, Kahsar-Miller M, et al. Prevalence of polycystic ovary syndrome in unselected black and white women of the southeastern United States: a prospective study. J Clin Endocrinol Metab 1998;83:3078–82.

[2] Ehrmann DA, Barnes RB, Rosenfield RL. Polycystic ovary syndrome as a form of functional ovarian hyperandrogenism due to dysregulation of androgen secretion. Endocr Rev 1995;16(3): 322–53.

[3] Dunaif A, Segal KR, Futterweit W, et al. Profound peripheral insulin resistance, independent of obesity, in polycystic ovary syndrome. Diabetes 1989;38(9):1165–74.

[4] Talbott E, Guzick D, Clerici A, et al. Coronary heart disease risk factors in women with polycystic ovary syndrome. Arterioscler Thromb Vasc Biol 1995;15(7):821–6.

[5] Talbott E, Clerici A, Berga SL, et al. Adverse lipid and coronary heart disease risk profiles in young women with polycystic ovary syndrome: results of a case-control study. J Clin Epidemiol 1998; 51(5):415–22.

[6] Talbott EO, Guzick DS, Sutton-Tyrrell K, et al. Evidence for association between polycystic ovary syndrome and premature carotid atherosclerosis in middle-aged women. Arterioscler Thromb Vasc Biol 2000;20(11):2414–21.

[7] Ehrmann DA, Barnes RB, Rosenfield RL, et al. Prevalence of impaired glucose tolerance and diabetes in women with polycystic ovary syndrome. Diabetes Care 1999;22(1):141–6.

[8] Legro RS, Kunselman AR, Dodson WC, et al. Prevalence and predictors of risk for type 2 diabetes mellitus and impaired glucose tolerance in polycystic ovary syndrome: a prospective, controlled study in 254 affected women. J Clin Endocrinol Metab 1999;84(1):165–9.

[9] Dahlgren E, Johansson S, Lindstedt G, et al. Women with polycystic ovary syndrome wedge resected in 1956 to 1965: a long-term followup focusing on natural history and circulating hormones. Fertil Steril 1992;57(3):505–13.

[10] Conway GS, Agrawal R, Betteridge DJ, et al. Risk factors for coronary artery disease in lean and obese women with the polycystic ovary syndrome. Clin Endocrinol (Oxf) 1992;37(2): 119–25.

[11] Kelly CJ, Speirs A, Gould GW, et al. Altered vascular function in young women with polycystic ovary syndrome. J Clin Endocrinol Metab 2002; 87(2):742–6.

[12] Paradisi G, Steinberg HO, Shepard MK, et al. Troglitazone therapy improves endothelial function to near normal levels in women with polycystic ovary syndrome. J Clin Endocrinol Metab 2003;88(2):576–80.

[13] Fogel RB, Malhotra A, Pillar G, et al. Increased prevalence of obstructive sleep apnea syndrome in obese women with polycystic ovary syndrome. J Clin Endocrinol Metab 2001;86(3):1175–80.

[14] Punjabi NM, Polotsky VY. Disorders of glucose metabolism in sleep apnea. J Appl Physiol 2005;99:1998–2007.

[15] Wolk R, Somers VK. Sleep and the metabolic syndrome. Exp Physiol 2007;92(1):67–78.

[16] Tasali E, Mokhlesi B, Van Cauter E. Obstructive sleep apnea and type 2 diabetes: interacting epidemics. Chest, in press.

[17] Ehrmann DA. Polycystic ovary syndrome. N Engl J Med 2005;352(12):1223–36.

[18] Nelson VL, Qin KN, Rosenfield RL, et al. The biochemical basis for increased testosterone production in theca cells propagated from patients with polycystic ovary syndrome. J Clin Endocrinol Metab 2001;86(12):5925–33.

[19] Barbieri RL, Makris A, Randall RW, et al. Insulin stimulates androgen accumulation in incubations of ovarian stroma obtained from women with hyperandrogenism. J Clin Endocrinol Metab 1986;62(5):904–10.

[20] Botwood N, Hamilton-Fairley D, Kiddy D, et al. Sex hormone-binding globulin and female reproductive function. J Steroid Biochem Mol Biol 1995;53(1–6):529–31.

[21] Buyalos RP, Geffner ME, Watanabe RM, et al. The influence of luteinizing hormone and insulin on sex steroids and sex hormone-binding globulin in the polycystic ovarian syndrome. Fertil Steril 1993;60(4):626–33.

[22] Nestler JE, Jakubowicz DJ, de Vargas AF, et al. Insulin stimulates testosterone biosynthesis by human thecal cells from women with polycystic ovary syndrome by activating its own receptor and using inositolglycan mediators as the signal transduction system. J Clin Endocrinol Metab 1998;83(6):2001–5.

[23] Fleming R, McQueen D, Yates RW, et al. Spontaneous follicular and luteal function in infertile women with oligomenorrhoea: role of luteinizing hormone. Clin Endocrinol (Oxf) 1995; 43(6):735–9.

[24] Joseph-Horne R, Mason H, Batty S, et al. Luteal phase progesterone excretion in ovulatory women with polycystic ovaries. Hum Reprod 2002;17(6):1459–63.

[25] Blank SK, McCartney CR, Marshall JC. The origins and sequelae of abnormal neuroendocrine function in polycystic ovary syndrome. Hum Reprod Update 2006;12(4):351–61.

[26] Maasilta P, Bachour A, Teramo K, et al. Sleep-related disordered breathing during pregnancy in obese women. Chest 2001;120(5):1448–54.

[27] Pien GW, Schwab RJ. Sleep disorders during pregnancy. Sleep 2004;27(7):1405–17.

[28] Regensteiner JG, Woodard WD, Hagerman DD, et al. Combined effects of female hormones and metabolic rate on ventilatory drives in women. J Appl Physiol 1989;66(2):808–13.

[29] Popovic RM, White DP. Upper airway muscle activity in normal women: influence of hormonal status. J Appl Physiol 1998;84(3) 1055–62.

[30] Driver HS, McLean H, Kumar DV, et al. The influence of the menstrual cycle on upper airway resistance and breathing during sleep. Sleep 2005;28(4):449–56.

[31] Gutendorf B, Westendorf J. Comparison of an array of in vitro assays for the assessment of the estrogenic potential of natural and synthetic estrogens, phytoestrogens and xenoestrogens. Toxicology 2001;166(1–2):79–89.

[32] Waldstreicher J, Santoro NF, Hall JE, et al. Hyperfunction of the hypothalamic-pituitary axis in women with polycystic ovarian disease: indirect evidence for partial gonadotroph desensitization. J Clin Endocrinol Metab 1988;66(1) 165–72.

[33] Strauss JF III. In: The synthesis and metabolism of steroid hormones. Philadelphia: Elsevier Saunders; 2004.

[34] Hollander LE, Freeman EW, Sammel MD, et al. Sleep quality, estradiol levels, and behavioral factors in late reproductive age women. Obstet Gynecol 2001;98(3):391–7.

[35] Netzer NC, Eliasson AH, Strohl KP. Women with sleep apnea have lower levels of sex hormones. Sleep Breath 2003;7(1):25–9.

[36] Dunaif A. Insulin resistance and the polycystic ovary syndrome: mechanism and implications for pathogenesis. Endocr Rev 1997;18(6): 774–800.

[37] Moran LJ, Noakes M, Clifton PM, et al. Dietary composition in restoring reproductive and metabolic physiology in overweight women with polycystic ovary syndrome. J Clin Endocrinol Metab 2003;88(2):812–9.

[38] Nestler JE. Metformin and the polycystic ovary syndrome. J Clin Endocrinol Metab 2001; 86(3):1430.

[39] Dunaif A, Scott D, Finegood D, et al. The insulin-sensitizing agent troglitazone improves metabolic and reproductive abnormalities in the polycystic ovary syndrome. J Clin Endocrinol Metab 1996;81(9):3299–306.

[40] Ehrmann DA, Schneider DJ, Sobel BE, et al. Troglitazone improves defects in insulin action, insulin secretion, ovarian steroidogenesis, and fibrinolysis in women with polycystic ovary syndrome. J Clin Endocrinol Metab 1997; 82(7):2108–16.

[41] Azziz R, Ehrmann D, Legro RS, et al. Troglitazone improves ovulation and hirsutism in the polycystic ovary syndrome: a multicenter, double blind, placebo-controlled trial. J Clin Endocrinol Metab 2001;86(4):1626–32.

[42] Dunaif A, Graf M, Mandeli J, et al. Characterization of groups of hyperandrogenic women with acanthosis nigricans, impaired glucose tolerance, and/or hyperinsulinemia. J Clin Endocrinol Metab 1987;65(3):499–507.

[43] Ehrmann DA, Sturis J, Byrne MM, et al. Insulin secretory defects in polycystic ovary syndrome: relationship to insulin sensitivity and family history of non-insulin-dependent diabetes mellitus. J Clin Invest 1995;96:520–7.

[44] Spiegel K, Knutson K, Leproult R, et al. Sleep loss: a novel risk factor for insulin resistance and type 2 diabetes. J Appl Physiol 2005;99(5): 2008–19.

[45] Gabir MM, Hanson RL, Dabelea D, et al. The 1997 American Diabetes Association and 1999 World Health Organization criteria for hyperglycemia in the diagnosis and prediction of diabetes. Diabetes Care 2000;23(8):1108–12.

[46] Legro RS, Gnatuk CL, Kunselman AR, et al. Changes in glucose tolerance over time in women with polycystic ovary syndrome: a controlled study. J Clin Endocrinol Metab 2005;90(6):3236–42.

[47] O'Meara NM, Blackman JD, Ehrmann DA, et al. Defects in beta-cell function in functional ovarian hyperandrogenism. J Clin Endocrinol Metab 1993;76(5):1241–7.

[48] Polonsky KS, Given BD, Hirsch LJ, et al. Abnormal patterns of insulin secretion in non-insulin-dependent diabetes mellitus. N Engl J Med 1988; 318:1231–9.

[49] Pirwany IR, Fleming R, Greer IA, et al. Lipids and lipoprotein subfractions in women with PCOS: relationship to metabolic and endocrine parameters. Clin Endocrinol (Oxf) 2001;54(4): 447–53.

[50] Legro RS, Azziz R, Ehrmann D, et al. Minimal response of circulating lipids in women with polycystic ovary syndrome to improvement in insulin sensitivity with troglitazone. J Clin Endocrinol Metab 2003;88(11):5137–44.

[51] Third Report of the National Cholesterol Education Program (NCEP) Expert Panel on Detection, Evaluation, and Treatment of High Blood Cholesterol in Adults (Adult Treatment Panel III) final report. Circulation 2002;106(25). 3143–3421.

[52] Ford ES. The metabolic syndrome and mortality from cardiovascular disease and all-causes: findings from the National Health and Nutrition Examination Survey II Mortality Study. Atherosclerosis 2004;173(2):309–14.

[53] Young T, Peppard PE, Taheri S. Excess weight and sleep-disordered breathing. J Appl Physiol 2005; 99(4):1592–9.

[54] Bixler EO, Vgontzas AN, Lin HM, et al. Prevalence of sleep-disordered breathing in women: effects of gender. Am J Respir Crit Care Med 2001;163(3 Pt 1):608–13.

[55] Young T, Palta M, Dempsey J, et al. The occurrence of sleep-disordered breathing among middle-aged adults. N Engl J Med 1993;328(17): 1230–5.

[56] Young T, Peppard PE, Gottlieb DJ. Epidemiology of obstructive sleep apnea: a population health perspective. Am J Respir Crit Care Med 2002; 165(9):1217–39.

[57] Young T, Skatrud J, Peppard PE. Risk factors for obstructive sleep apnea in adults. JAMA 2004; 291(16):2013–6.

[58] Shahar E, Redline S, Young T, et al. Hormone replacement therapy and sleep-disordered breathing. Am J Respir Crit Care Med 2003; 167(9):1186–92.

[59] Young T, Finn L, Austin D, et al. Menopausal status and sleep-disordered breathing in the Wisconsin Sleep Cohort Study. Am J Respir Crit Care Med 2003;167(9):1181–5.

[60] Vgontzas AN, Legro RS, Bixler EO, et al. Polycystic ovary syndrome is associated with obstructive sleep apnea and daytime sleepiness: role of insulin resistance. J Clin Endocrinol Metab 2001;86(2):517–20.

[61] Gopal M, Duntley S, Uhles M, et al. The role of obesity in the increased prevalence of obstructive

sleep apnea syndrome in patients with polycystic ovarian syndrome. Sleep Med 2002;3(5):401–4.

[62] Tasali E, Van Cauter E, Ehrmann DA. Relationships between sleep disordered breathing and glucose metabolism in polycystic ovary syndrome. J Clin Endocrinol Metab 2006; 91(1):36–42.

[63] Subramanian S, Desai A, Joshipura M, et al. Practice patterns of screening for sleep apnea in physicians treating PCOS patients. Sleep Breath 2007;11(4):233–7.

[64] Driver HS, Dijk DJ, Werth E, et al. Sleep and the sleep electroencephalogram across the menstrual cycle in young healthy women. J Clin Endocrinol Metab 1996;81(2):728–35.

[65] Liu K, Yee B, Philips C, et al. Sleep apnea and neuroendocrine function. Sleep Medicine Clinics 2007;2:225–36.

[66] Liu PY, Yee B, Wishart SM, et al. The short-term effects of high-dose testosterone on sleep, breathing, and function in older men. J Clin Endocrinol Metab 2003;88(8):3605–13.

[67] Zhou XS, Rowley JA, Demirovic F, et al. Effect of testosterone on the apneic threshold in women during NREM sleep. J Appl Physiol 2003;94: 101–7.

[68] White DP, Schneider BK, Santen RJ, et al. Influence of testosterone on ventilation and chemosensitivity in male subjects. J Appl Physiol 1985;59(5):1452–7.

[69] Cistulli PA, Grunstein RR, Sullivan CE. Effect of testosterone administration on upper airway collapsibility during sleep. Am J Respir Crit Care Med 1994;149(2 Pt 1):530–2.

[70] Harsch IA, Hahn EG, Konturek PC. Insulin resistance and other metabolic aspects of the obstructive sleep apnea syndrome. Med Sci Monit 2005;11(3):RA70–5.

[71] Babu AR, Herdegen J, Fogelfeld L, et al. Type 2 diabetes, glycemic control, and continuous positive airway pressure in obstructive sleep apnea. Arch Intern Med 2005;165(4):447–52.

[72] O'Connor C, Thornley KS, Hanly PJ. Gender differences in the polysomnographic features of obstructive sleep apnea. Am J Respir Crit Care Med 2000;161(5):1465–72.

[73] Vgontzas AN, Papanicolaou DA, Bixler EO, et al. Sleep apnea and daytime sleepiness and fatigue relation to visceral obesity, insulin resistance and hypercytokinemia. J Clin Endocrinol Metab 2000;85:1151–8.

[74] Vgontzas AN, Papanicolaou DA, Bixler EO, et al. Elevation of plasma cytokines in disorders of excessive daytime sleepiness: role of sleep disturbance and obesity. J Clin Endocrinol Metab 1997;82(5):1313–6.

[75] Vgontzas AN, Trakada G, Bixler EO, et al. Plasma interleukin 6 levels are elevated in polycystic ovary syndrome independently of obesity or sleep apnea. Metabolism 2006;55(8):1076–82.

SLEEP
MEDICINE
CLINICS

Sleep Med Clin 3 (2008) 47–60

Sleep Disturbed by Chronic Pain in Fibromyalgia, Irritable Bowel, and Chronic Pelvic Pain Syndromes

Joan L.F. Shaver, PhD, RN, FAAN

- Prevalence and somatic functional features of fibromyalgia, irritable bowel, and chronic pelvic pain
- Sleep in functional somatic syndromes
  Subjective sleep in functional somatic syndromes
  Objective sleep in functional somatic syndromes
- Sleep disruption in fibromyalgia, irritable bowel, and chronic pelvic pain: unique markers or not?
- Linking nonrestorative sleep patterns with pain
- The central processing component of pain

- The inflammatory/immune activation component in functional somatic syndromes
- Stress as context for pain hypersensitivity in fibromyalgia, irritable bowel, and chronic pelvic pain
  Predisposition, life-events, and emotional arousal
  Physiologic stress activation
- Linking sleep, stress and inflammatory/immune activation
- Summary
- References

Women are disproportionately prone to manifest a series of chronically widespread and regional painful, multisymptom syndromes, including fibromyalgia (FM), irritable bowel (IB), chronic pelvic pain (CPP), low back pain, temporomandibular joint disorder, an tension-type headache. Many times they meet criteria for more than one syndrome [1]. Pain hypersensitivity/sensitization and stress-immune dysregulation are evident across these syndromes in the context of emotional arousal and physiologic activation. Because no clear pathological indicators are available, these conditions are sometimes referred to as *functional somatic syndromes* (FSSs) [2,3] or *multisymptom illnesses* [4]. Without the availability of definitive diagnostic tests, these conditions are mainly diagnosed

through excluding other disease possibilities. In this article, FSSs refers to FM, IB, and CPP.

Across these FSSs, many other symptoms besides pain are reported [5], particularly sleep disturbances, unexplained and enduring fatigue, and activity intolerance. Poor sleep is commonly reported in chronic pain conditions; in studies of people presenting at outpatient chronic pain clinics, 65% to 70% reported poor sleep [6,7]. Poor sleep and higher pain intensity tend to be correlated [7]. A common view is that acute or chronic pain disturbs sleep, but in some contexts sleep disturbances or physiology during sleep may predispose to or precipitate chronic pain as part of underlying pathophysiology [8]. This article addresses some of the science related to three complex

University of Illinois at Chicago, College of Nursing, 845 South Damen (M/C 802), Chicago, IL 60612, USA
E-mail address: jshaver@uic.edu

1556-407X/08/$ – see front matter © 2008 Elsevier Inc. All rights reserved.
sleep.theclinics.com

doi:10.1016/j.jsmc.2007.10.007

painful FSSs and the reciprocal features of sleep and pain. Because pain is a potent correlate of poor sleep (ie, insomnia) and poor sleep is a correlate of fatigue, knowledge of other symptoms, general well-being, sleep, and pain related to these conditions is pertinent to informing diagnostics [1] and therapeutics [9–11] and comprehensively understanding their impact on quality of life for women.

Prevalence and somatic functional features of fibromyalgia, irritable bowel, and chronic pelvic pain

FM affects approximately 1% to 3% of the adult population with a prevalence estimated to be five to nine times higher in women than men [12]. A hallmark of FM is debilitating widespread (upper and lower and axial quadrants) musculoskeletal pain lasting at least 3 months with discrete points of tenderness (more than 10 of 18 sites). The pain profile is frequently accompanied by nonrestorative sleep, stiffness, and intense fatigue, among other symptoms. More than half of women who have FM meet criteria for chronic fatigue syndrome (CFS) (chronic fatigue and muscle and multiple joint pain without swelling or redness [13]) and for other FSSs. Many women are likely to report inability to concentrate, remember, or think properly, a condition that patients refer to as *fibro fog*. In the most severe FM cases, women have profound inability to perform activities of daily living and work.

For IB, categorized as a *functional gastrointestinal disorder*, prevalence estimates range from 3% to 20%, again with more women affected than men (2:1 in community settings and 3:1–4:1 in tertiary care settings) [14]. Hallmark features of IB are general abdominal pain or discomfort associated with altered bowel habits (diarrhea- or constipation-dominant or an alternating pattern of diarrhea and constipation) [14,15]. A high proportion of women meet criteria for both IB and FM [16]. One summary showed that approximately 32% to 77% of patients who had FM also had IB, and 32% to 65% of patients who had IB also had FM [17].

An accurate prevalence estimate for CPP is unavailable, although more than 9 million women in the United States are believed to experience some form of CPP [18]. According to a review by Stanford and colleagues [19] in 2007, 12% of outpatient gynecologic referrals, 10% to 12% of hysterectomies, and approximately 40% of gynecologic laparoscopies are for CPP. The American College of Obstetricians and Gynecologists definition is localized noncyclic pain lasting more than 6 months that causes a loss of function [20]. Often women who have CPP meet criteria for FM, IB, and

musculoskeletal disorders, such as trigger point pain and pelvic floor dysfunction [21].

A sizable number of women who have CPP are diagnosed with endometriosis, chiefly manifested as cyclic or noncyclic pain, often coinciding with dysmenorrheal (ie, painful menstruation), dyspareunia (ie, painful intercourse), and impaired fertility. Although broad sample heterogeneity across studies makes accurate prevalence estimates of CPP with endometriosis difficult to discern, reported prevalence rates range from 33% [22] to 70% [21]. Besides endometriosis, other reproductive tract conditions believed to contribute to CPP include adenomyosis, pelvic adhesions, pelvic inflammatory disease, congenital anomalies of the reproductive tract, and ovarian or tubal masses.

Evidence is emerging that, rather than being attributable to classic gynecologic conditions such as endometriosis, CPP more often manifests as pain of bladder origin, particularly interstitial cystitis. Without widely accepted definitional consensus, a symptom cluster of chronic urinary frequency, pelvic pain or pressure, and sensory urgency when all other causes of these symptoms have been reasonably ruled out is often used for diagnosis [23]. Estimates are that up to 85% of women who have CPP meet criteria for interstitial cystitis, with as many as 1 in 4.5 women in the United States having interstitial cystitis [19], roughly 10 times more often than men [24].

Sleep in functional somatic syndromes

Poor quality sleep is a prevalent feature of chronic pain in general and certainly with FM, IB, and CPP. As reviewed by Menefee and colleagues [25], sleep disturbance (mostly self-reported) is prevalently reported by people referred to pain clinics or rehabilitation programs for rheumatic conditions, arthritis, headache, and widespread chronic pain (mostly studied as FM). Evidence for the link between sleep and pain in these conditions is hindered by only a few studies incorporating objective or combined subjective and objective sleep measures, generally in reference to small samples. In reconciling data across studies, generalized results are confounded because perceptually assessed often does not match objectively assessed sleep quality [26–29].

Subjective sleep in functional somatic syndromes

Generally, in adults who have chronic pain, reported pain variables have correlated with more wakefulness (fewer hours of sleep, longer sleep latency, more and longer nighttime awakenings), lower perceived overall sleep quality, and shortened time asleep [6,30–32]. Compared with normative data, girls (aged 12–17 years) who had mixed chronic musculoskeletal pain conditions reported similar total sleep time and bedtimes, but significantly longer sleep onset latency and more night awakenings [33].

Poor and unrefreshing sleep is reported by large numbers of people who have FM. In various studies, upwards of 70% of people who had FM reported poor sleep quality and enduring fatigue [34–36]. Compared with people who have arthritis or healthy controls of similar age, individuals who have FM report more difficulty falling and staying asleep, premature awakening, fewer hours of sleep, and taking more sleep medications [4,37–39]. In a large nonrandom telephone survey, more midlife women who had FM (n = 442) than those who did not (n = 205) reported poor quality on almost all sleep factors [40]. A common dimension of FM is "unrefreshing sleep." In a large multicenter study, 76% of people who had FM reported feeling tired or unrefreshed on awakening [41].

Many women who have IB, although seemingly not as many as those who have FM, report poor sleep quality [27,42,43]. Using retrospective 7-day recall and daily diary ratings over two menstrual cycles, approximately one quarter of women who had IB (n = 82) reported sleep problems and, compared with controls (n = 35), had considerably higher levels of sleep disturbance [42]. When women were compared among groups of mild to moderate (n = 18), severe (n = 18), or no IB symptoms (n = 38), using the Pittsburgh Sleep Quality Inventory (PSQI), 56% of women who had severe IB versus 11% of control women were classified as experiencing poor sleep. The PSQI subcomponent scores showed that women who had severe IB differed from controls on reported sleep quality, efficiency, and disturbance, but no differences were found for sleep latency or duration, or use of sleep medication and daytime function [27]. In another study, two groups who had IB (n = 15 with IB-only, n = 16 with IB plus dyspeptic symptoms) had PSQI scores on every dimension significantly indicative of poorer sleep compared with controls (n = 23) [44].

Only one study of women who had CPP was found and it was focused on assessing in-depth self-reported sleep quality as part of overall quality-of-life assessment [45]. In this New Zealand mail questionnaire sent to 1160 randomly selected women aged 18 to 50 years, CPP was defined as recurrent or constant pain in the lower abdominal region lasting at least 6 months, unrelated to menstrual periods, intercourse, or pregnancy. Subgroups of women who had dysmenorrhea or dyspareunia or no pelvic pain from any source were compared with those experiencing CPP. Women who had CPP were more likely to report sleep problems compared with those experiencing no pelvic pain of any type (difficulty falling asleep, 17.8% versus 7.1%; frequency of awakening, 33.2% versus 24.2%; and nonrestorative sleep, 36.7% versus 17.1%). Women who had CPP had higher rates of other serious long-standing illnesses compared with those who did not; nearly 20% had associated genitourinary symptoms and 37.3% met criteria for IB. In addition, they were more likely to report pain, attributed to some feature other than CPP, and fatigue or both in the past 12 months [45].

Objective sleep in functional somatic syndromes

In chronic pain conditions, objective sleep measures using classic polysomnography scoring have shown a pattern of modestly lighter and less-consolidated (more fragmented) sleep, perhaps with more wakefulness and arousal [46] but no striking abnormalities that would match the extent of subjective poor sleep reports (Table 1). Compared with controls, people who have FM generally show more wakefulness (longer sleep onset latency, more wakefulness after sleep onset) with reduced sleep efficiency (time asleep/time in bed); somewhat lighter (more stage 1), less stage-2 or slow-wave sleep (SWS) (non–rapid eye movement [REM] stages 3 and 4 sleep); and less-stable sleep (more sleep stage changes and higher fragmentation index, particularly in the first half of the night) [28,37,47–51]. Studies of women who have IB have shown few polysomnographic sleep differences compared with healthy controls [27,44,52], although in one study, women who had IB showed significantly less SWS (4.5% ± 7.3% versus 19.3% ± 12.9%), increased stage 2 sleep (72.2% ± 6.6% versus 60.1% ± 16.8%), more sleep fragmentation, and a longer wake period after sleep onset [53]. Only one uncontrolled, small-sample overnight polysomnography study of women who had CPP (N = 11) was found. Using statistical comparisons with age-matched normative data (from 1974), women who had CPP had significantly more transitional (stage 1) but also more SWS sleep, with higher REM latencies and reduced REM sleep [54].

In summary, perceived poor and nonrestorative sleep is highly prevalent with FM; these features are evident with IB but perhaps in fewer women and not well established with CPP. The inconsistencies emanate from subject selection, normative variability within individuals making the comparative capture of sleep expression a challenge, and use of various derived sleep variables. Much more heterogeneity may be present within the samples than is known, including factors such as stage and

Table 1: **Summary of polysomnography sleep studies in women who have fibromyalgia, irritable bowel, and chronic pelvic pain syndromes[a]**

Reference	Study participants	Results	Comments
	Fibromyalgia		
Molony et al. [47]	7 FM 6 controls	More % stage 1 More miniarousals per hour	Miniarousal; brief NREM sleep interruption (5–19 seconds)
Anch et al. [48]	9 FM (6 women, 3 men) 11 controls (8 women, 3 men)	Less % Stage 1 Less % REM	
Jennum et al. [37]	20 FM 10 controls	Higher % arousal time Higher arousal index	Arousal; alpha activity in EEG longer than 3 seconds
Cote and Moldofsky [49]	10 FM 9 controls	More stage 1	FM; more sleepiness, fatigue, pain, and dysphoria
Shaver et al. [28]	11 FM 11 controls	First half of night: More stage 1 More stage changes Tendency to higher fragmentation index	Total night; no differences in sleep quality, depth, or continuity
Roizenblatt et al. [50]	40 FM 43 controls	More % stage 1 More alpha activity in stage 2 and SWS (first two sleep cycles)	
Landis et al. [51]	33 FM 37 controls	More % stage 1 Less % stage 2 Lower SE Longer SL to stage 2	No differences in deep sleep, WASO, REM, or REM latency
	Irritable bowel syndrome		
Elsenbruch et al. [44]	15 IB-only 16 IB with lower and upper dyspeptic symptoms 23 controls	No significant group differences	Poorer subjective sleep quality
Rotem et al. [53]	18 IB 20 women with mild benign snoring	Less SWS More Stage 2 High sleep fragmentation, arousals, more WASO	IB; more daytime sleepiness Epworth Sleepiness Scale score, more impaired quality of life not caused by baseline anxiety/depression differences
Robert et al. [52]	26 IB with depression 44 IB without depression (BDI $\geq$ 12) 21 controls	No differences Tendency to longer REM latency for IB with depression	Sample size as in the results, not the abstract
Heitkemper et al. [27]	18 IB moderate 18 IB severe 38 controls	Few differences Higher REM latency to stage 2 in IB groups	
	Chronic pelvic pain		
Dunlap et al. [54]	11 CPP No controls; compared with norms More % stage 1	More % stage 1 Less REM More SWS Longer REM latency	

Abbreviations: BDI, Beck Depression Inventory; CPP, chronic pelvic pain; FM, fibromyalgia; IB, irritable bowel; NREM, non-rapid eye movement; REM, rapid eye movement; SE, sleep efficiency; SL, sleep latency; SWS, slow-wave sleep; WASO, wakefulness after sleep onset.
[a] Compared with female controls unless otherwise noted.

severity of the FSS, cognitive emotional pain arousal, intensity of other bothersome symptoms, genetic propensities, and inherent sleep quality, mood, or stress reactivity tendencies. These factors warrant further investigation through which to subclassify these conditions and to more comprehensively delineate the links between sleep and pain in FSSs. Perhaps changes in sleep are subtle and require probing of the microstructure of sleep.

Sleep disruption in fibromyalgia, irritable bowel, and chronic pelvic pain: unique markers or not?

The sleep disturbances in FSSs are closely comparable to primary insomnia. In one polysomnography study of 26 individuals experiencing nonorganic pain compared with 25 subjects experiencing chronic primary insomnia, the type and extent of sleep disruption did not differ, despite whether pain was present at polysomnography [55]. Assessing preexisting or lifelong sleep quality is not typical in studies of chronic pain or FSSs, thus shedding little light on whether these conditions might be superimposed on inherently poor sleep quality.

The light, fragmented, and nonrestorative sleep associated with FSSs convey a pattern of aroused and unconsolidated sleep. More as a marker of sleep induction and maintenance, women who had FM and pain were reported to have fewer sleep spindles and reduced electroencephalogram (EEG) power in spindle frequency activity compared with controls of similar age [56].

The lack of concordance between self-reported and polysomnography variables, mostly studied in FM, has driven efforts to uncover sleep characteristics predictive of nonrestorative sleep. One characteristic is alpha EEG (7.5–11 Hz) intrusion into stages of non-REM delta sleep (called alpha–delta sleep), first reported in 1975 by Moldofsky and colleagues [57]. Other investigators, primarily using visual scoring methods or in a few cases spectral analysis, confirmed increased alpha activity in non-REM sleep in FM [29,58,59], whereas others did not [60] or only reported a trend for increased alpha activity [61]. People who had increased alpha activity showed no differences in pain, fatigue, or sleep quality compared with those who did not [59]. An alpha sleep pattern was described in various chronic pain contexts [62] and in some patients experiencing insomnia [63]. Some sleep alpha intrusion pattern subtypes have been described that seem to align more strongly with pain. Three patterns of alpha sleep were seen in women who had FM (n = 40) and those who did not (n = 43), namely (1) phasic alpha (simultaneous with delta

activity) in 50%; (2) tonic alpha (continuous throughout non-REM sleep) in 20%; and (3) low alpha activity in the remaining 30% who had FM and 87% of controls [50]. More women who had FM in the phasic alpha group reported worse pain after sleep (100% phasic alpha versus 58% low alpha or 25% tonic alpha). A similar pattern was seen for post–sleep tenderpoints [50]. Thus, a definitive role for alpha EEG intrusion into sleep in chronic pain conditions as it relates to the perception of nonrestorative sleep requires more study.

As potent disruptors of sleep, sleep-related disorders, such as restless leg syndrome (RLS), periodic limb movement disorder, and sleep apnea/hypopnea syndrome (SAHS), have been associated with FM. Obstructive sleep apnea and RLS have high rates of association in chronic pain conditions, including rheumatoid arthritis, headache, chronic back pain, and FM [25]. In polysomnography studies involving women or predominantly women who had FM, approximately 19% to 25% were found to have SAHS [64,65]. In an uncontrolled polysomnography study of 23 women from a rheumatology clinic who had FM, the median apnea/hypopnea index was 22 per hour, and 19 (83%) had an apnea/hypopnea index greater than 15. The one-night polysomnography sleep efficiency was low (76.5%) and the median arousal index was 23 per hour, which strongly correlated with the apnea/hypopnea index (r = 0.99, $P<.005$) [66]. In a large, nonrandom, telephone survey, more women who had FM were diagnosed with RLS (20.1% versus 0.5%), abnormal leg movements (10% versus 1%), and apnea (9% versus 0%) compared with those who did not [40]. Compared with a European study showing a 3.6% prevalence for RLS [67], this prevalence of 20% is much higher. Although individuals who have painful FSSs seem to have excessive vulnerability to sleep-related disorders, mixed and small sample sizes, clinic-based subject recruitment, and subject selection based on suspected sleep disorders obscure the clarity of this relationship. Studies incorporating careful assessment of sleep-related disorders and comparisons with other painful conditions and twin studies would be illuminating.

Linking nonrestorative sleep patterns with pain

Evidence linking sleep and pain has come from symptom assessment after manipulating sleep patterns or careful temporal reciprocal analysis of sleep and pain quality. A review of human experiments [68] concluded that total sleep or selective sleep-stage deprivation likely produces hyperalgesia in healthy subjects (mostly men; 5 of 8 studies)

[38,57,60,68–71], mostly seen on pressure assessment, and that consequences are strongest for SWS compared with REM sleep. In a study of selective SWS deprivation over 3 nights (without sleep length reductions) in healthy women (N = 12), the authors showed increased musculoskeletal discomfort (no change in other symptom clusters except vigor), tendency to reduced tenderpoint pain thresholds (including at two control sites), and heightened skinfold tenderness and an increased inflammatory flare to skin stimulus compared with baseline [60]. Experts have argued that disrupting sleep continuity is of greater importance to feelings of restoration than sleep length. However, Wesensten and colleagues [72] showed that any means of imposing sleep-stage deprivation will invariably elevate stage 1 (transitional) sleep, which might not have the recuperative properties of light sleep (stage 2) and SWS, thereby effectively reducing recuperative sleep duration. Not without challenges to interpretation and application to humans, in a 2006 review of sleep deprivation in animal studies, Lautenbacher and colleagues [8] concluded that REM sleep deprivation was consistently linked to nociceptive outcomes, potentially supporting a role for REM sleep in pain generation or modulation [68].

In both FM and IB, relationships have been observed among daytime pain and subsequent sleep, and night sleep with subsequent daytime pain. In women who had FM, analysis of prospective 30-day diary reports of sleep quality and pain intensity showed that higher daytime and concurrent pain led to poorer nighttime sleep, and a night of poor sleep was followed by a more painful day [73]. In women who had IB completing daily diaries over two menstrual cycles, regression analysis supported the hypothesis that on the day after a night of poor sleep, women reported worse ratings of gastrointestinal symptoms, although the opposite was not supported [42]. Which comes first—pain or poor sleep—remains unclear. Viewing them both as part of a common broader-based stress-related disturbance in a potential spiral of reinforcement seems pertinent for reasons discussed further in this article.

The central processing component of pain

Pain hypersensitivity is common across FM, IB, and CPP, and accompanied by altered pain processing mechanisms [74]. Pain is widespread (FM), regional or local (IB, bladder/pelvic), with hyperalgesia (noxious stimuli produce more and longer-lasting pain), allodynia (nonnoxious stimuli produce pain), and pain pressure points in tissues [75].

Pain pressure points tested in patients who have chronic pain (FM, whiplash, rheumatoid arthritis and endometriosis) showed generalized hypersensitivity across the groups, but those who had FM and whiplash showed the most pain sensitivity, as seen in lowest pain thresholds [74].

As reviewed by Clauw and Crofford [4] and Staud and Rodriguez [75], numerous studies confirm alterations in pain processing and hypersensitivity in FM, including reduced pain thresholds with mechanical, electrical, or thermal stimuli; altered invoked potentials in response to cutaneous stimuli and reduced blood flow to, or altered activation of, pain-related areas in the brain, as seen through functional brain imaging. In IB and other functional gastrointestinal disorders, pain hypersensitivity and sensitization are evident on balloon distention of the bowel [39,76]. Individuals who have IB declare pain at lower pressures (visceral hyperalgesia) or increased sensitivity even to normal intestinal pressures (ie, allodynia), and show a progressive increase in pain intensity and heightened somatic referral of visceral pain. People who have interstitial cystitis exhibit bladder hypersensitivity as reduced threshold for urinary first-sensation first-urge, and awake volume. Most interstitial cystitis bladder symptoms (urgency, frequency) are described as mild to moderate, with flares occurring in cycles, provoked by activation of seasonal allergies or physical or emotional stressors [77]. Pain signals from the bladder transmitted to the spinal cord can be perceived as pelvic pain in any location [19], which often obscures the bladder as generator.

Although commonly experienced in the suprapubic area, pain can be localized to the bladder, lower abdomen, urethra, lower back, vaginal area, perineum, scrotum, vulva, thighs, or rectum [24]. Pelvic discomfort or pain may be constant, intermittent (flare pattern), or triggered by stimuli such as menses, sexual activity, and ingestion of certain substances (eg, citrus fruits, chocolate, caffeine, alcohol, high-potassium foods) [24,77]. How endometriosis provokes CPP is not well understood. The relationship between the amount of endometrial tissue present in the pelvis and extent of pain is weak, implying that processes beyond the direct effects of endometrial tissue in the pelvis are involved [19].

Pain hypersensitivity is seen as a function of altered pain processing in the spinal cord and brain [4,74,78,79]. Excessive or relentless pain signals (neuronal or biochemical) from peripheral tissue invoke a series of changes in structure and function of spinal cord neurons that manifest in enhanced neuronal excitability, spontaneous nerve activity, expanded receptive fields, and augmented neuronal responses, such as abnormal temporal summation

One important receptor is the *N*-methyl-D-aspartic acid (NMDA) receptor, found at the postsynaptic membrane in dorsal horn neurons of the spinal cord. Further mechanisms in pain hypersensitivity involve altered conduction of pain signals to and from the brain through ascending and descending pathways, especially disinhibition of pain signals.

The locus of the pain and presumably the generator of the central pain processing changes are mainly somatic or visceral muscle or connective tissue, but the nature of tissue dysregulation is debated [74]. Although FM is considered a wide-spread pain phenomenon, women who have this syndrome often meet criteria for localized pain conditions such as IB, interstitial cystitis, headache, or temporomandibular disorder. This fuels speculation that FM is initiated by focal pain–generating mechanisms in peripheral tissue, perhaps caused by tissue injury. Overall, pain hypersensitivity might be a function of low-grade stress/inflammatory/immune activation shaped by environmental factors (physical or interpersonal) and person-specific propensities (physical or psychological). In all three FSSs, various inflammatory/immune changes are observed with or without obvious evidence of any classic instigators, such as infectious agents [79]. A complex picture of bidirectional connections is emerging between systems, including the nociceptive neural, inflammatory/immune, stress, and sleep/wake systems.

The inflammatory/immune activation component in functional somatic syndromes

In painful FSSs, inflammatory/immune activation indicators of the type to sensitize pain processing centrally are increasingly evident. For example, as reviewed by Nielsen and Henriksson [74] and Staud and Rodriguez [75], in people who have FM, neurotrophins (such as nerve growth factor) and tachykinins (such as substance P), which sensitize nociceptors, regulate inflammatory processes, and invoke cytokine expression, are elevated in cerebrospinal fluid, as are proinflammatory cytokines, such as interleukin (IL)-1ra, IL-8, and IL-6, in peripheral blood and skin [74,75]. A study of peripheral blood mononuclear cells in individuals who had IB (33 women, 22 men) showed that these subjects had significantly (P<.017) higher proinflammatory baseline cytokine levels, tumor necrosis factor, IL-1, and IL-6 compared with asymptomatic controls (23 women, 13 men). In IB subtypes, all levels of cytokines were highest in diarrhea-predominant IB [80]. Various mechanisms have been postulated to explain IB symptoms that include inflammatory/immune drivers and evidence that mucosal inflammation affects gut muscle function, with

heightened gut receptor sensitivity, degranulation of mast cells, and release of cytokines close to enteric nerves [81,82]. In interstitial cystitis, evidence of inflammatory/immune activation underlying visceral organ hypersensitization are emerging, such as reviews addressing mast cell activation [83] and peripheral and central neural up-regulation [84]. With endometriosis, pain is commonly believed to be invoked from host defense reactions to or bleeding from endometrial implants, with production of substances such as growth factors and cytokines by activated inflammatory cells; and pelvic floor nerve irritation or reactivity to the bleeding of endometrial implants or direct tissue infiltration [21].

Altered central neurochemicals relevant to modulating pain processing, including serotonin, epinephrine, and perhaps dopamine, might be part of FM abnormalities [85]. Reduced levels of serotonin, its precursor *L*-tryptophan, and its metabolites in blood or cerebral spinal fluid, have been observed in FM, although not consistently [4,78]. Believed to be antinociceptive, serotonin is produced by brainstem neurons and downwardly modulates pain signaling through inhibiting substance P in the spinal cord. However, low serotonin levels might pertain more to psychological distress coincidental in FM, for example, as shown in factors associated with a recently uncovered polymorphism for the serotonin transporter gene [86]. Additionally in FM, low cerebral spinal fluid levels of the principal metabolite of norepinephrine, methoxy-4-hydroxy-phenethylene, have been observed [4]. Norepinephrine is a neurotransmitter important for inhibiting descending pain-inhibitory neurons projecting to the spinal cord neurons [4]. Prolonged stress in animals leads to reduced output from dopaminergic neurons, resulting in hyperalgesia [25]. However, the relationship to humans and FM is not yet clear except that pain can be improved with the use of dopaminergic-active drugs in patients who have FM. The role that these neurochemicals play in pain hypersensitization still must be fully elucidated, but importantly they are also known to affect sleep and mood in the absence of pain.

Stress as context for pain hypersensitivity in fibromyalgia, irritable bowel, and chronic pelvic pain

Vulnerability to the enduring pain of FSSs is probably caused by a cascade of maladaptive emotional arousal and physiologic activation patterns evolving from normative processes for defending against harm or adapting to novel environmental circumstances. High life-strain (exposure to circumstances that are perceived as threatening or challenging) plus inherent emotional arousal and physiologic reactive propensities define the stress-relatedness of these conditions. Evidence of familial tendencies to develop these conditions suggests that certain individuals are vulnerable to developing FSSs [4]. Moreover, women can often pinpoint factors or events (stressors) believed to trigger noticeable symptoms, such as severe emotional stress, infection, injury, or exposure to toxic substances (eg, sick building, multiple chemical sensitivities, Gulf War Illness) [4]. In general, these factors are stressors capable of invoking activation of the stress inflammatory/immune (host defense) system.

Predisposition, life-events, and emotional arousal

Underlying the breakthrough to clinical manifestations of FSSs is evidence of preclinical predispositions related to perceived high-stress exposure or style of processing stressors (eg, life events). Based on investigations in Europe, predisposition to FM is related to reports of high exposure to or high perceived negativity related to life events, including major or daily hassles; sexual, physical, or emotional abuse; and a driven lifestyle (ie, excessively active mental or physical engagement) [87]. Life-event exposure has been associated with subsequent symptom severity in clinic patients who have IB, and on regression analysis using a community-based sample, total life stress was independently related to functional gastrointestinal disorders (IB or nonulcer dyspepsia) [88]. A study comparing women who had CPP, chronic low back pain, and no pain found that childhood physical abuse and stressful life events significantly impacted the occurrence of chronic pain in general, and childhood sexual abuse was correlated with CPP only [89]. Data from multiple studies support the connection between excess stressful life events and somatic symptoms, salient to the psychobiologic explanations of painful FSSs.

The clinical impression that FSSs and psychiatric disorders run concurrently [90,91] seems to be a bias derived from tertiary care sampling [92] and small and biased samples, using unblinded raters and nonstandard diagnostic interview methods [93]. With improved study designs, no excess vulnerability to psychiatric disorders has been found in people who have FSSs [4,94,95]. However, in primary care practices, estimates are that more than one half of all patients experiencing depression present with purely somatic symptoms, with pain the most prevalent [78]. In clinic-recruited women, those who had FM scored higher for depression and anxiety than those who had rheumatoid arthritis and multiple sclerosis [87]. Approximately 25% to 30% of patients who have

FM and who present for treatment have major depression [92] and high rates of familial major mood disorders [4]. In contrast, no significant differences in lifetime psychiatric diagnoses, including depression, anxiety, and somatization disorder, were found among participants who had FM or rheumatoid arthritis and pain-free normal controls [95].

Although perhaps not at a psychiatric level, emotional distress (stress arousal) is notably higher in people who have chronic pain [4] and women who have FM, IB, and CPP [27,28]. Among individuals recruited from the community, women who had FM and IB had significantly higher scores than controls on the Symptom Checklist 90R (SCL-90R), but in the high normative range and mostly with regard to depression, anxiety, and anger [28]. In British and New Zealand studies, women who had CPP had significantly lower scores on the mental health components of the SF-36 and declared higher symptom-related anxiety than those who had other forms of pelvic pain, such as dysmenorrhea or dyspareunia [45].

Dysphoria, particularly with depression and anxiety dimensions, coincides with chronic pain, including FSSs. Emotional distress is reciprocally related to chronic widespread pain, including observations that having one or the other is likely, over time, to result in the other appearing [4]. Whether a high emotive style predisposes to developing painful FSSs or is an outcome of having painful FSSs, thereby perpetuating the manifestation, or both, remains to be elucidated. Although psychiatric illness is often considered overlaid on FM (comorbid), dysphoria as part of a common underlying set of stress-related changes could worsen over time and be expressed as a psychiatric disorder.

Physiologic stress activation

The expression of emotional arousal translates to physiologic stress activation. During daily life, as individuals adapt to unusual and challenging environmental circumstances, common stress hormones, such as epinephrine, norepinephrine, and cortisol, rise and fall. A large portion of this activation occurs through the sympathetic nervous system and hypothalamic-pituitary-adrenal (HPA) axis with hypothalamic release of corticotropin-releasing hormone (CRH) invoking the release of ACTH, in turn driving cortisol from the adrenal glands. Activation of these stress hormones and others shift an individual toward an alerting catabolic state (break-down or energy use), which is adaptive when periodic with a short timeline of dissipation, returning to a more resting, anabolic state.

However, intense, frequent, or continuous activation can lead to sustained up-regulation of physiologic activation, which over time can dampen the reserve for physiologic adaptation and create weakened hormone modulation or response of tissue targets. Thus, a stress hyperactivated pattern can transition to a hypoactivated pattern, implying an exhausted or semiexhausted stress system. Some individuals who have FSSs (mostly studied in FM) exhibit indicators of stress hyporeactivity. Demitrack and Crofford [94] have argued that a "melancholic-type" major depression emanates from CRH and cortisol elevations, whereas "anergic-type" depression emanates from reduced activity of the HPA axis, with profound fatigue, bodily symptoms, and mood reactivity, similar to those in FM. These investigators show that this anergic pattern is also evident in the depressive phase of bipolar illness, seasonal affective disorder, and primary low thyroid conditions [94].

Stress ANS dysregulation and shifts toward sympathetic dominance are evident across FSSs, although broad generalizations are obscured by lack of controls for age, gender, and menstrual cycle phase; inadequate screening and designation of diagnostic subtypes; and a wide variety of ANS tests and measurements. People who have FM exhibit poor blood pressure regulation, particularly on changing positions or posture [96]. Seen also in IB, alterations in tests of ANS function are less obvious in women than men. In response to rectosigmoid balloon distention, people (particularly males) who had IB showed increased sympathetic and decreased parasympathetic reactivity compared with healthy controls [97]. However, when subtypes of IB symptoms were observed using multiple tests of function (ie, expiratory/inspiratory ratio, Valsalva maneuver, posture changes, and cold pressor) and measures of heart rate variability, women who had constipation-dominant IB had lower parasympathetic tone and higher ANS balance compared with those who had diarrhea-dominant IB [98].

Regarding stress hormones in FSSs, altered patterns have been described. People who have FM have been observed to display low 24-hour blood levels of free cortisol, and a vigorous ACTH but blunted cortisol response to injected CRH, indicating reduced responsiveness of the adrenal glands. Low blood levels of growth hormone, thyroid-stimulating hormone, thyroid hormones (free T_3 and T_4), insulin-like growth factor-1, and other factors are also evident [4,99], as is growth hormone during sleep in women who had FM [100]. The gut release of stress-related hormones affects colonic sensorimotor function (eg, corticotrophin-releasing factor [CRF]) and alters gastrointestinal sensation and motility [14]. On gut stimulation in patients who have IB, a nonselective CRH receptor antagonist administered peripherally improved gastrointestinal visceral perception, motility, and negative mood. Although almost no studies were found that involved probing stress system function in women who had CPP with endometriosis or interstitial cystitis, a clinic study of women who had CPP (n = 14) compared with those who were pain-free undergoing laparoscopy for infertility, showed that results of HPA challenge tests (CRH stimulation and dexamethasone) were similar to those for FM (ie, adequate hypothalamic pituitary [basal and stimulated ACTH] but reduced adrenal activation [salivary cortisol]) [101].

Maladaptive stress activation in the context of negative life events portends vulnerability to pain. Using psychosocial assessment in a population-based prospective cohort study, McBeth and Jones [102] identified 768 people who were at risk for chronic widespread pain but presently free of pain. Final participants (n = 241) underwent HPA axis functional assessment (ie, AM and PM salivary cortisol, post–low-dose dexamethasone suppression test). At the 15-month follow-up, 11.6% had developed new-onset chronic widespread pain, which was related to high odds ratios for an elevated cortisol in the post–dexamethasone suppression test and low morning and high evening cortisol levels.

Excess or sustained stress arousal/activation is likely a promulgator of inflammatory/immune activation and attendant cytokine expression. One consequential but still debatable concept is that a shift occurs in the relative balance of type 1/proinflammatory cytokines (eg, IL-12, tumor necrosis factor-alpha, interferon-gamma) and type 2/anti-inflammatory cytokines (eg, IL, transforming growth factor β). The balance of these cytokines can be shifted in either direction by factors such as stress emotional arousal; behavioral challenges such as sleep loss; or disruption or environmental challenges, including social or physical (eg, pathogens).

Linking sleep, stress and inflammatory/immune activation

In its primary form, similar to FSSs, insomnia is believed to be related to personality styles that are skewed toward stress-related hyperarousal (emotional) and hyperactivation (stress physiologic), in turn shaped by genetic makeup (family history tends to be a risk factor) and environmental factors. For example, compared with good sleepers, insomniacs score higher for psychological distress, (eg, on the Profile of Mood States and SCL-90R) [103], display higher norepinephrine and cortisol levels, metabolic rates [104] and heart rates during sleep and performance tasks [105], and experience sympathetic nervous system accentuation as measured with heart rate variability [106].

Aroused/activated individuals who have insomnia may be vulnerable to FSSs. When 3171 adults (25–65 years) free of chronic widespread pain at baseline were assessed 15 months later, 324 (10%) reported developing chronic widespread pain. Predictors were high baseline scores for sleep problems, somatization, and illness behaviors (seeking help). High scores in all three foci showed 12 times the odds of developing pain [107].

Stress affects sleep patterns, which are normally synchronized with stress hormones, and disrupting one reciprocally disturbs the other [108]. Chronic stress exposure and sleep loss synergistically increase vulnerability to neuron impairment particularly in the hypothalamus [108]. The early portion of nighttime sleep (more SWS) coincides with suppressed HPA axis activity, observed in the nadirs of ACTH and cortisol, but a peak in growth hormone. During the later portion of nighttime sleep (with more REM sleep), adrenal cortex activity escalates to reach maximal cortisol output shortly after awakening. Many shift workers, who report chronic sleep difficulties and in whom circadian hormone patterns often do not fully adapt, have higher risks for health issues, such as ischemic heart disease, gastrointestinal disorders, substance abuse, poor immune function, and infertility problems [108]. The influence of shiftwork in women is discussed by Shechter and colleagues elsewhere in this issue. Sleep and stress hormone patterns seem to be inextricably intertwined. For example, sleep loss leads to sustained elevated cortisol and sleep is affected by stress hormone manipulations, including the administration of CRH (less SWS and REM sleep), ACTH (delayed sleep onset, fragmented sleep, and less SWS), and cortisol (increased SWS and reduced REM sleep). In the context of FSSs, alterations in cortisol, as driven by enduring sleep loss, could impair HPA axis recovery dynamics challenged from other factors (eg, pain) and could worsen certain other outcomes, such as cognitive deficits and decreased carbohydrate tolerance. Thus, observed interactions between sleep and stress physiology make it plausible that sleep disturbance is part of a stress-related cascade that ultimately manifests as pain hypersensitization in FSSs [108].

As reviewed by Benca and Quintas [109], sleep has been considered integral to the inflammatory/immune components of host defense. Sleep is part of the acute-phase response to infection (eg, mediated by cytokines, especially IL-1, tumor necrosis factor-α, and IL-6). Increases in sleep accompany infectious illness and the amount of SWS (or non-REM) during infection has been related to mortality rates in animals. Although studies of sleep loss have shown conflicting outcomes on immune function parameters in humans because of the various outcome indicators and methods for depriving sleep that have been used, sleep loss is generally seen as detrimental to host defense.

Summary

Women are disproportionately prone to a spectrum of FSSs with pain, sleep, and stress inflammatory/immune dysregulation components. Poor and nonrefreshing sleep is prevalently reported, generally more intensively than can be detected as polysomnographic sleep abnormalities. On polysomnography, somewhat light and fragmented sleep and excess vulnerability to sleep-related disorders have been consistently observed, at least with FM. Further investigation is needed into how sleep is involved in the predisposition to or genesis or perpetuation of pain in women who have FSSs, including into the microstructure of sleep, and determining whether sleep-related disorders should be viewed as comorbid conditions that worsen the manifestations of FSSs or are part of the underlying FSSs dysfunction. A tense and highly vigilant inherent style of emotional interface with the environment in the context of exposure to stressors seems to convey vulnerability to insomnia and FSSs. Dysphoria, particularly with depression and anxiety dimensions, not necessarily of psychiatric intensity, coincides with FSSs. Whether a high emotive style, either as predispositional or integral to FSSs, worsens to meet psychiatric criteria remains to be clearly determined. Attendant with emotional distress, physiologic stress activation patterns of overactivation, perhaps transitioning to underactivation (eg, low cortisol), pertain with vulnerability to altered reactivity to stress system challenges (eg, position changes, heart rate variability); imbalanced or low levels of stress neuromodulators (eg, serotonin, norepinephrine, dopamine); and shifts toward stress-related inflammatory/immune activation (eg, inflammatory cytokines). Ultimately, a clinical syndrome of poor sleep, widespread or regional/local chronic pain, profound fatigue, dysphoria, and cognitive impairment ensues—a scenario that is enduring and in many cases irreversible. It is unknown whether poor sleep patterns ensue early as a function of individual stress-style, to predispose or contribute to other FSSs manifestations, and are potentially reinforced or worsen over the course of FSSs or emerge in conjunction with the stress/inflammatory/immune changes of FSSs, or perhaps both. In relation to sleep and pain, the constellation of both environmental risk (eg, stress exposures) and personal vulnerability factors (eg, inherent style, physiological mechanisms) that contribute to developing or the course of painful FSSs must be clarified. Explanations for these complex, multisymptom, painful FSSs and the salient sleep connections will be revealed through encompassing health ecologic (person/environmental) perspectives spanning multiple disciplinary worldviews.

References

[1] Yunus MB. Role of central sensitization in symptoms beyond muscle pain, and the evaluation of a patient with widespread pain. Best Pract Res Clin Rheumatol 2007;21(3):481–97.

[2] Masuko K, Nakamura H. Functional somatic syndrome: how it could be relevant to rheumatologists. Mod Rheumatol 2007;17(3):179–84.

[3] Rao SG, Bennett RM. Pharmacological therapies in fibromyalgia. Best Pract Res Clin Rheumatol 2003;17(4):611–27.

[4] Clauw DJ, Crofford LJ. Chronic widespread pain and fibromyalgia: what we know, and what we need to know. Best Pract Res Clin Rheumatol 2003;17(4):685–701.

[5] Bennett R. Fibromyalgia, chronic fatigue syndrome, and myofascial pain. Curr Opin Rheumatol 1998;10:95–103.

[6] Pilowsky I, Crettenden I, Townley M. Sleep disturbance in pain clinic patients. Pain 1985;23:27–33.

[7] Morin CM, Gibson D, Wade J. Self-reported sleep and mood disturbance in chronic pain patients. Clin J Pain 1998;14(4):311–4.

[8] Lautenbacher S, Kundermann B, Krieg JC. Sleep deprivation and pain perception. Sleep Med Rev 2006;10(5):357–69.

[9] Henningsen P, Zipfel S, Herzog W. Management of functional somatic syndromes. Lancet 2007;369(9565):946–55.

[10] Goldenberg DL. Pharmacological treatment of fibromyalgia and other chronic musculoskeletal pain. Best Pract Res Clin Rheumatol 2007;21(3):499–511.

[11] Mannerkorpi K, Henriksson C. Non-pharmacological treatment of chronic widespread musculoskeletal pain. Best Pract Res Clin Rheumatol 2007;21(3):513–34.

[12] Lawrence RC, Helmick CG, Arnett FC, et al. Estimates of the prevalence of arthritis and selected musculoskeletal disorders in the United States. Arthritis Rheum 1998;41(5):778–99.

[13] White KP, Harth M, Speechley M, et al. A general population study of fibromyalgia tender points in noninstitutionalized adults with chronic widespread pain. J Rheumatol 2000;27(11):2677–82.

[14] Foxx-Orenstein A. IBS–review and what's new. MedGenMed 2006;8(3):20.

[15] Drossman DA. Irritable bowel syndrome. Gastroenterologist 1994;2:315–26.

[16] Chang L. The association of functional gastrointestinal disorders and fibromyalgia. Eur J Surg Suppl 1998;583:32–6.

[17] Sperber AD, Atzmon Y, Neumann L, et al. Fibromyalgia in the irritable bowel syndrome: studies of prevalence and clinical implications. Am J Gastroenterol 1999;94(12):3541–6.

[18] Mathias SD, Kuppermann M, Liberman RF, et al. Chronic pelvic pain: prevalence, health-related quality of life, and economic correlates. Obstet Gynecol 1996;87(3):321–7.

[19] Stanford EJ, Dell JR, Parsons CL. The emerging presence of interstitial cystitis in gynecologic patients with chronic pelvic pain. Urology 2007;69(4 Suppl):53–9.

[20] ACOG Committee on Practice Bulletins—Gynecology. ACOG Practice Bulletin Clinical Management Guidelines for Obstetrician–Gynecologists Number 51, March 2004. Obstet Gynecol 2004;103:589–605.

[21] Practice Committee of the American Society for Reproductive Medicine. Treatment of pelvic pain associated with endometriosis. Fertil Steril 2006;86(5 Suppl):S18–27.

[22] Guo SW, Wang Y. The prevalence of endometriosis in women with chronic pelvic pain. Gynecol Obstet Invest 2006;62(3):121–30.

[23] Hanno PM. Interstitial cystitis-epidemiology, diagnostic criteria, clinical markers. Rev Urol 2002;4(Suppl 1):S3–8.

[24] Teichman JM, Parsons CL. Contemporary clinical presentation of interstitial cystitis. Urology 2007;69(4 Suppl):41–7.

[25] Menefee LA, Cohen MJ, Anderson WR, et al. Sleep disturbance and nonmalignant chronic pain: a comprehensive review of the literature. Pain Med 2000;1(2):156–72.

[26] Edinger JD, Krystal AD. Subtyping primary insomnia: is sleep state misperception a distinct clinical entity? Sleep Med Rev 2003;7(3):203–14.

[27] Heitkemper M, Jarrett M, Burr R, et al. Subjective and objective sleep indices in women with irritable bowel syndrome. Neurogastroenterol Motil 2005;17(4):523–30.

[28] Shaver JL, Lentz M, Landis CA, et al. Sleep, psychological distress, and stress arousal in women with fibromyalgia. Res Nurs Health 1997;20(3):247–57.

[29] Drewes AM. Pain and sleep disturbances. Clinical, experimental and methodological aspects with special reference to the fibromyalgia syndrome and rheumatoid arthritis. Rheumatology 1999;38:1035–8.

[30] Haythornthwaite JA, Hegel MT, Kerns RD. Development of a sleep diary for chronic pain patients. J Pain Symptom Manage 1991;6(2):65–72.

[31] Smith MT, Haythornthwaite JA. How do sleep disturbance and chronic pain inter-relate? Insights from the longitudinal and cognitive-behavioral clinical trials literature. Sleep Med Rev 2004;8(2):119–32.

[32] McCracken LM, Iverson GL. Disrupted sleep patterns and daily functioning in patients with chronic pain. Pain Res Manag 2002;7(2):75–9.

[33] Meltzer LJ, Logan DE, Mindell JA. Sleep patterns in female adolescents with chronic musculoskeletal pain. Behav Sleep Med 2005;3(4): 193–208.

[34] White KP, Speechley M, Harth M, et al. Co-existence of chronic fatigue syndrome with fibromyalgia syndrome in the general population. A controlled study. Scand J Rheumatol 2000; 29(1):44–51.

[35] Wolfe F, Hawley DJ, Wilson K. The prevalence and meaning of fatigue in rheumatic disease. J Rheumatol 1996;23(8):1407–17.

[36] Theadom A, Cropley M, Humphrey KL. Exploring the role of sleep and coping in quality of life in fibromyalgia. J Psychosom Res 2007;62(2): 145–51.

[37] Jennum P, Drewes AM, Andreasen A, et al. Sleep and other symptoms in primary fibromyalgia and in healthy controls. J Rheumatol 1993; 20(10):1756–9.

[38] Drewes AM, Nielsen KD, Arendt-Nielsen L, et al. The effect of cutaneous and deep pain on the electroencephalogram during sleep—an experimental study. Sleep 1997;20(8):632–40.

[39] Price DD, Zhou Q, Moshiree B, et al. Peripheral and central contributions to hyperalgesia in irritable bowel syndrome. J Pain 2006;7(8): 529–35.

[40] Shaver JL, Wilbur J, Robinson FP, et al. Women's health issues with fibromyalgia syndrome. J Womens Health (Larchmt) 2006; 15(9):1035–45.

[41] Wolfe F, Smythe HA, Yunus MB, et al. The American College of Rheumatology 1990 Criteria for the Classification of Fibromyalgia. Report of the Multicenter Criteria Committee [see comments]. Arthritis Rheum 1990;33: 160–72.

[42] Jarrett M, Heitkemper M, Cain KC, et al. Sleep disturbance influences gastrointestinal symptoms in women with irritable bowel syndrome. Dig Dis Sci 2000;45(5):952–9.

[43] Zimmerman J. Extraintestinal symptoms in irritable bowel syndrome and inflammatory bowel diseases: nature, severity, and relationship to gastrointestinal symptoms. Dig Dis Sci 2003; 48(4):743–9.

[44] Elsenbruch S, Thompson J, Harnish MJ, et al. Behavioral and physiological sleep Characteristics in women with irritable bowel syndrome. Am J Gastroenterol 2002;97(9):2306–14.

[45] Grace V, Zondervan K. Chronic pelvic pain in women in New Zealand: comparative wellbeing, comorbidity, and impact on work and other activities. Health Care Women Int 2006; 27(7):585–99.

[46] Staedt J, Windt H, Hajak G, et al. Cluster arousal analysis in chronic pain-disturbed sleep. J Sleep Res 1993;2(3):134–7.

[47] Molony RR, MacPeek DM, Schiffman PL, et al. Sleep, sleep apnea and the fibromyalgia syndrome. J Rheumatol 1986;13(4):797–800.

[48] Anch AM, Lue FA, MacLean AW, et al. Sleep physiology and psychological aspects of the fibrositis (fibromyalgia) syndrome. Can J Psychol 1991;45(2):179–84.

[49] Cote KA, Moldofsky H. Sleep, daytime symptoms, and cognitive performance in patients with fibromyalgia. J Rheumatol 1997;24(10):2014–23.

[50] Roizenblatt S, Moldofsky H, Benedito-Silva AA, et al. Alpha sleep characteristics in fibromyalgia. Arthritis Rheum 2001;44(1):222–30.

[51] Landis CA, Lentz MJ, Tsuji J, et al. Pain, psychological variables, sleep quality, and natural killer cell activity in midlife women with and without fibromyalgia. Brain Behav Immun 2004;18(4): 304–13.

[52] Robert JJ, Orr WC, Elsenbruch S. Modulation of sleep quality and autonomic functioning by symptoms of depression in women with irritable bowel syndrome. Dig Dis Sci 2004; 49(7–8):1250–8.

[53] Rotem AY, Sperber AD, Krugliak P, et al. Polysomnographic and actigraphic evidence of sleep fragmentation in patients with irritable bowel syndrome. Sleep 2003;26(6):747–52.

[54] Dunlap KT, Yu L, Fisch BJ, et al. Polysomnographic characteristics of sleep disorders in chronic pelvic pain. Prim Care Update Ob Gyns 1998;5(4):195.

[55] Schneider-Helmert D, Whitehouse I, Kumar A, et al. Insomnia and alpha sleep in chronic nonorganic pain as compared to primary insomnia. Neuropsychobiology 2001;43(1):54–8.

[56] Landis CA, Lentz MJ, Rothermel J, et al. Decreased sleep spindles and spindle activity in midlife women with fibromyalgia and pain. Sleep 2004;27(4):741–50.

[57] Moldofsky H, Scarisbrick P, England R, et al. Musculoskeletal symptoms and non-REM sleep disturbance in patients with "fibrositis syndrome" and healthy subjects. Psychosom Med 1975;37(4):341–51.

[58] Branco J, Atalaia A, Paiva T. Sleep cycles and alpha-delta sleep in fibromyalgia syndrome. J Rheumatol 1994;21(6):1113–7.

[59] Carette S, Oakson G, Guimont C, et al. Sleep electroencephalography and the clinical response to amitriptyline in patients with fibromyalgia. Arthritis Rheum 1995;38(9):1211–7.

[60] Lentz MJ, Landis CA, Rothermel J, et al. Effects of selective slow wave sleep disruption on musculoskeletal pain and fatigue in middle aged women. J Rheumatol 1999;26(7):1586–92.

[61] Manu P, Lane TJ, Matthews DA. Chronic fatigue and chronic fatigue syndrome: clinical epidemiology and aetiological classification. Ciba Found Symp 1993;173:23–31.

[62] Wittig RM, Zorick FJ, Blumer D, et al. Disturbed sleep in patients complaining of chronic pain. J Nerv Ment Dis 1982;170(7):429–31.

[63] Schneider-Helmert D, Kumar A. Sleep, its subjective perception, and daytime performance in insomniacs with a pattern of alpha sleep. Biol Psychiatry 1995;37(2):99–105.

[64] Hamm C, Derman S. Sleep parameters in fibrositis/fibromyalgia syndrome (FS). Arthritis Rheum 1989;32(Suppl):S70.

[65] Chen L, Baqir M. Increased incidence of sleep apnea in fibromyalgia patients. Arthritis Rheum 2004;50:S494.

[66] Shah MA, Feinberg S, Krishnan E. Sleep-disordered breathing among women with fibromyalgia syndrome. J Clin Rheumatol 2006;12(6): 277–81.

[67] Ohayon MM, Roth T. Prevalence of restless legs syndrome and periodic limb movement disorder in the general population. J Psychosom Res 2002;53(1):547–54.

[68] Kundermann B, Krieg JC, Schreiber W, et al. The effect of sleep deprivation on pain. Pain Res Manag 2004;9(1):25–32.

[69] Older SA, Battafarano DF, Danning CL, et al. The effects of delta wave sleep interruption on pain thresholds and fibromyalgia-like symptoms in healthy subjects; correlations with insulin-like growth factor I. J Rheumatol 1998;25: 1180–6.

[70] Arima T, Svensson P, Rasmussen C, et al. The relationship between selective sleep deprivation, nocturnal jaw-muscle activity and pain in healthy men. J Oral Rehabil 2001;28(2):140–8.

[71] Onen SH, Alloui A, Gross A, et al. The effects of total sleep deprivation, selective sleep interruption and sleep recovery on pain tolerance thresholds in healthy subjects. J Sleep Res 2001;10(1):35–42.

[72] Wesensten NJ, Balkin TJ, Belenky G. Does sleep fragmentation impact recuperation? A review and reanalysis. J Sleep Res 1999;8(4):237–45.

[73] Affleck G, Urrows S, Tennen H, et al. Sequential daily relations of sleep, pain intensity, and attention to pain among women with fibromyalgia. Pain 1996;68:363–8.

[74] Nielsen LA, Henriksson KG. Pathophysiological mechanisms in chronic musculoskeletal pain (fibromyalgia): the role of central and peripheral sensitization and pain disinhibition. Best Pract Res Clin Rheumatol 2007;21(3):465–80.

[75] Staud R, Rodriguez ME. Mechanisms of disease: pain in fibromyalgia syndrome. Nat Clin Pract Rheumatol 2006;2(2):90–8.

[76] Moshiree B, Price DD, Robinson ME, et al. Thermal and visceral hypersensitivity in irritable bowel syndrome patients with and without fibromyalgia. Clin J Pain 2007;23(4):323–30.

[77] Evans RJ, Sant GR. Current diagnosis of interstitial cystitis: an evolving paradigm. Urology 2007;69(4 Suppl):64–72.

[78] Abeles AM, Pillinger MH, Solitar BM, et al. Narrative review: the pathophysiology of fibromyalgia. Ann Intern Med 2007;146(10): 726–34.

[79] Staud R. Future perspectives: pathogenesis of chronic muscle pain. Best Pract Res Clin Rheumatol 2007;21(3):581–96.

[80] Liebregts T, Birgit A, Christoph B, et al. Immune activation in patients with irritable bowel syndrome. Gastroenterology 2007;132:913–20.

[81] Azpiroz F, Bouin M, Camilleri M. Mechanisms of hypersensitivity in IBS and functional disorders. Neurogastroenterol Motil 2007;19(1 Suppl): 62–88.

[82] Khan WI, Collins SM. Gut motor function: immunological control in enteric infection and inflammation. Clin Exp Immunol 2006; 143(3):389–97.

[83] Sant GR, Kempuraj D, Marchand JE, et al. The mast cell in interstitial cystitis: role in pathophysiology and pathogenesis. Urology 2007; 69(4 Suppl):34–40.

[84] Nazif O, Teichman JM, Gebhart GF. Neural up-regulation in interstitial cystitis. Urology 2007; 69(4 Suppl):24–33.

[85] Wood PB. Stress and dopamine: implications for the pathophysiology of chronic widespread pain. Med Hypotheses 2004;62(3):420–4.

[86] Offenbaecher M, Bondy B, de Jonge S, et al. Possible association of fibromyalgia with a polymorphism in the serotonin transporter gene regulatory region. Arthritis Rheum 1999; 42(11):2482–8.

[87] Van Houdenhove B, Neerinckx E, Onghena P, et al. Daily hassles reported by chronic fatigue syndrome and fibromyalgia patients in tertiary care: a controlled quantitative and qualitative study. Psychother Psychosom 2002;71(4):207–13.

[88] Locke GR III, Weaver AL, Melton LJ III, et al. Psychosocial factors are linked to functional gastrointestinal disorders: a population based nested case-control study. Am J Gastroenterol 2004;99(2):350–7.

[89] Lampe A, Doering S, Rumpold G, et al. Chronic pain syndromes and their relation to childhood abuse and stressful life events. J Psychosom Res 2003;54(4):361–7.

[90] Clark S, Campbell SM, Forehand ME, et al. Clinical characteristics of fibrositis. II. A "blinded," controlled study using standard psychological tests. Arthritis Rheum 1985; 28(2):132–7.

[91] Shaver JL. Fibromyalgia syndrome in women. Nurs Clin North Am 2004;39(1):195–204.

[92] Aaron LA, Bradley LA, Alarcon GS, et al. Psychiatric diagnoses in patients with fibromyalgia are related to health care-seeking behavior rather than to illness. Arthritis Rheum 1996;39(3): 436–45.

[93] Yunus MB. Psychological aspects of fibromyalgia syndrome: a component of the dysfunctional spectrum syndrome. Baillieres Clin Rheumatol 1994;8(4):811–37.

[94] Demitrack MA, Crofford LJ. Evidence for and pathophysiologic implications of hypothalamic-pituitary-adrenal axis dysregulation in

fibromyalgia and chronic fatigue syndrome. Ann N Y Acad Sci 1998;840:684–97.

[95] Ahles TA, Khan SA, Yunus MB, et al. Psychiatric status of patients with primary fibromyalgia, patients with rheumatoid arthritis, and subjects without pain: a blind comparison of DSM-III diagnoses. Am J Psychiatry 1991;148(12):1721–6.

[96] Martinez-Lavin M, Hermosillo AG, Rosas M, et al. Circadian studies of autonomic nervous balance in patients with fibromyalgia: a heart rate variability analysis. Arthritis Rheum 1998; 41:1966–71.

[97] Tillisch K, Mayer EA, Labus JS, et al. Sex specific alterations in autonomic function among patients with irritable bowel syndrome. Gut 2005;54(10):1396–401.

[98] Heitkemper M, Jarrett M, Cain KC, et al. Autonomic nervous system function in women with irritable bowel syndrome. Dig Dis Sci 2001;46(6):1276–84.

[99] Crofford LJ. Neuroendocrine abnormalities in fibromyalgia and related disorders. Am J Med Sci 1998;315:359–66.

[100] Landis CA, Lentz MJ, Rothermel J, et al. Decreased nocturnal levels of prolactin and growth hormone in women with fibromyalgia. J Clin Endocrinol Metab 2001;86(4):1672–8.

[101] Heim C, Ehlert U, Rexhausen J, et al. Psychoendocrinological observations in women with chronic pelvic pain. Ann N Y Acad Sci 1997; 821:456–8.

[102] McBeth J, Jones K. Epidemiology of chronic musculoskeletal pain. Best Pract Res Clin Rheumatol 2007;21(3):403–25.

[103] Shaver JL, Johnston SK, Lentz MJ, et al. Stress exposure, psychological distress, and physiological stress activation in midlife women with insomnia. Psychosom Med 2002;64(5):793–802.

[104] Bonnet MH, Arand DL. 24-Hour metabolic rate in insomniacs and matched normal sleepers. Sleep 1995;18(7):581–8.

[105] Roehrs T, Merlotti L, Petrucelli N, et al. Experimental sleep fragmentation. Sleep 1994;17(5): 438–43.

[106] Bonnet MH, Arand DL. Heart rate variability in insomniacs and matched normal sleepers. Psychosom Med 1998;60(5):610–5.

[107] Gupta A, Silman AJ, Ray D, et al. The role of psychosocial factors in predicting the onset of chronic widespread pain: results from a prospective population-based study. Rheumatology (Oxford) 2007;46(4):666–71.

[108] Van Reeth O, Weibel L, Spiegel K, et al. Interactions between stress and sleep: from basic research to clinical situations. Sleep Med Rev 2000;4:201–19.

[109] Benca RM, Quintas J. Sleep and host defenses: a review. Sleep 1997;20(11):1027–37.

ELSEVIER
SAUNDERS

SLEEP
MEDICINE
CLINICS

Sleep Med Clin 3 (2008) 61–71

Breast Cancer and Fatigue

Wayne A. Bardwell, PhD, MBA[a,b], Sonia Ancoli-Israel, PhD[a,b,c,*]

Fatigue is a common and frequently disabling symptom in patients who have cancer and in cancer survivors [1,2]. Fatigue also is often a presenting symptom at cancer diagnosis [3–5]. Cancer fatigue differs from other manifestations of fatigue in that it generally is not alleviated by sleep or rest, typically is of greater duration and severity, often is associated with high levels of distress, and is disproportionate to the level of exertion [6–11]. Cancer-related fatigue often co-occurs with other troublesome symptoms such as pain, sleep disturbance, and depression [12–14]. Thus, the impact of cancer fatigue on health-related quality of life can be substantial, reducing the patient's engagement in work and in personal and social activity [2,15–17]. Some studies have reported that fatigue in patients who have cancer has a greater negative impact on quality of life than all other symptoms, including nausea, pain, and depression [2,18].

Treatment of cancer-related fatigue has been recently identified as a priority by the National Institutes of Health [19].

Specific to breast cancer, fatigue is reported by a substantial majority of patients during their initial treatment (surgery, radiation, and/or chemotherapy). In addition, although estimates vary widely, approximately 33% of individuals who have breast cancer report persistent fatigue up to 10 years into survivorship [6,20,21].

Fatigue is a rather nebulous symptom; hence, numerous definitions of this construct are found in the literature [6,22]. A further complication is that patients who have breast cancer and breast cancer survivors commonly complain of both sleepiness and fatigue [23]. These terms are often used interchangeably, and both have been linked with decrements in various aspects of health-related quality of life and with the restriction of daytime

This work was supported by NCI CA112035, NCI CA85264, CBCRP 11GB-0049, CBCRP 11IB-0034, NIA AG08415, M01 RR00827, the Research Service of the Veterans Affairs San Diego Healthcare System; Lance Armstrong Foundation, and Susan G. Komen Foundation POP0504026.
[a] Department of Psychiatry, University of California, San Diego, 9500 Gilman Drive, La Jolla, CA 92093, USA
[b] Moores University of California San Diego, Cancer Center, 3855 Health Sciences Drive #0658, La Jolla, CA 92093, USA
[c] Veterans Affairs San Diego Healthcare System, 3500 La Jolla Village Drive, San Diego, CA 92161, USA
* Corresponding author. Department of Psychiatry, University of California, San Diego, 116A, VASDHS, 3350 La Jolla Village Drive, San Diego, CA 92161.
E-mail address: sancoliisrael@ucsd.edu (S. Ancoli-Israel).

activities. Nonetheless, there are important differences in these concepts.

Sleepiness involves a propensity to fall asleep, whether at bedtime or during the day at times when wakefulness is desired (eg, daytime sleepiness). Sleepiness is thought to be the overt manifestation of an underlying physiologic need for sleep and can be measured subjectively (eg, with the Epworth Sleepiness Scale) or quantified objectively using daytime tests (eg, the Maintenance of Wakefulness Test or the Multiple Sleep Latency Test). By comparison, fatigue is a poorly understood but highly prevalent complaint in patients who have breast and other cancers. Fatigue includes physical and psychologic features as well as cultural and social factors. Thus, the conceptual borders of fatigue are defined imprecisely, overlapping with related concepts such as lack of energy or vigor, lethargy, feeling tired, decreased strength, and trouble concentrating [24]. One definition of cancer-related fatigue is: "a subjective state of overwhelming and sustained exhaustion and decreased capacity for physical and mental work that is not relieved by rest" [25]. Another accepted definition is "a persistent and subjective sense of tiredness that interferes with usual functioning" [3,22,26]. Both definitions include the subjective phenomenologic experience of fatigue as well as its observable impact on usual levels of functioning. As is the case with pain, fatigue is a complaint that almost always is evaluated using self-report scales [6,24]. Therefore, by default, fatigue ultimately is defined by the instruments employed for its measurement. The next section provides an overview of several types of scales for assessing fatigue.

Assessment of fatigue

Numerous self-report instruments are used to assess fatigue in general as well as cancer-related fatigue (Table 1). In the past, fatigue commonly was assessed as one component of a symptom checklist or a quality-of-life or mood scale (ie, as an item or subscale of items on an instrument having the primary purpose of measuring symptoms, mood, or quality of life) [6,34]. Thus, the approach to measurement of this construct historically has been unidimensional. Examples of scales that use this unidimensional approach to the measurement of fatigue are the Symptom Distress Scale [35], Rotterdam Symptom Checklist [36], Profile of Mood States Fatigue subscale [33] and the Medical Outcomes Study 36-Item Short-Form Health Survey Vitality (Energy/Fatigue) subscale [28].

More recently, research into the multidimensional nature of general (not cancer-specific) fatigue

has resulted in the development of instruments that often yield an overall total fatigue score as well as subscale scores for various dimensions of fatigue (eg, physical, mental, emotional). Vigor, a construct thought to be related to, but not necessarily the opposite of, fatigue also has been assessed on mood measures (eg, the Profile of Mood States Vigor subscale) [33] and on multidimensional fatigue scales (eg, the Multidimensional Fatigue Symptom Inventory Vigor subscale) [30].

Fatigue assessment also has been expanded through the development of instruments either designed for or specifically normed on particular patient groups. For example, the Fatigue Symptom Inventory (FSI) [37] and the Multidimensional Fatigue Symptom Inventory (MFSI) [30], although appropriate for assessing fatigue in nonpatient populations, were originally normed on patients who had breast cancer [30]. The 83-item MFSI yields a total fatigue score as well as subscale scores for general, mental, emotional, and physical fatigue and for vigor. A 30-item short form of this instrument (MFSI-SF) also has shown excellent psychometric properties and includes the same subscales as the full version of the MFSI [31]. The Functional Assessment of Cancer Therapy—Fatigue scale was designed to assess fatigue specifically in patients who have cancer [17].

One drawback to all these questionnaires is that they capture information from only one time point. Ecological momentary assessment—data collected several times a day, over several days—confirms that the level of fatigue reported varies throughout the day [38]. Newer approaches to the measurement of fatigue may be needed.

A recent focus of research into fatigue has been on the development of a clinical syndrome (symptom-cluster) approach to defining and assessing cancer-related fatigue [25,26]. For this purpose, a structured clinical interview has been devised (the Diagnostic Interview Guide for Cancer-Related Fatigue [25]), using the proposed International Classification of Disease-10 criteria for cancer-related fatigue (Box 1) [34]. This approach holds promise for improving the sensitivity and specificity of the assessment of cancer-related fatigue. For example, Andrykowski and colleagues [26] evaluated a group of 288 women who were receiving adjuvant treatment for early-stage (stage 0 to stage II) breast cancer. The authors observed that 10% of these patients met all criteria for cancer-related fatigue immediately after surgery, increasing to 26% after completion of the initial course of adjuvant treatment [26]. They reported that the cause of cancer-related fatigue is multifactorial, and their results supported the use of this case-definition approach to define cancer-related

Table 1: **Frequently used self-report instruments for assessing cancer-related fatigue**

Self-report instrument	Items	Measurement focus/scoring	Time frame
Fatigue Severity Scale (FSS) [27]	9	Series of statements about life domains that affect or bring on fatigue. Rated using a 7-point response format (1= strongly disagree; 7 = strongly agree). Yields a total fatigue severity score.	During the past 2 weeks
Functional Assessment of Cancer Therapy—Fatigue Scale (FACT-F) [17]	41 (13 of which assess fatigue)	Addresses concerns or problems associated with cancer-related fatigue. Rated on a 5-point scale indicating how true each statement was for the respondent during the last week (0 = not at all true; 4 = very true). Yields a total fatigue score.	During the past week
Medical Outcomes Study (MOS) 36-item Short Form Health Survey (SF-36) [28,29]	4	The SF-36 is designed to assess physical and mental health-related disability. Includes four items comprising the Vitality (energy/fatigue) subscale. Scored from 0 (more fatigue) to 100 (more energy). Yields a total fatigue score.	During the past 4 weeks
Multidimensional Fatigue Symptom Inventory (MFSI) [30] Multidimensional Fatigue Symptom Inventory Short Form (MFSI-SF) [31]	83 30	A series of statements designed to assess the principal manifestations of fatigue. Used in various patient and nonpatient groups; normed for women who have breast cancer. Rated on a 5-point scale indicating how true each statement was for the respondent (0 = not at all true; 4 = extremely true). Yields general, physical, emotional, and mental fatigue and vigor subscales and a total fatigue score.	During the past week
Piper Fatigue Scale [32]	27	22 fatigue-related items scored using 11-point Likert scales, plus five open-ended questions. Yields behavioral-severity, affective meaning, sensory, and cognitive-mood subscales and a total fatigue score.	Current
Profile of Mood States (POMS)Fatigue-Inertia Subscale; [33] Profile of Mood States Short Form (POMS-SF) Fatigue-Inertia Subscale [33]	65 (7 fatigue items) 30 (5 fatigue items)	Adjective checklist assessing various psychologic parameters including fatigue-inertia. Rated on a 5-point scale indicating how true each statement was for the respondent (0 = not at all true; 4 = extremely true). Yields a total fatigue score.	During the past week

fatigue [26]. To date, however, this approach has been used only in limited settings [6].

Fatigue before treatment

Several studies have now shown that women who have breast cancer complain of fatigue even before the start of treatment [5,39]. Ancoli-Israel and colleagues [5] found that women diagnosed as having breast cancer had increased fatigue, disturbed sleep, and increased daily dysfunction before the start of chemotherapy, and that patients who had fatigue, poor sleep, and depression before chemotherapy experienced more fatigue and poorer quality of life during chemotherapy than women who had fewer symptoms before treatment [40]. These data suggest that fatigue is not just a result of radiation or chemotherapy but rather is multifactorial.

Box 1: **Diagnostic interview guide for cancer-related fatigue using the proposed ICD-10 criteria for cancer-related fatigue [25,34]**

1. Six (or more) of the following symptoms have been present every day or nearly every day during the same 2-week period in the past month, and at least one of the symptoms is significant fatigue (item 1):

    a. Significant fatigue, diminished energy, or increased need to rest disproportionate to any recent change in activity level
    b. Complaints of generalized weakness or limb heaviness
    c. Diminished concentration or attention
    d. Decreased motivation or interest to engage in usual activities
    e. Insomnia or hypersomnia
    f. Experience of sleep as unrefreshing or nonrestorative
    g. Perceived need to struggle to overcome inactivity
    h. Marked emotional reactivity (eg, sadness, frustration, or irritability) to feeling fatigued
    i. Difficulty completing daily tasks attributed to feeling fatigued
    j. Perceived problems with short-term memory
    k. Postexertional malaise lasting several hours

2. The symptoms cause clinically significant distress or impairment in social, occupational, or other important areas of functioning.
3. There is evidence from the history, physical examination, or laboratory findings that the symptoms are a consequence of cancer or cancer therapy.
4. The symptoms are not primarily a consequence of comorbid psychiatric disorders such as major depression, somatization disorder, somatoform disorder, or delirium.

Fatigue during treatment

The most widespread and distressing symptom of cancer and its initial adjuvant treatment (chemotherapy, radiotherapy, and/or biologic response modifier therapy) is fatigue [1,16,41]. Estimates of cancer-related fatigue during initial treatment range from approximately 60% to 90% [2,42–45], with the highest reported frequency in patients undergoing chemotherapy (80%–96%) [43,46] compared with those treated with radiation (60%–93%) [16,42,47]. For example, in the study by Andrykowski and colleagues [26], patients undergoing adjuvant chemotherapy were more than two times more likely than patients receiving adjuvant radiation therapy to report cancer-related fatigue during treatment.

Bower [6] has suggested that a key mechanism in the fatigue experienced during adjuvant radiation treatment may be the activation of proinflammatory cytokines. In her longitudinal study of 49 patients receiving adjuvant radiotherapy for early-stage breast or prostate cancer, she found a positive relationship between cumulative cytokine exposure and fatigue (J.E. Bower and colleagues, unpublished data, 2007). Although in earlier studies the findings on the role of inflammation in radiation treatment-related fatigue were inconsistent, the Bower study, which involved five assessment points before and during radiation treatment, provides some of the strongest evidence to date of the possible mechanistic role of inflammation vis-à-vis fatigue in cancer patients.

Fatigue during survivorship

Although most common during the treatment phase, fatigue also affects a substantial subpopulation of individuals who have breast cancer for months and even years into survivorship [3,20]. Approximately 30% of breast cancer survivors experience moderate to severe fatigue after completion of initial treatment [3,20,48], and fatigue in these survivors has been shown to endure for up to 10 years postdiagnosis [3].

The functioning/quality-of-life impact of this enduring fatigue is significant and has been associated with decrements in physical activity [3,49,50]. Thus, although increased physical activity has been shown to alleviate symptoms of fatigue, greater fatigue nonetheless is associated with lower levels of physical activity. This finding suggests a possible self-perpetuating cycle of increasing fatigue leading to decreasing physical activity leading to even greater fatigue, and so on.

Underlying mechanisms of fatigue

The etiology of fatigue, whether experienced during initial treatment or during survivorship, is far from being characterized definitively. The underlying mechanisms probably vary from patient to patient, and the candidate causes surely co-vary considerably. This variability adds to the complexity of understanding this rather vague but common and potentially disabling complaint. In addition to the usual suspects, such as dysphoric mood, disrupted sleep, and anemia, recent studies have suggested some possible novel mechanisms (eg, inflammation, immune system dysregulation). Thus, fatigue is multiply determined, with a likely mixture of both biologic and psychologic underpinnings [3]. For example, evidence implicates anemia, ATP, links in the hypothalamic-pituitary-adrenal axis, cytokines, circadian rhythms, and vagal afferents [8,9,11,51–54].

Because most previous studies of cancer fatigue involved cross-sectional research designs, the direction of causality between these candidate risk factors and the experience of cancer-related fatigue cannot be determined with certainty. Nonetheless, the literature suggests important possible links between fatigue and a wide range of potential underlying mechanisms.

Depression

Fatigue is a common component of, and one of several key diagnostic criteria for, major depressive disorder, dysthymia, and other clinical mood disorders [55]. A substantial body of research has examined the interplay of fatigue and mood in patients who have chronic medical illnesses. One might assume that fatigue and mood would worsen in tandem as disease severity progresses. Findings are conflicting, however, even when disease severity is taken into account [24,56].

It is difficult to determine the direction of causation between mood and fatigue, particularly in patients dealing with chronic medical conditions, such as breast cancer. Nonetheless, depression or general psychologic distress has been associated with cancer-related fatigue in many studies [20,26,57–60]. For example, in a pre-/posttreatment study of 288 women undergoing treatment for early-stage breast cancer, a significant association was observed between cancer-related fatigue and major depressive disorder [26]. Nearly one in five of the patients reporting cancer-related fatigue after treatment also reported symptoms consistent with a diagnosis of major depressive disorder. By comparison, only approximately 1 in 20 patients who did not report cancer-related fatigue experienced major depression [26]. In addition, a history of major depressive disorder was linked in this study with cancer-related fatigue after initial treatment [26].

In a recent cross-sectional analysis of 2613 women who had a history of early-stage (stages I ≥ 1 cm], II, or IIIA) breast cancer, the present authors reported that cancer-specific factors (ie, cancer stage at diagnosis, type of initial treatment received, ongoing use of tamoxifen, and number of months since breast cancer diagnosis) were unimportant in understanding the risk for fatigue [61]. Rather, worse physical health, less exercise, and more depressive symptoms were the risk factors most strongly linked with fatigue in these women who had completed initial treatment within the previous 4 years [61].

Thus, the evidence linking mood disturbance and cancer-related fatigue is variable. It is difficult to tease out the effects of the medical illness versus those of mood symptoms on fatigue in the chronically medically ill [24,56]. Nonetheless, the fact that four of five patients who have breast cancer–related fatigue do not experience a concurrent major depressive disorder suggests that mood and fatigue in cancer are overlapping but far from fully redundant concepts [26].

Personality characteristics

In their study, Andrykowski and colleagues [26] observed that a tendency to catastrophize over fatigue predicted greater cancer-related fatigue after treatment. They also observed weaker evidence for a link between symptom-focused coping (compared with a tendency to accommodate to the cancer) accompanied by a sense of helplessness and an elevated risk for developing cancer-related fatigue [26]. Links between lower levels of optimism and greater levels of fatigue also have been reported previously [61]. Thus, various aspects of personality have been associated with fatigue in patients who have cancer and in cancer survivors.

Sleep

Sleep disturbances, particularly difficulty falling or staying asleep, are common in patients who have cancer [23]; the prevalence rates of sleep difficulty in patients who have newly diagnosed breast cancer are between 30% and 50% [62]. Insomnia complaints have been reported to be chronic (> 6 months) for a majority of patients who have cancer [63], but these sleep problems often are neglected [62]. Specific sleep disorders such as sleep-disordered breathing and restless legs syndrome also are common in patients who have cancer (for full recent reviews see [64,65]). Although not many studies have addressed the relationships between sleep disruption and fatigue in breast cancer, results suggest that relationships between these two constructs are stronger before and during treatment than after treatment. Part of the difficulty in determining the relationship between sleep and fatigue is that both can be a result of multiple factors such as mood, pain, inflammation, hot flashes, other medical illnesses, and medications. This abundance of factors makes casual relationships difficult to distinguish.

The rates of sleep disturbances (30%–75%) in patients who have newly diagnosed or recently treated cancer [23,64] are about twice as high as in the general population [66]. Objective sleep estimates suggest that patients who have breast cancer already complain of sleep problems and of fatigue before the start of chemotherapy [5], sleeping for only 77% of the night. Disturbed sleep before treatment correlates with fatigue, depressive symptoms, and functional outcome [5]. Although the causal relationship between sleep and these factors cannot be determined from these data, pretreatment sleep disturbance predicted more fatigue, more depressive symptoms, and worse quality of life throughout the chemotherapy [67,68].

As shown in Table 2, some inflammatory markers are abnormally elevated or reduced during chemotherapy, and at times the elevated levels are associated with fatigue. Elevated inflammatory markers also are associated with more disrupted sleep during chemotherapy [69]. Savard and colleagues [70], when examining the relationship between insomnia and the immune system in breast cancer survivors, found that after successful treatment of the insomnia with behavioral therapies, participants also had improved levels of some inflammatory markers.

Hot flashes, reported by 40% to 70% of breast cancer survivors, have been associated with more disturbed sleep, specifically with increased wakefulness and decreased stage 2 sleep and with more stage shifts to lighter sleep around the time of hot flashes [71]. In other studies of breast cancer

survivors, self-reporting of insomnia was not a sig nificant predictor of fatigue up to 4 years after diag nosis [61]. Similarly, in a separate analysis that used insomnia as the outcome variable, fatigue was no associated significantly with insomnia [72].

The present authors [61,72] recently reported a 4-year repeated-measures analysis of risk factors for self-reported insomnia in this same group of breast cancer survivors. Using three different methods of statistical analysis (multinomial logistic regression, mixed modeling, and a generalized estimating equation), they still were unable to observe a significant association between insomnia and fatigue in survivors [73].

As described later, however, treatment studies have shown that treating insomnia in patients who have breast cancer often improves fatigue as well. Additional studies are needed to help elucidate the relationship between poor sleep and fatigue.

Anemia

Low white blood cell count and low levels of hemo globin commonly are thought to be causative factors in fatigue. Although probably playing a role, they do not account for all of the variance in cancer-related fatigue [43,74], and results regarding low concentra tion of hemoglobin have been mixed [75–77].

Inflammation

A relatively new area of investigation involves the role of inflammation as a causative factor in breast cancer fatigue. A recent quantitative review of the literature on inflammation and fatigue in patients who had cancer by Schubert and colleagues [75] examined 18 studies of moderately high

Table 2: Inflammatory markers and fatigue

Inflammatory marker	Study [reference]	Relationship with fatigue
IL-1ra	Bower et al [49]	+
	Collado-Hidalgo et al [98]	+
IL-1β	Savard et al [70]	+
	Bower et al [49]	Not significant
IL-6	Wratten et al [99]	+
	Mills et al [74]	Not significant
	Collado-Hidalgo et al [98]	Not significant
sIL-6r	Collado-Hidalgo et al [98]	+
sTNF-RII	Bower et al [49]	+
	Collado-Hidalgo et al [98]	Not significant
Neopterin	Bower et al [49]	+
ICAM-1	Wratten et al [99]	+
	Mills et al [74]	Not significant
VEGF	Mills et al [74]	+
INF-gamma	Savard et al [70]	+

Abbreviations: ICAM-1, intercellular adhesion molecule I; IL, interleukin; IL-1ra, interleukin-1 receptor agonist; INF, inter feron; sIL-6r, soluble interleukin-6 receptor; sTNF-RII, soluble tumor necrosis factor receptor II; VEGF, vascular endothelia growth factor.

methodological quality that involved 1037 patients averaging 58 participants per study). A significant positive association was observed between cancer-related fatigue and circulating levels of various markers of inflammation. When individual inflammatory markers were examined, fatigue was positively associated with interleukin (IL)-6, IL-1 receptor agonist, and neopterin, but not with IL-β or tumor necrosis factor-α [75].

As shown in Table 2, of the 18 studies mentioned in the previous paragraph, 8 were conducted in patients who had breast cancer or in breast cancer survivors. Of these studies, three found no significant association between inflammatory markers and fatigue [76–78]. The other five studies did observe significant links between inflammation and fatigue, but findings regarding the specific inflammatory markers varied. Thus, although findings remain inconsistent, several studies suggest a role for underlying inflammation in breast cancer–related fatigue.

Treatment of fatigue in patients who have breast cancer and in breast cancer survivors

Clinical trials of treatment regimens for the alleviation and management of cancer-related fatigue have been limited compared with those focused on the alleviation of pain and suffering [3]. Treatment of cancer-related fatigue can be complex because of the links observed between fatigue and various physical and psychologic variables. Thus, a multidisciplinary approach to the treatment and management of cancer-related fatigue is likely to be necessary for many cancer patients and survivors [79], and treatments must be individualized based on underlying pathology [80].

To recap, in two large studies 4 and 5 years after diagnosis or treatment of breast cancer, survivors' fatigue was most strongly linked with depressive symptoms, pain, and sleep disturbance [20] and with worse physical health, less physical activity, and depressive symptoms [61]. Depressed mood, cardiovascular problems, and cancer treatment modality also were linked with ongoing fatigue [20]. Thus, several possible underlying factors have been implicated in cancer-related fatigue, many of which respond well to conventional treatments.

Pharmacotherapy

Clinical trials of pharmacotherapeutic agents for cancer-related fatigue have emerged only during the past 20 to 25 years, probably because fatigue commonly has been considered as a rather ubiquitous or inevitable sequela of cancers and their treatment [11]. Since then, various pharmacotherapeutic agents have been used in the treatment of cancer-related fatigue. These include psychostimulants,

antidepressants, erythropoiesis-stimulating agents, and cytokine antagonists, among others.

Psychostimulants such as methylphenidate have been used in various settings with the goal of improving energy levels in patients having illness-related fatigue. Although methylphenidate improved cancer-related fatigue in open-label studies [81,82], there was not a significant therapeutic effect in a placebo-controlled trial [11,83]. Dexmethylphenidate, however, did show significant effects on fatigue in a placebo-controlled trial in non-anemic patients who had cancer [11,84].

Modafinil, an agent that promotes wakefulness, has been studied only recently for its effects on cancer-related fatigue but has shown promising results in a couple of studies, including one with breast cancer survivors [11,85,86].

Antidepressants have been shown to reduce fatigue as well as other symptoms of depression in various patient groups. The atypical antidepressant bupropion has been shown to improve cancer-related fatigue in two open-label case-series studies, but placebo-controlled trials are needed [11,87,88]. At least two recent studies in patients who have breast cancer and other patients undergoing initial treatment for cancer have not been as promising. Although the authors were able to demonstrate an effect of the selective serotonin reuptake inhibitor paroxetine on other depressive symptoms, no significant effect was observed in reported levels of fatigue [89,90].

Erythropoiesis-stimulating agents (eg, epoetin alfa) have been used to increase hemoglobin concentration with a positive effect on fatigue in diverse populations of patients who have cancer, including breast cancer [11,91]. Not all patients who have breast cancer experience anemia during initial treatment, however, and there is some evidence that use of erythropoietin-α may be linked with worse outcomes (disease progression, thromboembolic complications) [92].

Because of the growing evidence for links between inflammation and fatigue (see Table 2), a potentially promising area of clinical research is on the use of cytokine antagonists for the reduction of fatigue [6]. In patients who had advanced cancer, Monk and colleagues [93] observed that the use of etanercept, which works by reducing the effects of tumor necrosis factor, safely and effectively reduced their reported levels of fatigue.

Physical activity

Exercise is probably the most thoroughly evaluated treatment for cancer-related fatigue, and there is strong evidence for its use, primarily from studies during initial treatment of patients who had cancer [94]. Although somewhat counterintuitive, increasing physical activity has been associated with significant improvements in fatigue in many studies. For example, Schneider and colleagues [95] recently observed that individualized, prescribed physical activity of moderate intensity resulted in significant reductions in cancer-related fatigue during initial treatment and even into survivorship.

Cognitive-Behavioral Therapies

As reviewed by Fiorentino and Ancoli-Israel [96], cognitive behavioral therapy for insomnia (CBT-I) has been shown to be both efficacious and suitable in the breast cancer population. CBT-I uses a tailored approach to treating insomnia, addressing the specific needs of patients who have breast cancer by targeting fatigue. In addition, as reviewed by Theobald [97], treating insomnia in patients who have cancer with a combination of pharmacologic and nonpharmacologic therapy may have a positive impact on the insomnia itself and also on related symptoms, including pain, fatigue, and psychologic distress.

Summary and future directions

Although research into the cause, course, and treatment of cancer-related fatigue is relatively new, much progress has been made in recent years; however, considerable opportunities remain. Some well-powered studies have examined risk factors for fatigue in patients who have breast cancer and in breast cancer survivors, but most studies examining underlying mechanisms have involved small to very small sample sizes. Although a few studies employing repeated assessments have been conducted, most have been cross-sectional in design. Thus, more longitudinal studies that involve assessment of patients who have cancer before and after completion of initial treatment and into survivorship are needed. Although multiple factors have been linked with cancer-related fatigue, the factors that predispose, precipitate, or exacerbate/maintain the patients' experience of fatigue are yet to be determined. For example, longitudinal studies examining and comparing the effects of chemotherapy- and radiation-induced inflammation on functioning during survivorship are warranted. Also, additional studies using statistical analytic techniques that can evaluate hypotheses about causal pathways are needed. These studies will require multiple assessments of established or promising biomarkers of fatigue. Such studies also should assess fatigue using multidimensional scales normed on and/or tailored to patients who have breast cancer.

A case-definition approach, using a structured clinical interview, has much promise for improving the assessment of cancer-related fatigue. This improvement should be very much in line with the greater sensitivity and specificity of diagnosis of mood disorders by means of a structured clinical interview compared with the use of pencil-and-paper scales. In addition, further evaluation is needed of the scientific value of the criteria for cancer-related fatigue, including the comparison of functioning in patients who meet the case definition criteria versus those who do not.

References

[1] Lawrence DP, Kupelnick B, Miller K, et al. Evidence report on the occurrence, assessment and treatment of fatigue in cancer patients. J Natl Cancer Inst Monogr 2004;32:40–50.

[2] Curt GA, Breitbart W, Cella D, et al. Impact of cancer-related fatigue on the lives of patients: new findings from the Fatigue Coalition. Oncologist 2000;5:353–60.

[3] Ganz PA, Bower JE. Cancer related fatigue: a focus on breast cancer and Hodgkin's disease survivors. Acta Oncol 2007;46:474–9.

[4] Ganz PA, Moinpour CM, Pauler DK, et al. Health status and quality of life in patients with early stage Hodgkin's disease treated on Southwest Oncology Group Study 9133. J Clin Oncol 2003;21:3512–9.

[5] Ancoli-Israel S, Liu L, Marler MR, et al. Fatigue, sleep, and circadian rhythms prior to chemotherapy for breast cancer. Support Care Cancer 2006;14:201–9.

[6] Bower JE. Cancer-related fatigue: links with inflammation in cancer patients and survivors. Brain Behav Immun 2007;21:863–71.

[7] Poulson MJ. Not just tired. J Clin Oncol 2001;19:4180–1.

[8] Morrow GR, Hickok JT, Andrews PL, et al. Reduction in serum cortisol after platinum based chemotherapy for cancer: a role for the HPA axis in treatment-related nausea? Psychophysiology 2002;39:491–5.

[9] Morrow GR, Andrews PL, Hickok JT, et al. Fatigue associated with cancer and its treatment. Support Care Cancer 2002;10:389–98.

[10] Ahlberg K, Ekman T, Gaston-Johansson F, et al. Assessment and management of cancer-related fatigue in adults. Lancet 2003;362:640–50.

[11] Carroll JK, Kohli S, Mustian KM, et al. Pharmacologic treatment of cancer-related fatigue. Oncologist 2007;12(Suppl 1):43–51.

[12] Armstrong TS, Cohen MZ, Eriksen LR, et al. Symptom clusters in oncology patients and implications for symptom research in people with primary brain tumors. J Nurs Scholarsh 2004;36:197–206.

[13] Barton-Burke M. Cancer-related fatigue and sleep disturbances. Further research on the prevalence of these two symptoms in long-term cancer survivors can inform education, policy, and clinical practice. Am J Nurs 2006;106:72–7.

[14] Dodd MJ, Miaskowski C, Lee KA. Occurrence of symptom clusters. J Natl Cancer Inst Monogr 2004;32:76–8.

[15] Broeckel JA, Jacobsen PB, Horton J, et al. Characteristics and correlates of fatigue after adjuvant chemotherapy for breast cancer. J Clin Oncol 1998;16:1689–96.

[16] Cella D, Davis K, Breitbart W, et al. Cancer-related fatigue: prevalence of proposed diagnostic criteria in a United States sample of cancer survivors. J Clin Oncol 2001;19:3385–91.

[17] Yellen SB, Cella DF, Webster K, et al. Measuring fatigue and other anemia-related symptoms with the Functional Assessment of Cancer Therapy (FACT) measurement system. J Pain Symptom Manage 1997;13:63–74.

[18] Vogelzang NJ, Breitbart W, Cella D, et al. Patient, caregiver, and oncologist perceptions of cancer-related fatigue: results of a tripart assessment survey. The Fatigue Coalition. Semin Hematol 1997;34:4–12.

[19] Patrick DL, Ferketich SL, Frame PS, et al. National Institutes of Health State-of-the-Science Conference Statement: symptom management in cancer: pain, depression, and fatigue, July 15–17, 2002. J Natl Cancer Inst 2003;95:1110–7.

[20] Bower JE, Ganz PA, Desmond KA, et al. Fatigue in breast cancer survivors: occurrence, correlates, and impact on quality of life. J Clin Oncol 2000; 18:743–53.

[21] Bower JE, Ganz PA, Desmond KA, et al. Fatigue in long-term breast carcinoma survivors: a longitudinal investigation. Cancer 2006;106:751–8.

[22] Jacobsen PB. Assessment of fatigue in cancer patients. J Natl Cancer Inst Monogr 2004;32:93–7.

[23] Ancoli-Israel S, Moore PJ, Jones V. The relationship between fatigue and sleep in cancer patients: a review. Eur J Cancer Care (Engl) 2001;10:245–55.

[24] Bardwell WA, Moore P, Ancoli-Israel S, et al. Fatigue in obstructive sleep apnea: driven by depressive symptoms instead of apnea severity? Am J Psychiatry 2003;160:350–5.

[25] Cella D, Peterman A, Passik S, et al. Progress toward guidelines for the management of fatigue. Oncology (Williston Park) 1998;12: 369–77.

[26] Andrykowski MA, Schmidt JE, Salsman JM, et al. Use of a case definition approach to identify cancer-related fatigue in women undergoing adjuvant therapy for breast cancer. J Clin Oncol 2005;23:6613–22.

[27] Krupp LB, LaRocca NG, Muir-Nash J, et al. The fatigue severity scale. Application to patients with multiple sclerosis and systemic lupus erythematosus. Arch Neurol 1989;46:1121–3.

[28] Ware JE, Sherbourne CD. The MOS 36-item short-form health survey (SF-36). Med Care 1992;30:473–83.

[29] Ware JE, Snow KK, Kosinski M, et al. SF-36 health survey: manual and interpretation guide. Lincoln (RI): Quality-Metric Incorporated; 2000.

[30] Stein KD, Martin SC, Hann DM, et al. A multidimensional measure of fatigue for use with cancer patients. Cancer Pract 1998;6:143–52.

[31] Stein KD, Jacobsen PB, Blanchard CM, et al. Further validation of the multidimensional fatigue symptom inventory-short form. J Pain Symptom Manage 2004;27:14–23.

[32] Piper BF, Dibble SL, Dodd MJ, et al. The revised piper fatigue scale: psychometric evaluation in women with breast cancer. Oncol Nurs Forum 1998;25:677–84.

[33] McNair PM, Lorr M, Droppleman LF. POMS manual: profile of mood states. San Diego (CA): Educational and Industrial Testing Service; 1992.

[34] Sadler IJ, Jacobsen PB. Progress in understanding fatigue associated with breast cancer treatment. Cancer Invest 2001;19:723–31.

[35] McCorkle R, Quint-Benoliel J. Symptom distress, current concerns and mood disturbance after diagnosis of life-threatening disease. Soc Sci Med 1983;17:431–8.

[36] de Haes JC, van Knippenberg FC, Neijt JP. Measuring psychological and physical distress in cancer patients: structure and application of the Rotterdam Symptom Checklist. Br J Cancer 1990;62:1034–8.

[37] Hann DM, Jacobsen PB, Azzarello LM, et al. Measurement of fatigue in cancer patients: development and validation of the Fatigue Symptom Inventory. Qual Life Res 1998;7:301–10.

[38] Dimsdale JE, ncoli-Israel S, Ayalon L, et al. Taking fatigue seriously, II: variability in fatigue levels in cancer patients. Psychosomatics 2007; 48:247–52.

[39] Cimprich B. Pretreatment symptom distress in women newly diagnosed with breast cancer. Cancer Nurs 1999;22:185–94.

[40] Ancoli-Israel S, Liu L, Cooke JR, et al. Women with breast cancer who experience fatigue, depression and poor sleep before chemotherapy have more fatigue and poorer quality of life during chemotherapy. Sleep Med 2007;8: S50.

[41] Bower JE. Prevalence and causes of fatigue after cancer treatment: the next generation of research. J Clin Oncol 2005;23:8280–2.

[42] Irvine D, Vincent L, Graydon JE, et al. The prevalence and correlates of fatigue in patients receiving treatment with chemotherapy and radiotherapy. A comparison with the fatigue experienced by healthy individuals. Cancer Nurs 1994;17:367–78.

[43] Blesch KS, Paice JA, Wickham R, et al. Correlates of fatigue in people with breast or lung cancer. Oncol Nurs Forum 1991;18:81–7.

[44] Cella D. The Functional Assessment of Cancer Therapy-Anemia (FACT-An) Scale: a new tool for the assessment of outcomes in cancer anemia and fatigue. Semin Hematol 1997;34:13–9.

[45] Cella DF, Tulsky DS, Gray G, et al. The Functional Assessment of Cancer Therapy

scale: development and validation of the general measure. J Clin Oncol 1993;11:570–9.

[46] Meyerowitz BE, Watkins IK, Sparks FC. Quality of life for breast cancer patients receiving adjuvant chemotherapy. Am J Nurs 1983;83:232–5.

[47] Nail LM, Winningham M. Fatigue. In: Groenwald SL, Frogge MH, Goodman M, et al, editors. Cancer nursing: principles and practice. Boston: Jones and Bartlett; 1993.

[48] Lindley C, Vasa S, Sawyer WT, et al. Quality of life and preferences for treatment following systemic adjuvant therapy for early-stage breast cancer. J Clin Oncol 1998;16:1380–7.

[49] Bower JE, Ganz PA, Aziz N, et al. Fatigue and proinflammatory cytokine activity in breast cancer survivors. Psychosom Med 2002;64:604–11.

[50] Berger AM, Higginbotham P. Correlates of fatigue during and following adjuvant breast cancer chemotherapy: a pilot study. Oncol Nurs Forum 2000;27:1443–8.

[51] Cleeland CS, Bennett GJ, Dantzer R, et al. Are the symptoms of cancer and cancer treatment due to a shared biologic mechanism? A cytokine-immunologic model of cancer symptoms. Cancer 2003;97:2919–25.

[52] Lee BN, Dantzer R, Langley KE, et al. A cytokine-based neuroimmunologic mechanism of cancer-related symptoms. Neuroimmunomodulation 2004;11:279–92.

[53] Parker AJ, Wessely S, Cleare AJ. The neuroendocrinology of chronic fatigue syndrome and fibromyalgia. Psychol Med 2001;31:1331–45.

[54] Payne JK. A neuroendocrine-based regulatory fatigue model. Biol Res Nurs 2004;6:141–50.

[55] American Psychiatric Association. Diagnostic and statistical manual of mental disorders. 4th edition. Washington, DC: (DSM-IV) American Psychiatric Association Press; 1994.

[56] Bardwell WA, Ancoli-Israel S, Dimsdale JE. Comparison of the effects of depressive symptoms and apnea severity on fatigue in patients with obstructive sleep apnea: a replication study. J Affect Disord 2007;97:181–6.

[57] Andrykowski MA, Curran SL, Lightner R. Off-treatment fatigue in breast cancer survivors: a controlled comparison. J Behav Med 1998;21:1–18.

[58] Jacobsen PB, Donovan KA, Weitzner MA. Distinguishing fatigue and depression in patients with cancer. Semin Clin Neuropsychiatry 2003;8:229–40.

[59] Goldstein D, Bennett B, Friedlander M, et al. Fatigue states after cancer treatment occur both in association with, and independent of, mood disorder: a longitudinal study. BMC Cancer 2006;6:240.

[60] Smets EM, Visser MR, Willems-Groot AF, et al. Fatigue and radiotherapy: (A) experience in patients undergoing treatment. Br J Cancer 1998;78:899–906.

[61] Bardwell WA, Dimsdale JE, Pierce JP. Risk factors for fatigue in women treated for early-stage

breast cancer [abstract]. Psychooncology 2007; 16(S1):21–2.

[62] Savard J, Morin CM. Insomnia in the context of cancer: a review of a neglected problem. J Clin Oncol 2001;19:895–908.

[63] Davidson JR, MacLean AW, Brundage MD, et al. Sleep disturbance in cancer patients. Soc Sci Med 2002;54:1309–21.

[64] Liu L, Ancoli-Israel S. Sleep disorders—clinical science. In: Cleeland C, Fischer DG, Dunn A, editors. Cancer symptom science. Cambridge (UK): Cambridge University Press; 2007 [in press].

[65] Fiorentino L, Ancoli-Israel S. Sleep dysfunction in patients with cancer. Curr Treat Options Neurol 2007;9:337–46.

[66] Berger AM, Parker KP, Young-McCaughan S, et al. Sleep wake disturbances in people with cancer and their caregivers: state of the science. Oncol Nurs Forum 2005;32:E98–126.

[67] Liu L, Parker B, Dimsdale J, et al. Pre-treatment subjective sleep quality predicts fatigue, mood, and quality of life in breast cancer patients during chemotherapy [abstract]. Sleep 2006; 29(Suppl):A309.

[68] Ancoli-Israel S, Liu L, Parker BA, et al. Sleep quality before treatment predicts fatigue, depression and quality of life in breast cancer patients during chemotherapy. Breast Cancer 2006;100.

[69] Mills PJ, Parker B, Jones V, et al. The effects of standard anthracycline-based chemotherapy on soluble ICAM-1 and vascular endothelial growth factor levels in breast cancer. Clin Cancer Res 2004;10:4998–5003.

[70] Savard J, Simard S, Ivers H, et al. Randomized study on the efficacy of cognitive-behavioral therapy for insomnia secondary to breast cancer, part II: immunologic effects. J Clin Oncol 2005; 23:6097–106.

[71] Savard J, Davidson JR, Ivers H, et al. The association between nocturnal hot flashes and sleep in breast cancer survivors. J Pain Symptom Manage 2004;27:513–22.

[72] Bardwell WA, Casden D, Rock CL, et al. The relative importance of specific risk factors for insomnia in women treated for early-stage breast cancer. Psycho-Oncology, in press.

[73] Bardwell WA, Natarajan L, Dimsdale J, et al. Cancer-specific factors do not predict chronic insomnia in breast cancer survivors (BCS) [abstract]. Podium presentation for the 2007 Sleep Conference. Sleep, in press.

[74] Mills PJ, Parker B, Dimsdale JE, et al. The relationship between fatigue and quality of life and inflammation during anthracycline-based chemotherapy in breast cancer. Biol Psychol 2005;69:85–96.

[75] Schubert C, Hong S, Natarajan L, et al. The association between fatigue and inflammatory marker levels in cancer patients: a quantitative review. Brain Behav Immun 2007;21:413–27.

[76] Geinitz H, Zimmermann FB, Stoll P, et al. Fatigue, serum cytokine levels, and blood cell counts during radiotherapy of patients with breast cancer. Int J Radiat Oncol Biol Phys 2001;51:691–8.

[77] Gelinas C, Fillion L. Factors related to persistent fatigue following completion of breast cancer treatment. Oncol Nurs Forum 2004;31:269–78.

[78] Pusztai L, Mendoza TR, Reuben JM, et al. Changes in plasma levels of inflammatory cytokines in response to paclitaxel chemotherapy. Cytokine 2004;25:94–102.

[79] Smets EM, Visser MR, Willems-Groot AF, et al. Fatigue and radiotherapy: (B) experience in patients 9 months following treatment. Br J Cancer 1998;78:907–12.

[80] Morrow GR, Shelke AR, Roscoe JA, et al. Management of cancer-related fatigue. Cancer Invest 2005;23:229–39.

[81] Hanna A, Sledge G, Mayer ML, et al. A phase II study of methylphenidate for the treatment of fatigue. Support Care Cancer 2006;14:210–5.

[82] Bruera E, Driver L, Barnes EA, et al. Patient-controlled methylphenidate for the management of fatigue in patients with advanced cancer: a preliminary report. J Clin Oncol 2003;21:4439–43.

[83] Bruera E, Valero V, Driver L, et al. Patient-controlled methylphenidate for cancer fatigue: a double-blind, randomized, placebo-controlled trial. J Clin Oncol 2006;24:2073–8.

[84] Lower E, Fleischman S, Cooper A, et al. A phase III, randomized placebo-controlled trial of the safety and efficacy of d-MPH as a new treatment of fatigue and "chemobrain" in adult cancer patients [abstract]. J Clin Oncol 2005;23(16S):8000.

[85] Morrow GR, Gillin JC, Hickok JT, et al. The positive effect of the psychostimulant modafinil on fatigue from cancer that persists after treatment is completed [abstract]. J Clin Oncol 2005;23(16S):8012.

[86] Kaleita TA, Wellisch D, Grahan CA, et al. Pilot study of modafinil for treatment of neurobehavioral dysfunction and fatigue in adult patients with brain tumors [abstract]. J Clin Oncol 2005;23(16S):1503.

[87] Moss EL, Simpson JS, Pelletier G, et al. An open-label study of the effects of bupropion SR on fatigue, depression and quality of life of mixed-site cancer patients and their partners. Psychoncology 2006;15:259–67.

[88] Cullum JL, Wojciechowski AE, Pelletier G, et al. Bupropion sustained release treatment reduces fatigue in cancer patients. Can J Psychiatry 2004;49:139–44.

[89] Morrow GR, Hickok JT, Roscoe JA, et al. Differential effects of paroxetine on fatigue and depression: a randomized, double-blind trial from the University of Rochester Cancer Center Community Clinical Oncology Program. J Clin Oncol 2003;21:4635–41.

[90] Roscoe JA, Morrow GR, Hickok JT, et al. Effect of paroxetine hydrochloride (Paxil) on fatigue and depression in breast cancer patients receiving chemotherapy. Breast Cancer Res Treat 2005;89:243–9.

[91] Demetri GD, Gabrilove JL, Blasi MV, et al. Benefits of epoetin alfa in anemic breast cancer patients receiving chemotherapy. Clin Breast Cancer 2002;3:45–51.

[92] Leyland-Jones B, Semiglazov V, Pawlicki M, et al. Maintaining normal hemoglobin levels with epoetin alfa in mainly nonanemic patients with metastatic breast cancer receiving first-line chemotherapy: a survival study. J Clin Oncol 2005;23:5960–72.

[93] Monk JP, Phillips G, Waite R, et al. Assessment of tumor necrosis factor alpha blockade as an intervention to improve tolerability of dose-intensive chemotherapy in cancer patients. J Clin Oncol 2006;24:1852–9.

[94] Bower JE. Management of cancer-related fatigue. Clin Adv Hematol Oncol 2006;4:828–9.

[95] Schneider CM, Hsieh CC, Sprod LK, et al. Effects of supervised exercise training on cardiopulmonary function and fatigue in breast cancer survivors during and after treatment. Cancer 2007;110:918–25.

[96] Fiorentino L, Ancoli-Israel S. Insomnia and its treatment in women with breast cancer. Sleep Med Rev 2006;10:419–29.

[97] Theobald DE. Cancer pain, fatigue, distress, and insomnia in cancer patients. Clin Cornerstone 2004;6:S15–21.

[98] Collado-Hidalgo A, Bower JE, Ganz PA, et al. Inflammatory biomarkers for persistent fatigue in breast cancer survivors. Clin Cancer Res 2006;12:2759–66.

[99] Wratten C, Kilmurray J, Nash S, et al. Fatigue during breast radiotherapy and its relationship to biological factors. Int J Radiat Oncol Biol Phys 2004;59:160–7.

ELSEVIER
SAUNDERS

SLEEP
MEDICINE
CLINICS

Sleep Med Clin 3 (2008) 73–80

Sleep Disruption During Pregnancy

Eileen P. Sloan, MD, PhD, FRCPC[a,b,*]

Sleep disruption is one of the most frequently reported complaints of pregnant women [1,2]. Its high prevalence has likely resulted in disturbed sleep being considered a normal part of pregnancy and therefore not warranting investigation or treatment. However, for a proportion of women, disturbed sleep is problematic and has a profound impact on daytime function and mood. This article discusses the potential impact of sleep disruption during pregnancy and the postpartum period. Areas of clinical concern are addressed, including the medical and psychiatric complications of insomnia, and the potential effect of primary sleep disorders on the fetus are discussed.

According to a report on sleep in woman published a decade ago by the National Sleep Foundation that surveyed 1012 women between ages 30 and 60 years, 79% reported that sleep was or had been disturbed during pregnancy [3]. Women who were currently or had been recently pregnant were more likely to report frequent insomnia (64%) compared with premenopausal or menopausal women. Of women reporting sleep disturbance during pregnancy, 70% reported that it interfered with daily functioning on at least a few

days per month, this figure again being higher than for women in the other categories. For what proportion this disruption represented a serious problem is unclear. A major drawback of this survey is that it did not include women in younger age groups, and therefore multiparous women may have been more represented. Furthermore, not all women were pregnant at the reporting and were therefore providing retrospective accounts of their sleep during pregnancy. The extent to which the sample represents the general population could also be questioned, although it does provide information about the extent of subjective sleep disruption during pregnancy.

How does pregnancy affect sleep?

Objective changes

Sleep is a highly structured and well-organized activity that follows a circadian (approximately 24 hours) rhythm and is regulated by the interplay of biologic processes, such as temperature and melatonin, and environmental (eg, daylight) factors. The initial part of the sleep cycle is spent in light (stages 1 and 2) sleep, followed by deep or slow-wave sleep

[a] Department of Psychiatry, University of Toronto, 600 University Avenue, Toronto, Ontario, M5G 1X5, Canada
[b] Maternal/Infant Mental Health Program, Mount Sinai Hospital, Tonronto, Ontario, Canada
* Department of Psychiatry, University of Toronto, Perinatal Mental Health Clinic, Mount Sinai Hospital, 600 University Avenue, Toronto, Ontario, M5G 1X5, Canada
E-mail address: esloan@mtsinai.on.ca

doi:10.1016/j.jsmc.2007.10.009

(SWS) (stages 3 and 4). Approximately 90 minutes after sleep onset, rapid eye movement sleep (REM) is attained. This cycle is repeated throughout the night, with the amount of deep sleep decreasing as the night progresses, and the amount of REM sleep increasing. The amount of time spent in each stage of sleep depends on age (eg, young children have a high percentage of SWS, whereas elderly individuals have little SWS and large amounts of light sleep). Other factors, however, affect sleep architecture, including medications, psychiatric and medical illness, and primary sleep disorders.

Pregnancy has been shown to significantly impact sleep architecture, quantity, and quality. Molin and colleagues [4], Santiago and colleagues [5], and Lee [6] have published comprehensive reviews, with this article highlighting the most salient points.

Few studies have examined changes in sleep architecture during pregnancy and, although the findings are not fully consistent, they indicate more disturbed sleep as pregnancy progresses. Non-pregnant women of child-bearing age have total sleep times on average of 7 to 9 hours per night, with 55% of the time spent in light sleep, 20% in SWS, and 20% to 25% in REM sleep. The pioneering study of Karacan and colleagues [7] published in 1968 reported a decrease in stage 3 and 4 sleep in the third trimester but no significant change in REM sleep across pregnancy. They hypothesized that this lightening of sleep may represent anticipation of disruption after the infant's arrival. Alternatively, they suggested it could be a manifestation of a subclinical depression and that SWS suppression may be a marker for the later development of postpartum depression.

Driver and Shapiro [8] recorded polysomnographs in a series of five primiparous women at two points during pregnancy and at 3 months post partum and found an increase in time awake as pregnancy progressed. REM sleep decreased from week 17 onward. In contrast with the findings of Karacan and colleagues [7], these investigators noted that SWS, stage 4 in particular, increased from early to late pregnancy. They postulated that the SWS increase suggested the restorative role that sleep plays during a time of increased energy demands from the fetus. However, both studies used small sample sizes, and parity may be an important factor in changes in sleep during pregnancy.

A prospective study by Brunner and colleagues [9] of 29 women (16 multiparous and 13 primiparous) before and during pregnancy found that total sleep time increased in the first trimester by a mean of 34 minutes. However, sleep efficiency (the amount of time in bed actually spent sleeping) decreased in the first trimester, normalized in the second trimester, and decreased again in the third trimester. The drop in total sleep time continued at 1 month post partum, at which time sleep efficiency had dropped from 93% prepregnancy to a mean of 81% (normal sleep efficiency is >90%). SWS was significantly lower during pregnancy relative to prepregnancy and postpartum values. This finding contradicts the theory that this stage of sleep plays a restorative function during pregnancy because otherwise an increase would be anticipated. Compared with primiparas, multiparas had lower sleep efficiency at all time points, except post partum, suggesting that prior pregnancy and childrearing has a lasting disruptive impact on sleep. The lower postpartum sleep efficiency in the primiparous group can be understood to be stress related; at 3 months post partum, this group's sleep efficiency had improved, although not back to the prepregnancy baseline, but similar to that for the multiparas.

Another study comparing the sleep of primiparous (n = 8) and multiparous (n = 11) women during the second trimester, 1 week before delivery, and then 1 week and 6 weeks post partum using actigraphy yielded different results [10]. The sleep of primiparous women was generally poorer although the same amount of sleep was obtained by each group post partum. During the second trimester, the primiparous group had more wake after sleep onset, spent more time in bed, and had less efficient sleep. At 1 week post partum, they had fewer sleep episodes per day and spent less time in bed. During the first week post partum, women overall got 1.5 hours less sleep than during the last week of pregnancy, experienced three times more sleep episodes in 24-hours, and showed increased day-to-day variability. By 6 weeks post partum wake after sleep onset for both groups was lower than even during pregnancy, and total sleep time had increased by an average of an hour although it was not back to the levels noted in the second trimester.

Although a discrepancy exists in which aspects of sleep change across pregnancy, these studies highlight that substantial changes accompany pregnancy, and most studies suggest that sleep becomes lighter and more disrupted as pregnancy progresses. These changes seem to persist into the postpartum period.

Subjective changes

An important factor is to what extent disrupted sleep during pregnancy impacts quality of life, mood, and ability to cope with other aspects of pregnancy. Few studies have sought to determine this using subjective reports and sleep logs. They indicate that a large percentage of women note alterations in their sleep (between 66% and 94%) [11,12]. During the first trimester, subjective sleep quality decreases and the number of nocturnal awakenings increases. Daytime sleepiness is more problematic. During the second trimester, women report that sleep normalizes, although 19% of women continue to experience difficulties at this stage [11]. By the third trimester, women experience worsening insomnia, increased daytime sleeping, and decreased alertness. The reasons women cited for the increased sleep disturbances were mainly urinary frequency, backache, fetal movement, abdominal discomfort, leg cramps, and heartburn.

A survey of sleep disruption across pregnancy in 127 women found that 97% identified themselves as having disrupted sleep, but only a third felt they had a "sleep disorder" [13], although the impact this had on daytime function, mood, and quality of life was not assessed. Some women may resign themselves to poor sleep, believing it prepares them for the child's arrival, or they may believe that no treatment is available anyway. Alternatively, certain women may be vulnerable to the effects of sleep disruption. When the impact of sleep deprivation on performance in volunteer subjects is examined, wide variability on the effects of prolonged sleep deprivation is noted, with some subjects having a "catastrophic response" and others being minimally impacted [14]. A percentage of women may be biologically or psychologically predisposed to the detrimental effects of disrupted sleep. Factors such as a prior history of an affective disorder, lack of a social support network, poor coping skills, and difficulty adjusting to the impending role of motherhood may be important.

Factors contributing to changes in sleep

Many factors contribute to sleep disruption during pregnancy, including endocrine changes, such as increased progesterone and prolactin levels; increased size, fetal movement, and bladder distension; diaphragmatic elevation; gastrointestinal discomfort and vomiting; and temperature fluctuations. Progesterone levels, for example, increase across pregnancy. Progesterone has been shown to have somnogenic properties in animal models when applied to the preoptic area of the forebrain [15], and in men and women when administered exogenously [16,17]. Increased daytime somnolence in the later stages of pregnancy from increased progesterone levels could, therefore, be anticipated. The sharp and sudden drop in progesterone levels at delivery probably contributes to decreased sleep quantity and quality, along with the many other issues facing new mothers.

The possibility should be considered that a primary sleep disorder, such as obstructive sleep apnea (OSA) or restless legs syndrome (RLS), may develop during pregnancy and contribute to sleep deprivation.

The prevalence of OSA is approximately 5% in nonpregnant women of reproductive age [18], the risk increasing substantially with obesity [19]. Some of the changes in respiratory physiology during pregnancy, such as decreased functional residual capacity secondary to elevation of the diaphragm and relaxation of the costochondral muscles [20], changes in the airway mucosa resulting in nasopharyngeal edema [21], and hyperventilation with increased sensitivity to carbon dioxide [22–24], may predispose to obstructive or central apneic events. Conversely, progesterone and being somnogenic stimulate respiratory activity so that a lower risk for sleep-disordered breathing would be expected. Some investigators have found no decrease in nocturnal arterial oxygen saturation during pregnancy [25,26], whereas others report significantly more nocturnal desaturation in pregnant women compared with controls [27,28]. A polysomnographic study of 10 pregnant women who were referred for suspected OSA during the third trimester and at 3 months post partum found a significant reduction in the apnea–hypopnea index post partum in REM and non-REM sleep, increase in mean arterial oxygen saturation post partum, and decrease in arterial blood pressure [29].

The risk for OSA in women who are obese prepregnancy was shown to be significantly higher than in those who are nonobese. Maasilta and colleagues [30] found that the former group experienced 1.7 events per hour versus 0.2 events per hour in the nonobese group ($P < .05$), and 5.3 events per hour of 4% oxygen desaturation versus 0.2 events per hour ($P < .005$). The obese women snored 32% of the time, whereas the nonobese group snored only 1% of the time ($P < .001$).

The relationship among snoring, pregnancy-induced hypertension, and intrauterine growth restriction has been examined. In a sample of 502 women who were asked the day after delivery if they had snored during the last week of pregnancy, 23% reported that they had. Hypertension and lower Apgar scores were significantly more common in this group compared with those who did not snore [31]. Several case series indicate that sleep apnea may be associated with intrauterine growth restriction, especially if other complications such as maternal obesity and diabetes mellitus are present [31,32]. Most of these case series relied on clinical examination rather than polysomnography, and the numbers are small. Given the increasing rates of obesity, this important topic must be further examined. Sleep-disordered breathing during pregnancy is discussed in more detail in the article by Edwards and Sullivan elsewhere in this issue.

In women who had preeclampsia, the control of partial upper airway obstruction and snoring through the use of nasal continuous positive airway pressure (CPAP) resulted in a significant decrease in blood pressure [33]. This area also requires further investigation with large prospective and longitudinal studies. Current evidence raises concerns about potentially serious consequences of sleep apnea and upper airway resistance during pregnancy, but the prevalence of these disorders remain to be determined.

The subjective sensation or restlessness in the legs, usually occurring in the evening, in RLS and the involuntary contraction of the anterior tibialis muscle during sleep in periodic leg movements syndrome (PLMS) increase during pregnancy and can have a significant impact on sleep continuity [34,35]. Questionnaire studies show that women cite restless legs as a common cause of sleep disruption during pregnancy [2,12]. Complaints of leg cramps during waking should raise the possibility of PLMS, especially in women experiencing daytime sleepiness or fatigue.

The potential impact of insomnia during pregnancy

Insomnia undoubtedly has a significant impact on psychosocial, occupational, and health factors in the general population, and contributes to increased rates of health care use. People who have insomnia have 60% higher health care costs [36,37], increased rates of absenteeism [38], and increased social disability [37]. It is associated with increased daytime fatigue and impaired cognitive and psychomotor performance [39]. Sleep-deprived subjects are very poor at assessing the detrimental impact of the deprivation on their performance, even when the mistakes being made are catastrophic [14].

Insomnia is a common feature of major depressive disorder, but patients who have persistent insomnia are at significant risk for developing depression [40–42], even when a medical cause exists for the insomnia, such as sleep apnea. Breslau and colleagues [41] found that in subjects aged 21 to 30 years and those who had insomnia at the outset of the study, the relative risk for developing new onset depression during a 3.5-year follow-up was four times (95% CI, 2.2–7.0) that for those experiencing no sleep disturbance. The relative risk for new-onset anxiety disorders and drug abuse was higher in the groups who had insomnia. Using a questionnaire study of almost 8000 members of the general population, Ford and Kamerow [40] found that those reporting insomnia at baseline and follow-up had a 39.8 times greater risk for depression than those reporting no insomnia (95% CI, 19.8–80). Therefore, women who have marked sleep disruption during pregnancy and in the weeks post partum may be at higher risk for postpartum mood disorders.

The questions arise as to what is *marked* or *significant* when assessing sleep disruption, especially in a population for whom the disruption is expected and inevitable when nurturing a newborn, and how women who are particularly vulnerable are identified. This area has not been addressed. Paradoxically, scales used in the assessment of postpartum depression eliminate somatic factors such as insomnia and fatigue [43,44], arguing that they are normal features of pregnancy and childbirth. However, a study by Ross and colleagues [45] indicated that women in the postpartum period may be more likely to articulate their distress with these symptoms (eg, insomnia) rather than admit feeling depressed.

An association between sleep disruption and mood is reported in a questionnaire-based study of 124 primiparous women [46]. Participants completed questionnaires on sleep and depressive symptoms (the General Sleep Disturbance Scale and the Center for Epidemiological Studies Depression Scale, respectively) during the last month of pregnancy and at 1, 2, and 3 months post partum. Sleep disturbance and depressive symptoms were associated at prepartum and at 3 months post partum; the women reporting more depressive symptoms had a higher frequency of sleep disturbance, difficulty falling asleep, early awakening, and greater daytime tiredness. As these authors stress, a complaint of trouble falling asleep may be the most relevant screening question in relation to a woman's risk for postpartum depression. This finding is important given that the screening tools for postpartum depression omit questions regarding sleep/insomnia.

The risk for new-onset mania or recurrence of a preexisting illness during the postpartum period is significant. Women who have a history of bipolar affective disorder have a twofold increase in risk for symptom exacerbation during the immediate postpartum period. Furthermore, women who have no history of bipolar affective disorder have a sevenfold increase in risk for admission in the puerperium compared with nonpostpartum and nonpregnant women [47]. Sleep disruption that results from caring for a neonate likely plays an important role in the development or recurrence of postpartum psychiatric illness. Sleep disruption often heralds the onset of a manic or hypomanic episode in patients who have bipolar illness [48].

Patients who have insomnia often use alcohol and over-the-counter remedies. The National Sleep Foundation report found that 7% of pregnant women used over-the-counter medications and 7% used alcohol at some point in the pregnancy to help them sleep, whereas 4% used prescription medications for this purpose [3]. Although these figures are significantly lower than those for premenopausal and menopausal/postmenopausal women (with some degree of underreporting likely), the use of these sleep aids during pregnancy or in the postpartum period could have significant consequences.

Aside from psychiatric sequelae, several physiologic changes result from sleep deprivation. Insomnia has been shown to be associated with immune down-regulation. Several studies have shown a positive correlation between natural killer cell activity and insomnia in patients experiencing insomnia with and without depression [49,50]. A recent study examined the relationship between self-reported sleep variables and circulating serum cytokine levels during each trimester of pregnancy in 35 women and 43 nonpregnant women [51]. Results showed that sleep was subjectively more disturbed in the pregnant group. Interleukin 10 in this group was significantly higher in all trimesters, as was C-reactive protein, an indicator of systemic inflammation. Subjectively reported sleep disruption was associated with increases in tumor necrosis factor α in the pregnant women and C-reactive protein in those who were not. These associations indicate that sleep disruption during pregnancy influences immune function, but whether this is relevant to other disorders of pregnancy, such as preeclampsia or premature delivery, remains unclear.

Sleep disturbance has also been shown to have a stimulatory effect on the activity of the hypothalamic-pituitary-adrenal axis and a suppressive effect on the growth hormone axis [52]. Whether any of these changes are relevant for pregnancy or the postpartum woman remains to be determined, as does the effect of insomnia on other endocrine and hormonal factors.

Treatment of pregnancy-related sleep disruption

Essentially all women complain of sleep disruption in late pregnancy and post partum, and therefore the question remains how to determine whether the disruption is significant. First, the author believes that primary caregivers must inquire about it, because women may not complain or may discount it as a natural consequence of pregnancy. The simple step of asking a woman how she is sleeping allows women experiencing sleep disruption to be more forthright about their situation. Women are reluctant to complain about any aspect of new motherhood—a "taboo" that society encourages—and therefore introducing the issue for them can be an important step.

Inquiring about sleep is particularly pertinent in patients who have a history of a mood disorder (depression or bipolar disorder). A thorough history of the complaint should be taken, including prepregnancy sleep patterns and history of insomnia or other sleep problems (eg, narcolepsy). Potential medical causes should be considered (eg, medications, thyroid problems, psychiatric illness) and treated when appropriate. Primary sleep disorders should be ruled out. OSA should be considered if women complain of excessive daytime sleepiness, snoring, witnessed apneas, morning headaches, a history of intrauterine growth restriction, presence of hypertension, or diabetes. Significant respiratory disturbance can be treated with CPAP, which has been shown to be safe during pregnancy [33,53]. Milder respiratory disturbances may respond to the use of an oral appliance or conservative measures such as sleeping on one's side (positional therapy, which many pregnant women already use).

RLS/PLMS should be considered if patients complain of leg cramps or restless legs during the day or evening, they experience excessive daytime sleepiness, or the bed-partner reports that the patient kicks her legs during sleep. RLS and PLMS are typically treated pharmacologically (eg, levadopa, pramipexole, gabapentin). The safety of these drugs during pregnancy has not been determined and therefore should not be initiated, and clinical experience shows that pregnant women are reluctant to start medication in these cases (ie, when safety data is not available). Other treatment options include codeine and clonazepam. The safety profile of the latter, particularly in the first trimester and around delivery, must be discussed with the woman so she can make an informed choice. A relationship exists between low serum ferritin levels and RLS/PLMS, and iron supplementation should be instituted. Implementing conservative measures, such as reducing caffeine intake, massaging the legs, and wearing supportive stockings in bed, may be beneficial. Anecdotal reports by women who have RLS suggest that stretching exercises in the evening are beneficial, as is a warm bath before retiring. Some patients who have RLS/PLMS also find taking a calcium/magnesium supplement in the evening helpful.

During the postpartum period, the sleep of women who have a history of a mood disorder must be protected. Prolongation of their hospital stay to enable the new mother to recover from the impact of labor and birth may be beneficial [54,55]. The author's service routinely requests that these women remain in the hospital for 5 days and 5 nights, with the baby spending each night at the nursing station so that the new mother can get as consolidated a night's sleep as possible. The patient's partner and other family members should be encouraged to play an active role in overnight feeding. Emphasizing the potential impact of a depressive or manic episode on the child can help alleviate the guilt that women often experience with this practice.

When no primary cause for the sleep disruption can be determined, attention to sleep hygiene factors should be highlighted, such as maintaining a regular sleep-wake schedule, avoiding caffeinated beverages, reducing the amount of fluids consumed in the evening, and ensuring the temperature in the bedroom is comfortable. Women should be encouraged to eliminate daytime napping if it seems to have a detrimental impact on their nocturnal sleep.

Most women are likely to resist the use of sleeping medications, but when insomnia has a severe effect, the use of a sleep aid may be warranted. Dimenhydrinate can be sedating and has been shown to be safe during pregnancy. Some evidence shows that the antidepressant trazodone may be beneficial for reducing sleep-onset latency and improving sleep quality [56]. The American Academy of Pediatrics states that data are too limited to provide a recommendation on the use of this and other sedating antidepressants, such as mirtazapine, during pregnancy [57]. A study by Einarson and colleagues [58] of subjects matched for age, smoking, and alcohol use found no difference in pregnancy outcome (including rate of major malformations and gestational age at birth) between patients taking nefazodone (no longer available in Canada) and trazodone during the first trimester and those taking other nonteratogenic antidepressants or drugs (eg, sumatriptan, dextromethorphan). Both antidepressant groups, however, showed a trend toward a higher rate of spontaneous abortions, although the difference was not statistically significant. The doses of trazodone and nefazodone used in the study are not stated but presumably were within the range typically used for depression. Lower doses are typically prescribed when treating insomnia (eg, trazodone, 50–100 mg, at night), and therefore, these agents may be associated with less risk when used for this purpose. The effect of these antidepressants in improving insomnia during pregnancy has not been considered, and whether the lower does would result in a higher rate of spontaneous abortion is unknown.

The tricyclic antidepressant, amitriptyline, has considerable sedating properties. It does not seem to have teratogenic effects and is considered safe in pregnancy for treating depression [57]. When used to treat insomnia, it is also given in lower doses than for depression.

Benzodiazepines are frequently used to treat insomnia in the general population. However, their use should be limited during pregnancy because they can induce sedation, withdrawal signs (including restlessness, hypertonia, irritability, seizures, and abdominal distension), and floppy baby syndrome (eg, muscular hypotonia, low Apgar scores, neurologic depression) in the neonate [57]. These effects can last up to 3 months. Although analysis of pooled data from cohort studies suggests that fetal exposure to benzodiazepines during the first trimester is not associated with major malformations or oral cleft, pooled data from case-control studies showed a small but significant risk for these events [59]. The authors of this analysis emphasize, however, that the number of reports was small and that most cases for analyses of oral cleft and major malformations were derived from only three studies. Studies included in the analysis did not use consistent definitions of *major malformations*, and the authors did not delineate and which benzodiazepines were included in the studies was not delineated. No congenital defects have been associated with lorazepam or alprazolam [57]. Lorazepam is recommended because it lacks active metabolites and seems to have less risk for inducing a withdrawal syndrome in the neonate.

Use of the newer nonbenzodiazepine hypnotic preparations—zopiclone, zolpidem, and zaleplon—during pregnancy has received little research attention. Pregnancy outcomes in 40 women who were exposed to zopiclone during the first trimester were compared with those of a nonexposed group [60]. No increase was seen in outcome of pregnancy, including the rate of major malformations in the two groups, therefore the authors concluded that zopiclone is not a major teratogen. Until larger-scale studies of these drugs are available, their use during pregnancy should be limited.

No reports have been published on the efficacy of nonpharmacologic approaches to managing insomnia during pregnancy. Cognitive therapy involves identifying dysfunctional beliefs and attitudes about sleep and replacing them with more adaptive beliefs. This modality has been shown to be effective in the treatment of insomnia in the general population and its effects are sustained over time [61]. The efficacy of relaxation techniques, stimulus control therapy, and other nonpharmacologic interventions—all of which require minimal training—for treating insomnia during pregnancy has not been assessed.

No data are available on the safety and efficacy of herbal preparations, such as valerian, during pregnancy.

Summary

Fortunately, the sleep disruption that occurs during pregnancy and in the postpartum period will not result in significant long-term sequelae for most women. However, data from the general population indicate that it will be problematic for a proportion of women and will likely predispose them to mood and anxiety disorders and chronic insomnia with its consequences, although the extent of this is unknown. The impact of sleep disruption, if any, on the developing fetus must be researched further. The impact of insomnia in women in high-risk groups (eg, obese, hypertensive, previous history of depression and insomnia) also must be addressed. The extent to which women self-medicate with over-the-counter sleep aids or alcohol must also be further assessed, and the pharmacologic management of severe insomnia requires greater consideration. No studies examine the efficacy of nonpharmacologic measures and techniques that can be implemented during the postpartum period—a time of even more marked sleep disruption—and beyond.

References

[1] Lee K, DeJoseph JF. Sleep disturbances, vitality and fatigue among a select group on employed childbearing children. Birth 1992;19:208–13.

[2] Hertz G, Fast A, Feinsilver S, et al. Sleep in normal late pregnancy. Sleep 1992;15:246–51.

[3] National Sleep Foundation. Women and sleep. Available at: http://www.sleepfoundation.org/atf/cf/%7BF6BF2668-A1B4-4FE8-8D1A-. Accessed January 14, 2007.

[4] Molin ML, Broch L, Zak R, et al. Sleep in women across the life cycle from adulthood through menopause. Sleep Med Rev 2003;7(2):155–77.

[5] Santiago JR, Nolledo MS, Kinzler W, et al. Sleep and sleep disorders during pregnancy. Ann Intern Med 2001;134:396–408.

[6] Lee KA. Alterations in sleep during pregnancy and postpartum: a review of 30 years of research. Sleep Med Rev 1998;2(4):231–42.

[7] Karacan I, Wayne H, Harman AW, et al. Characteristics of sleep patterns during late pregnancy and the postpartum periods. Am J Obstet Gynecol 1968;101:579–86.

[8] Driver HS, Shapiro CM. A longitudinal study of sleep stages in young women during pregnancy and postpartum. Sleep 1992;15:449–53.

[9] Brunner DP, Munch M, Biedermann K, et al. Changes in sleep and sleep electroencephalogram during pregnancy. Sleep 1994;7:576–82.

[10] Signal TL, Gander PH, Sangall MR, et al. Sleep duration and quality in healthy nulliparous and multiparous women across pregnancy and post-partum. Aust N Z J Obstet Gynaecol 2007; 47:16–22.

[11] Lee K, Zaffke ME, McEnany G. Parity and sleep patterns during and after pregnancy. Obstet Gynecol 2000;95:14–8.

[12] Schweiger MS. Sleep disturbance in pregnancy. A subjective survey. Am J Obstet Gynecol 1972; 114:879–82.

[13] Mindell JA, Jacobson BJ. Sleep disturbances during pregnancy. J Obstet Gynecol Neonatal Nurs 2000;29:590–7.

[14] Hauri PJ. Cognitive deficits in insomnia patients. Acta Neurol Belg 1997;97:113–7.

[15] Kimura M, Zhang SQ, Inoue S. Pregnancy associated sleep changes in the rat. Am J Physiol 1996; 271:R1063–9.

[16] Merryman W, Boiman R, Barnes L, et al. Progesterone-induced changes in sleep in male subjects. J Clin Endocrinol 1954;14:1567–9.

[17] Little BC, Matta RJ, Zahn TP. Physiological and psychological effects of progesterone in man. J Nerv Ment Dis 1974;159:256–62.

[18] Young TB, Palta J, Dempsey J. Occurrence of sleep disordered breathing among middle-aged adults. N Engl J Med 1993;328:1230–5.

[19] Sloan EP, Shapiro CM. Obstructive sleep apnea in a consecutive series of obese women. Int J Eat Disord 1995;17(2):167–73.

[20] Weinberger SE, Weiss ST, Cohen WR. State of the art: pregnancy and the lung. Am Rev Respir Dis 1980;121:559–81.

[21] Elkus R, Popovich J. Respiratory physiology in pregnancy. Clin Chest Med 1992;13:555–65.

[22] Prowse CM, Gaensler EA. Respiratory and acid-base changes during pregnancy. Anesthesiology 1965;26:381–92.

[23] Contreras G, Guttierrez M, Beroiza T, et al. Ventilatory drive and respiratory muscle function in pregnancy. Am Rev Respir Dis 1991;144:837–41.

[24] Bromwell LG, West P, Kryger MH. Breathing during sleep in normal pregnancy women. Am Rev Respir Dis 1986;133:38–41.

[25] Nikkola E, Ekblad U, Ekholm E, et al. Sleep in multiple pregnancy: breathing patterns, oxygenation and periodic leg movements. Am J Obstet Gynecol 1996;174:1622–5.

[26] Trakada G, Tsapanos V, Spiropoulos K. Normal pregnancy and oxygenation during sleep. Eur J Obstet Gynecol Reprod Biol 2003;109(2):128–32.

[27] Feinsilver SH, Hertz G. Respiration during sleep in pregnancy. Clin Chest Med 1992;13:637–44.

[28] Bourne T, Ogilvie AJ, Vickers R, et al. Nocturnal hypoxemia in late pregnancy. Br J Anaesth 1995; 75:678–82.

[29] Edwards N, Blyton DM, Hennessy A, et al. Severity of sleep disordered breathing improves following parturition. Sleep 2005;28(6): 737–41.

[30] Maasilta P, Bachour A, Terama K. Sleep-related disordered breathing in obese women. Chest 2001;120:1448–54.

[31] Franklin KA, Holmgren PA, Jonsson F. Snoring, pregnancy-induced hypertension and growth retardation of the fetus. Chest 2000;117:137–41.

[32] Charbonneau M, Falcone T, Cosio MG, et al. Obstructive sleep apnea during pregnancy. Therapy and implications for health. Am Rev Respir Dis 1991;144:461–3.

[33] Edwards N, Blyton DM, Kirjavainen T, et al. Nasal continuous positive airway pressure reduces sleep-induced blood pressure increments in preeclampsia. Am J Respir Crit Care Med 2000;162:252–7.

[34] Garcia-Borreguero D, Egatz R, Winklemann J, et al. Epidemiology of restless legs syndrome: the current status. Sleep Med Rev 2006;10(3):153–67.

[35] Goodman DS, Brodie C, Ayida GA. Restless leg syndrome in pregnancy. Br Med J 1988;29:1101–2.

[36] Mellinger GD, Balter MB, Ulenhuth EH. Insomnia and its treatment: prevalence and correlates. Arch Gen Psychiatry 1985;42:225–32.

[37] Simon GE, VonKorff M. Prevalence, burden and treatment of insomnia in primary care. Am J Psychiatry 1997;154:1417–23.

[38] Kuppermann M, Lubeck DP, Mazonson PD. Sleep problems and their correlates in a working populations. J Gen Intern Med 1995;10:25–32.

[39] Lichstein KL, Means MK, Noe SL. Fatigue and sleep disorders. Behav Res Ther 1997;35:733–40.

[40] Ford DE, Kamerow DB. Epidemiologic study of sleep disturbance and psychiatric disorder: an opportunity for prevention? JAMA 1989;262:1479–84.

[41] Breslau N, Roth T, Rosenthal L. Sleep disturbance and psychiatric disorders: a longitudinal epidemiological study of young adults. Biol Psychiatry 1996;39:411–8.

[42] Gillin JC. Are sleep disturbances risk factors for anxiety, depressive and addictive disorders? Acta Psychiatr Scand 1998;98:39–43.

[43] Cox JL, Holden JM, Sagavosky R. Detection of postnatal depression: development of the 10-item Edinburgh Postnatal Depression Scale. Br J Psychiatry 1987;150:782–6.

[44] Sugawara M, Sakamoto S, Kitamura T. Structure of depressive symptoms in pregnancy and the postpartum period. J Affect Disord 1999;54:161–9.

[45] Ross LE, Gilbert Evans SE, Sellers EM, et al. Measurement issues in postpartum depression part 2: assessment of somatic symptoms using the Hamilton Rating Scale for Depression. Arch Womens Ment Health 2003;6:59–64.

[46] Goyal D, Gay CL, Lee KA. Patterns of sleep disruption and depressive symptoms in new mothers. J Perinat Neonatal Nurs 2007;21(2):123–9.

[47] Sharma V, Mazmanian D. Sleep loss and postpartum psychosis. Bipolar Disord 2003;5(2):98–105.

[48] Wehr TA, Sack DA, Rosenthal NE. Sleep reduction as a final common pathway in the genesis of mania. Am J Psychiatry 1987;144:201–4.

[49] Irwin M, Smith TL, Gillin JC. Electroencephalographic sleep and natural killer activity in depressed patients and control subjects. Psychosom Med 1992;54:10–21.

[50] Cover H, Irwin M. Immunity and depression: Insomnia, retardation and reduction of natural killer cell activity. J Behav Med 1994;17:217–23.

[51] Okun ML, Coussons-Read ME. Sleep disruption during pregnancy: how does it influence serum cytokines? J Reprod Immunol 2007;73(2):158–65.

[52] Vgontzas AN, Mastorakos G, Bixler EO, et al. Sleep deprivation effects on the activity of the hypothalamic-pituitary-adrenal and growth axes: potential clinical implications. Clin Endocrinol 1999;51:205–15.

[53] Gillleminault C, Kreutzer M, Chang J. Pregnancy sleep-disordered breathing and treatment with nasal continuous positive airway pressure. Sleep Med 2004;5:43–51.

[54] Steiner M, Fairman J, Jansen K, et al. Can postpartum depression be prevented? Presented at the Marce Society Biennial Scientific Meeting, Sydney, Australia, September 25–27, 2002.

[55] Gardner DL. Fatigue in postpartum women. Appl Nurs Res 1991;4(2):57–62.

[56] Van Bemmel AL, Havermans RG, Van Diest R. Effects of trazodone on EEG sleep and clinical state in major depression. Psychopharmacology 1992;107:569–74.

[57] American Academy of Pediatrics Committee on Drugs. Use of psychoactive medication during pregnancy and possible effects on the fetus and newborn. Pediatrics 2000;105(4):880–7.

[58] Einarson A, Bonari L, Voyer-Lavigne S, et al. A multicentre prospective controlled study to determine the safety of trazodone and nefazodone sue during pregnancy. Can J Psychiatry 2003; 48(2):106–10.

[59] Dolovitch LR, Addis A, Vaillancourt JM, et al. Benzodiazepine use in pregnancy and major malformations or oral cleft: meta-analysis of cohort and case-control studies. B Med J 1998; 317(7162):839–44.

[60] Diav-Citrin O, Okotore B, Lucarelli K, et al. Pregnancy outcome following first-trimester exposure to zopiclone: a prospective controlled cohort study. Am J Perinatol 1999;16:157–60.

[61] Morin CM, Culbert JP, Schwartz SM. Nonpharmacological interventions for insomnia: a meta-analysis of treatment efficacy. Am J Psychiatry 1994;151:1172–80.

ELSEVIER
SAUNDERS

SLEEP
MEDICINE
CLINICS

Sleep Med Clin 3 (2008) 81–95

Sleep-Disordered Breathing in Pregnancy

Natalie Edwards, PhD*, Colin E. Sullivan, MD, PhD

Recent data suggest that pregnancy is a strong risk factor for the development of sleep-disordered breathing (SDB) and that when SDB occurs in pregnancy, it is a potentially significant factor in the development of systemic hypertension. This article summarizes current data regarding the link between SDB and pregnancy and explores potentially important questions that need further research.

Knowledge regarding the spectrum of sleep breathing disorders and the clinical correlates and outcomes in women who have SDB is only emerging, and equivalent knowledge regarding SDB in pregnancy is in its infancy. Nonetheless, it is becoming clear that SDB in pregnancy has many extremely important implications, including its impact on maternal cardiorespiratory and metabolic

David Read Laboratory, Department of Medicine, The University of Sydney, NSW, 2006, Australia
* Corresponding author.
E-mail address: ne@med.usyd.edu.au (N. Edwards).

1556-407X/08/$ – see front matter © 2008 Elsevier Inc. All rights reserved.   doi:10.1016/j.jsmc.2007.10.010
sleep.theclinics.com

control, fetal well-being, and resultant neonatal and child health. Indeed, based on emerging data, the link between SDB and cardiovascular control may be even stronger during pregnancy than in the nonpregnant patient. The impact of maternal well-being during pregnancy on long-term outcomes of the offspring is now well established, with intrauterine health linked to such long-term outcomes as childhood and adult obesity, adult cardiovascular risk, and adult metabolic control [1–3]. Thus, in pregnancy, in addition to considering the direct effects of SDB on the mother, one must consider the implications for placental function, the fetus, the neonate, the child, and the future adult.

Gender differences in sleep-disordered breathing

Before an in-depth discussion of SDB in pregnancy, this section briefly reviews the emerging understanding of SDB in women in general.

Obstructive sleep apnea (OSA) is characterized by repetitive episodes of partial or complete upper airway obstruction during sleep. These repetitive episodes lead to recurring hypoxemia and hypercapnia, cyclic hemodynamic fluctuations, and frequent arousals from sleep. As a result, sleep consolidation and cardiovascular control are compromised significantly.

Clear evidence demonstrates an independent association between SDB and cardiovascular disease. The most robust association among cardiovascular risk factors is with systemic hypertension; it has been well established that sleep apnea is independently causal in the nonpregnant population. The first important gender difference in SDB is that the association with cardiovascular risk factors, and hypertension in particular, is significantly stronger in women than in men, regardless of menopausal status [4], and the association with other cardiovascular risk factors, including coronary artery disease, also is stronger [5]. The knowledge of this link between female gender and adverse cardiovascular outcomes is not new. In one of the first epidemiologic studies of snoring, published in 1980, there was evidence that women who exhibit snoring and sleep apnea, although representing only a fraction of the total population that has these sleep breathing disorders, have a higher vascular risk than do men [6].

The second important difference between female and male SDB is that women are likely to have a different spectrum of symptoms and are more likely to present with fatigue, and/or symptoms of poor sleep at night rather than with the classical male symptom of excessive daytime sleepiness [7].

The third important difference is that the pattern of SDB is more likely to vary from the classical repetitive episodes of complete obstruction often described in male subjects who have sleep apnea. Rather, the female pattern of SDB may be dominated by what currently is regarded as a syndrome variant, the "high upper airway resistance syndrome." Because so much of the knowledge about SDB is dominated by the classical pattern of frank apnea, and because current methods used to diagnose sleep apnea are not efficient in detecting partial upper airway obstruction (excluding the invasive and uncomfortable use of esophageal pressure manometry) and high upper airway resistance, it is likely that the extent and consequences of SDB in women have been underestimated greatly. It is important to note the parallel with the emerging understanding of SDB in infants and young children, in whom an apnea hypopnea index (the number of apneas and hypopneas per hour of sleep, AHI) of greater than 1 is considered abnormal. In this group evidence has demonstrated a clear link between resolution (with adenotonsillectomy) of this low level of SDB (characterized by obstructed breathing but in the absence of frank obstructive events and maintenance of almost normal arterial oxyhemoglobin saturation) and clear clinical benefits. Similarly, early studies showed that the equivalent level of disease severity in women (for which the term "high upper airway resistance syndrome" was coined) is associated with marked impairment of daytime function and that reversal of the SDB with the use of nasal continuous positive airway pressure (CPAP) significantly improved daytime function [8]. In this context it is important to acknowledge the concept proposed by Lugaresi and colleagues [6] of a continuum from mild snoring through heavy obstructed snoring, long cycles of hypopnea, and finally repetitive complete obstructive apneas.

Prevalence of sleep-disordered breathing in women

Clinically, male gender is still regarded as one of the strongest risk factors associated with obstructive sleep apnea. Nonetheless, the prevalence of SDB in young women of childbearing age is still relatively high. In an important way, the fact that sleep apnea is so common in men may have overshadowed its prevalence in women. This erroneous view was the reason that the early study of the prevalence of sleep apnea in a rural community had a disproportionately small number of females [9]. This study, published in 1993, was one of the first epidemiologic studies in which objective overnight data were recorded. Investigators were surprised to ind that, even in that small sample, the prevalence of SDB was remarkably high. With the publication of the Wisconsin sleep cohort study, reported in the early 1990s [10], it became clear that the prevalence of obstructive sleep apnea (as defined by an AHI of at least five events per hour) in young women was substantially higher than previously predicted, occurring in 6.5% to 8.5% of women in later child-bearing years. By any standard, this is a very high prevalence. There have been relatively few studies of the prevalence of OSA in the general female population younger than 30 years of age. One study that specifically assessed the prevalence in a group of women of childbearing age (20–44 years) is that of Bixler and colleagues [11], who reported that only 0.6% of women met their criteria for OSA with an AHI of at least 15 events per hour of sleep. When they changed their criteria to an AHI of at least 10 per hour of sleep and included day-time symptoms, specifically excessive daytime sleepiness, the prevalence was still only 0.7%. When interpreting these data, however, one must remember that the spectrum of symptoms associated with SDB in women do not reflect those reported in men and that, regardless of the severity of apnea, women are far less likely than men who have comparable apnea severity to report excessive daytime sleepiness [7]. Considering the implications of these data, the most relevant outcome of the Bixler study is that it identified a substantial proportion (8.2%) of the female participants in their cohort who reported regular snoring and also had an AHI of greater than 1 per hour of sleep, regardless of the lack of the traditional association with excessive daytime sleepiness.

As in the male population, obesity poses a considerable risk for the development of obstructive sleep apnea in women, with an estimated 37% of obese women having OSA [12]. In assessing these data, the prevalence of at least mild SDB in young women of childbearing potential seems to be in the order of 6% to 8% of the population; as obesity rates increase, so too, the prevalence of SDB inevitably will increase.

Physiology of pregnancy and sleep-disordered breathing

Given the relatively high prevalence of at least mild SDB in women who are of childbearing age, what is its prevalence during pregnancy? Although there are case reports in the literature of OSA during pregnancy from as early as 1978, until relatively recently pregnancy was considered as likely to be protective against the development of SDB. Nonetheless, a number of the physiologic changes that occur during pregnancy may be conducive to the development of SDB.

Progesterone and estrogen

Circulating estrogen and progesterone concentrations increase markedly during pregnancy. Since the 1940s progesterone has been recognized as a powerful respiratory stimulant [13], with more recent evidence suggesting that this effect is mediated through estrogen-dependent receptors [14]. Because of progesterone's properties as a powerful respiratory stimulant, its substantial increase during pregnancy was thought to confer protection against SDB [15,16]. Indeed, there have been two recent studies on the influence of menstrual cycle on sleep-related breathing: the authors of this article and their colleagues reported a luteal-phase improvement in OSA severity during rapid-eye-movement (REM) sleep [17], and Driver and colleagues [18] found a trend for a lower respiratory disturbance index in women who did not have significant SDB during the luteal phase, when progesterone is high, compared with the follicular phase. The increased respiratory drive and thus reduced arterial CO_2 of pregnancy (typically in the order of 35 Torr), coupled with the apneic threshold for CO_2 at sleep onset, are known, however, to be a potential source of respiratory instability at sleep onset [19].

In considering the physiologic impact of progesterone, one should recognize a number of additional effects that it may have in causing the development or exacerbation of SDB. Currently there is some uncertainty as to the impact of progesterone on upper airway drive. Driver and colleagues [18] found that upper airway resistance was lower during the luteal phase than during the follicular phase in a group of 11 women who had ovulatory cycles and no SDB. Further, Popovic [20] found that peak phasic and tonic genioglossus activity was greatest during the luteal phase of the menstrual cycle in 12 normal premenopausal women, supporting a protective role for progesterone. There is evidence, however, that, following priming with repetitive episodes of hypoxia (on a 2-minute hypoxia/2-minute normoxia schedule), there is marked suppression of upper airway dilator muscle activity during the luteal phase of the menstrual cycle [21]. These data suggest that under normal conditions, progesterone does lead to increased upper airway muscle activity; however, after priming with repetitive hypoxia, this enhanced upper airway muscle activity may be reversed.

Progesterone does, however, have a marked impact on diaphragmatic drive, significantly increasing phrenic nerve activity [22]. Thus, in the face of increasingly negative upper airway pressure, and when drive to the upper airway may not be augmented (and, indeed, might be inhibited), the propensity for collapse almost certainly is aggravated. Progesterone reduces the integrity of the vascular endothelium leading to fluid leakage from the intravascular to the extravascular space, leading to tissue edema [23] that has the potential to reduce the size of the upper airway significantly.

In addition to the relative changes in the drive to diaphragmatic and upper airway muscular groups, changes in patency of the upper airway are of particular importance during pregnancy. Increased circulating estrogen concentrations that are associated with pregnancy lead to vascular relaxation, particularly in the upper portion of the upper airway. Rhinitis is a common occurrence in pregnancy, with at least 45% of women complaining of rhinitis during the last trimester of pregnancy [24].

Relaxin and the upper airway

Another hormonal change during pregnancy that is likely to have a significant impact on upper airway patency is the hormone relaxin, a member of the family of insulin-like growth factors. This hormone is released specifically during pregnancy and originally was described for its effect on maternal pubic ligament laxity [25]. Although relaxin has a diverse range of effects throughout the body, its importance in maternal SDB is its role as both a muscle relaxant and a powerful vasodilator [26]. Both these properties may increase the propensity for collapse by increasing collapsibility and by decreasing upper airway caliber (by a mechanism similar to that proposed for estrogen), respectively.

Lung volume and upper airway caliber

In considering upper airway caliber, it also is important to note that physical intrusion of the gravid uterus into the maternal thoracic cavity, particularly in the supine position, may have an impact on the maternal upper airway. Maternal functional residual capacity is decreased up to 15% by the third trimester of pregnancy [27], and evidence suggests that passive reductions in lung volume are associated with substantial reductions in pharyngeal cross-sectional area [28].

Empiric evidence for reduced upper airway dimensions in pregnancy

Although in theory a decrease in the internal luminal diameter of the maternal upper airway would be expected, relatively few empiric studies have investigated this phenomenon systematically. The Mallampati grade, which visually assesses the size of the Faucial pillars, the soft palate, and the base of the uvula [29], is a reasonably reliable predictor of severity of SDB. Mallampati scores range from 1,

in which the entire posterior pharynx is easily visualized, to 4, in which no posterior structures can be seen; a high score is associated with more severe SDB [30]. The first study to have assessed upper airway size in pregnancy was performed in 1995 [31] when the Mallampati score was compared in 242 normal pregnant women at 12 weeks' gestation and again at 38 weeks' gestation. There was a 34% increase in the number of women who had Mallampati scores of 4 (indicating substantial narrowing of the upper airway) at 38 weeks' gestation compared with those at 12 weeks' gestation.

Subsequently, Izci and colleagues [32] compared upper airway caliber among three groups of women: normal nonpregnant women, normal pregnant women at 36 weeks' gestation, and preeclamptic women (diagnosed according to standard international criteria [33]). In this study, the change in the calibers of the upper airway, as measured using acoustic reflectance, with change in position from seated to supine was significantly greater in pregnant than in nonpregnant women. As expected, women who had pre-eclampsia had significantly reduced upper airway caliber in all positions. (The substantial issue of SDB in pre-eclampsia is discussed later). In a further study using the same technique [34], the oropharyngeal junction area and the mean pharyngeal cross-sectional area of the upper airway in normal pregnant women was found to be significantly smaller than in age- and prepregnancy body mass index (BMI)–matched nonpregnant women. Furthermore, the mean postpartum pharyngeal area in the pregnant sample was significantly greater in both the seated and supine positions.

The importance of the caliber of the upper airway in determining the propensity for the development of SDB is highlighted by several studies that have demonstrated a clear link between the internal size of the upper airway and the presence of SDB [35–37].

Snoring in pregnancy

To date few studies have systematically investigated the incidence or prevalence of SDB during pregnancy. The very first questionnaire studies of disordered breathing during sleep in pregnancy indicated that the prevalence of snoring increased incrementally, from small increases during the first trimester to substantial increases during the last trimester. The reported prevalence of snoring as measured by questionnaire during pregnancy varied substantially and almost certainly depends to a large extent on the definition used: that is, whether the questionnaire specifies a minimum number of days per week that snoring is noticed (regularity or whether a certain level of snoring (intensity) is the target question.

Although the prevalence of habitual snoring in nonpregnant women reportedly ranges from 4% to 17% [34,38,39], the prevalence of snoring at least sometimes during pregnancy increases from 39% in the first trimester to 66% in the third trimester. The prevalence of women reporting "always snoring" increases from 7% in the first trimester of pregnancy to 13% in the third trimester. The prevalence of snoring "often or always" during the third trimester, as reported in the study by Izci and colleagues [34], was 41%, which decreased to 17% 3 months postpartum. In a Chinese population, the prevalence of snoring increased from 30% in the first trimester to 41% in the second trimester and to 46% in the third trimester [40]. The design of these studies seems to have had a substantial impact on the reported prevalence of snoring during pregnancy. For example, in two of the studies that specifically assessed self-reported snoring every night during pregnancy, the retrospective study found a prevalence of 7% [41], whereas a similar but prospective study found a prevalence of 3% [42].

Prevalence of sleep-disordered breathing in pregnancy

From these studies it is clear that snoring increases incrementally throughout pregnancy. Emerging evidence also suggests an increased incidence of OSA during pregnancy and exacerbation of pre-existing SDB, particularly during the later stages of pregnancy. In a study of a small cohort of women who presented with SDB during the last trimester of pregnancy, the authors [43] found a marked improvement in severity of apnea up to 3 months following parturition. Although 7 of these 10 women still had a degree of SDB according to standard criteria (AHI > 5), the disorder had resolved completely in 30% of them, with each having postnatal AHI of less than 5 events per hour (the mean antenatal AHI in these three women was substantial, at 21 events per hour). These data suggest that late pregnancy is associated with exacerbation of SDB and also suggest compellingly that in some women late pregnancy can be associated with development of the disorder.

Pregnancy itself seems to be associated with OSA, and the later stages of pregnancy are most closely linked with the development and/or precipitation of the disorder. The proposal that late pregnancy is associated with the development or precipitation of SDB was first suggested in 1989 [44] with a case report in which a 27-year-old primigravida first developed symptoms of loud snoring and excessive daytime sleepiness at 6 months' gestation and subsequently was diagnosed as having severe OSA.

A recent longitudinal questionnaire study of symptoms of SDB (as measured by the Multivariable Apnea Prediction Index) [42] found cumulative increases in apnea symptom score from 14 weeks until delivery. Although 1.3% of participants in this study reported witnessed apneas on at least 3 nights per week at 14 weeks' gestation, by 28 to 29 weeks' gestation this figure had increased to 15% of the cohort. As yet, there have been no studies of the prevalence of SDB in pregnancy using objective measures during sleep.

Obesity and sleep-disordered breathing in pregnancy

Because obesity is a key factor in the development of SDB, any evaluation of SDB must include a parallel examination of obesity. The prevalence of obesity in the general population has continued to increase during recent years, and this trend is reflected in the increasing prevalence of obesity during pregnancy. In a recently published large study of 66,221 women in the United States, the prevalence of pregravid obesity (defined as a BMI greater than 29 kg/m^2) increased from 13% immediately before pregnancy in 1993 to 22% immediately before pregnancy in 2002/2003 [45]. In a recent Australian study, the prevalence of overweight or obesity (with a BMI greater than 25 kg/m^2) was 34% [46].

The risks associated with obesity during pregnancy are numerous and include increased risk of pre-eclampsia, hypertension, and gestational diabetes [46,47], as well as increased complications during delivery, including increased cesarean section rate. Obesity is one of the strongest risk factors for the development of OSA in the nonpregnant population (reviewed in Ref. [48]), and some studies suggest that it may increase the risk for SDB during pregnancy [49]. The now well-established link between type II diabetes, the metabolic syndrome, and OSA leads to the question: how much does unrecognized SDB in pregnancy contribute to the SDB-related adverse outcomes such as hypertension and gestational diabetes?

Prevalence of sleep-disordered breathing in pre-eclampsia

Pre-eclampsia is a condition arising in pregnancy that is characterized by abrupt hypertension, hyperalbuminuria, and edema of the hands, feet, and face. Occurring in the third trimester, pre-eclampsia is the most common complication of pregnancy and affects about 7% of all pregnancies. There is accumulating evidence suggesting that pre-eclampsia is associated with an even higher risk of developing SDB than normal pregnancy or that SDB precipitates pre-eclampsia.

In the first published description of sleep in pre-eclampsia, Ekholm and colleagues [50] reported an increased level of movement during sleep in women who had pre-eclampsia compared with that in normal pregnancy. Although this study did not report on breathing, it is likely that the increased movement was associated at least in part with upper airway dysfunction during sleep. The authors of this article have studied a large number of women who had pre-eclampsia and found that SDB, in the form of either apneas and hypopneas [51] or partial upper airway flow limitation [52,53], occurs universally during sleep in these women. Similarly, other studies have confirmed the correlation between SDB and pre-eclampsia [41,54,55].

Maternal complications of sleep-disordered breathing in pregnancy

The increased prevalence of SDB, particularly during the latter stages of pregnancy, should alert clinicians to the potential impact that this disorder has on maternal, fetal, and neonatal outcomes. There is a clear interaction between many of the common disorders of pregnancy and SDB, including gestational diabetes mellitus, pre-eclampsia, hypertension, and fetal growth restriction. The now well-described acute hemodynamic oscillations, including repetitive episodes of hypotension and bradycardia followed by marked transient hypertension and tachycardia that are associated with obstructive apneic cycles in the both the male [56] and the nonpregnant female patient [17],

also occur in pregnancy but are exaggerated (Fig. 1) [51].

Vascular responses to sleep-disordered breathing in pregnancy

It now is recognized that sleep apnea induces marked changes in vascular responsiveness. The authors of this article were among the first to show that endothelial function is compromised in patients who have SDB in a study in which they demonstrated that the response to hypoxia changed from a normal vasodilator pattern (reflected in maintenance of arterial blood pressure despite increased cardiac output) to a potent pressor pattern in subjects who had documented SDB [57]. Subsequently it has been shown that subjects who have SDB have a specific abnormality of the endothelial vasodilator system [58,59]. Although the mechanism of endothelial dysfunction in SDB is not known currently, it probably is a combination of repetitive hypoxia [60,61], hypercapnia, and increases in circulating inflammatory mediators [62]. An important subsequent finding is that the impaired flow-mediated vascular relaxation (an endothelial-mediated event) is much greater in women than in men who have SDB of comparable severity [63], but the impact of the menstrual cycle on flow-mediated vascular responses was not investigated. The authors showed that the menstrual cycle had an important influence in determining vascular responses to apnea in 13 women who had SDB [17]. There was significant augmentation of pressor responses during the luteal phase compared with the follicular phase of the menstrual cycle, even though the luteal phase was associated with an improvement in apnea severity, particularly during REM sleep. Progesterone has been proposed as the candidate mediator of these effects. Similarly,

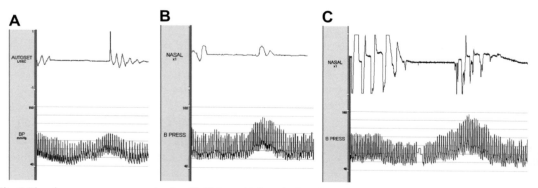

Fig. 1. Blood pressure responses (scale, 40–180 mm Hg) to similar obstructive respiratory events (*A*) in a nonpregnant patient, (*B*), in the same patient during pregnancy, and (*C*) in a patient who has pre-eclampsia, showing augmentation of the pressor response during pregnancy and even further exacerbation in pre-eclampsia. (*Data from* Edwards N, Blyton DM, Kirjavainen TT, et al. Hemodynamic responses to obstructive respiratory events during sleep are augmented in women with preeclampsia. Am J Hypertens 2001;14(11):1090–5.)

The authors examined the blood pressure response to individual apneic events in the last trimester of pregnancy and some months postpartum and showed that this response was potentiated in the last trimester of pregnancy (see Fig. 1) [51].

The sympathetic nervous system and sleep-disordered breathing in pregnancy

In considering the impact of SDB during pregnancy on cardiovascular health, the role of the autonomic nervous system, which plays an integral role in the response to OSA, is relevant. Although both acute (associated with apneic cycles during sleep) and chronic (persisting into the daytime) sympathetic hyperactivity are hallmarks of the autonomic nervous system response to OSA in the nonpregnant patient (reviewed in Ref. [64]), these changes have not been investigated during pregnancy. Pregnancy is associated with a biphasic change in relative autonomic balance, with increased parasympathetic tone and decreased sympathetic tone during the first trimester, parasympathetic/sympathetic balance similar to the nonpregnant state during the second trimester, and relative sympathetic hyperactivity during the third trimester [65]. Given the close association between SDB and sympathetic hyperactivity in the nonpregnant population, the presence of SDB during the third trimester of pregnancy probably further exacerbates the pre-existing sympathetic hyperactivity and is particularly relevant in women who have pre-eclampsia.

Pre-eclampsia is associated with widespread endothelial dysfunction, which has the effect of increasing the hypertensive response to pressor-inducing stimuli, first described in response to angiotensin [66] and now recognized to include a number of other pressor-inducing stimuli, including sympathetic mediators [67]. In pre-eclamptic women who have coexisting SDB (as discussed later), the increased sympathetic hyperactivity is almost certainly associated with significant exacerbation of hypertension. Pressor responses to obstructive respiratory events during sleep are enhanced significantly in women who have pre-eclampsia [51].

Gestational hypertension and sleep-disordered breathing

Given the augmentation of vascular responses and sympathetic hyperactivity in response to SDB in pregnancy, chronic maternal blood pressure control is almost certainly compromised significantly. One study that overwhelmingly demonstrated the link between OSA and the development of hypertension is the Sleep Heart Health study, a prospective study that has shown that sleep apnea at baseline predicts the onset of systemic hypertension, independently

of confounding factors [68]. Although hypertension was described in many of the early studies of sleep apnea, and a causal link was suggested when marked reductions in blood pressure followed treatment of sleep apnea with tracheostomy [69], it has taken a long time for a definitive link to be established. A major reason for this delay has been the confounding of data by the presence of obesity. This confounding is no longer an issue, because sleep apnea has been shown to cause hypertension independently of obesity, and indeed, it is likely that sleep apnea contributes to the link between obesity and hypertension [70]. Recent data indicate that sleep apnea is a very common finding in patients who have difficult-to-control hypertension and that the use of CPAP to control the sleep apnea leads to marked improvement in blood pressure control [71].

Available evidence is persuasive for a strong link between SDB and hypertension in pregnancy. The first case description in which SDB was associated with hypertension in pregnancy was in 1996 with the report of a pre-eclamptic patient also presenting with SDB [72]. In the first epidemiologic description suggesting a link between hypertension and SDB, the prevalence of hypertension was significantly higher in women who reported snoring (retrospectively) during their pregnancy [41].

Compellingly, a recent retrospective questionnaire study of SDB in pregnancy showed that the adjusted odds ratio of hypertensive disease in pregnancy in women who reported witnessed apnea during their pregnancy (arguably the strongest evidence for SDB in this population) was 8.0 [54]. These data are supported by other recent preliminary data from a case-controlled study showing that the adjusted odds ratio of having SDB is 7.5 in a population of women who had gestational hypertension [73].

Sleep-disordered breathing and pre-eclampsia: the ischemic placenta

Although there is a causal link between SDB in pregnancy and the development of gestational hypertension, the link with pre-eclampsia is less clear. Pre-eclampsia is a disease in which hypertension is accompanied by renal, hepatic, and hematologic compromise. As already reviewed, the prevalence of SDB in pre-eclampsia is remarkably high, but this prevalence does not necessarily indicate that SDB is causal in the pathogenesis of pre-eclampsia. Indeed, it is more likely that there are a series of interactions between the two diseases, with neither being clearly causal in the development of the other.

Incompatibility of maternal versus paternal genetic material is a current favored hypothesis [74], and an ischemic placenta seems to be at the center of the pathophysiology. Partial maternal rejection of the implanting placenta and growing fetus sets up a cascade of events that eventually lead to the pathologic and clinical findings of the disease. Although clinical signs of the disease do not become evident until after the twentieth week of gestation, the primary pathologic mechanism occurs early in the first trimester of pregnancy, with failure of normal placental implantation resulting from shallow trophoblastic invasion into the maternal spiral arteries [75]. There is consequent failure of the normal remodeling of the spiral arteries of the uterus into low-resistance, high-flow vessels; instead, these vessels maintain low-flow, high-resistance properties that are characteristic of the nonpregnant state, thereby inducing a state of uteroplacental hypoperfusion with compromised blood flow to the placenta and developing fetus. As fetal growth continues and the demands on the placental unit increase, the placental ischemic/hypoxic injury accelerates and leads to localized production of inflammatory mediators and cytokines, which spill over into the maternal circulation and produce widespread maternal endothelial damage [76]. The maternal blood vessels become leaky, and there is widespread edema, renal damage, proteinuria, and a sustained increase in peripheral vascular resistance. The normal operation of vascular endothelium in maintaining relaxed resistance blood vessels is damaged, and specifically, nitric oxide production, the major local vascular dilator, is abnormally reduced.

Pre-eclampsia, sleep-disordered breathing, and hemodynamic control

It has been known for some time that women who have pre-eclampsia lose the normal diurnal blood pressure pattern and the normal nocturnal dip in blood pressure [77]. The development of SDB in pre-eclampsia associated with upper airway changes serves to exacerbate the clinical condition further, with increasing nocturnal hypertension and increased release of inflammatory mediators that are associated with the pathophysiology of SDB [78]. Of particular importance in the development of SDB is the reduced internal luminal diameter of the upper airway [32,34]. The reduction in upper airway size is almost certainly a consequence of the widespread peripheral edema that occurs in pre-eclampsia. Fluid shift associated with the supine position may be an important additional factor. A recent physiologic study of tissue fluid shift demonstrated a change in upper airway resistance associated with lower-body positive pressure [79], demonstrating how fluid shift can have a significant impact on the upper airway caliber. The causal association between SDB, hypertension, and other clinical factors associated with pre-eclampsia has been demonstrated with the use of nocturnal nasal CPAP, which reversed upper airway dysfunction during sleep in pre-eclampsia [53]. In this study, nocturnal blood pressure increments were minimized successfully by the application of CPAP, and there also was an improvement in peripheral edema and a significant reduction in serum uric acid concentration, an important index of the severity of pre-eclampsia [80].

It is important to emphasize that the patients the authors [53] studied did not have frank obstructive apnea nor significant nocturnal desaturation, but flow limitation with minor increments in end tidal CO_2 concentrations increasing in the order of 4 to 6 Torr (as would be expected with prolonged partial upper airway obstruction). Thus, the effector mechanism of the worsening hypertension in sleep in these women could not have been simply the occurrence of repetitive apnea and hypoxia but rather was the setting of the vascular system. In pre-eclampsia, the peripheral resistance vessels do not have the normal vasodilator mechanisms and are highly responsive, so that any further pressor stimulus (such as a hypercapnia-induced, brainstem-mediated increase in peripheral sympathetic tone) is likely to have a very large effect. Emerging data suggest a similar level of endothelial dysfunction in nonpregnant patients who have OSA [81].

The link between endothelial dysfunction and hypertension in SDB undoubtedly involves the production of inflammatory mediators, including cytokines (Fig. 2). Sleep apnea has been shown to induce an inflammatory state [78], and it is likely that a range of inflammatory mediators are involved. One important mediator, tumor necrosis factor-alpha (TNF-α), may be a candidate for some of these effects. This cytokine has been shown to have an independent link to hypertension and pre-eclampsia [82] and to be elevated in sleep apnea. In pre-eclampsia, the release of TNF-α almost certainly is linked to placental ischemia, and in an animal model of placental ischemia, TNF-α release has been shown to mediate systemic hypertension [83].

Pregnancy in its own right markedly increases the pressor response to apnea. With SDB-induced changes in circulating cytokines and inflammatory mediators and with altered endothelial function, it is clear that the circulatory responses are potentially critical in pregnancy. These findings underscore the concept that the pressor response to SDB is the important determinant of changes in vascular function.

A

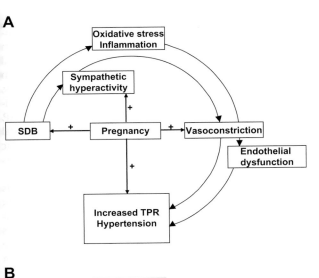

B

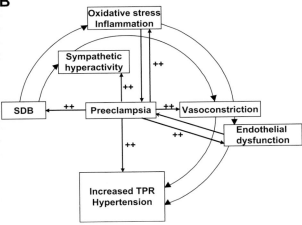

Fig. 2. The interactions between sleep-disordered breathing (SDB) and hypertension (*A*) in normal pregnancy and (*B*) in pre-eclamptic pregnancy. Although a normal third-trimester pregnancy is associated with increased sympathetic activity, increased vasoconstrictor response, and increased hypertensive response to obstructive respiratory events during sleep, these responses are increased significantly in pre-eclampsia. Furthermore, endothelial dysfunction and inflammatory responses that occur in SDB interact synergistically with the pre-eclamptic disease process, which itself is primarily a disease of endothelial dysfunction and inflammation produced by placental ischemia. TPR, total peripheral resistance.

Sleep-induced hemodynamics in pre-eclampsia

Other findings from the authors' studies of sleep in pre-eclampsia relate to maternal cardiovascular and hemodynamic control and are relevant to disease progression and maternal and fetal outcomes. The hemodynamic profile in women who have pre-eclampsia includes intravascular volume depletion, increased peripheral vascular resistance, and reduced cardiac output [84]. In a polysomnographic study of 24 women who had pre-eclampsia and 15 normal pregnant women, the authors demonstrated that sleep is associated with exacerbation of adverse hemodynamics. A marked increase in systemic vascular resistance and suppression of maternal cardiac output probably contributed to further placental ischemia in pre-eclampsia [85]. These adverse changes were alleviated with the use of nocturnal nasal CPAP treatment. The mechanism of changes in systemic vascular resistance and cardiac output probably is related to the previously described small increments in arterial CO_2 resulting from SDB and leading to brainstem-mediated increases in peripheral noradrenergic tone. The resultant increase in peripheral vascular tone thereby increases cardiac afterload, which in turn reduces cardiac output. Reversal of sleep-induced upper airway obstruction minimizes mild hypercapnia, thereby improving the hemodynamic profile.

A further pathophysiologic role of upper airway obstruction that may be associated with an adverse impact on the maternal hemodynamic profile is the impact on atrial natriuretic peptide (ANP). From early studies it became clear that pre-eclampsia is associated with significant intravascular volume contraction and that this volume contraction is associated with restricted fetal growth and poorer fetal outcomes [84]. Studies in male apneic subjects showed that increasingly negative intrathoracic pressures are associated with increased release of

ANP [86]. As a potent diuretic hormone, ANP may contribute substantially to intravascular depletion in women who have pre-eclampsia and SDB. Studies have demonstrated elevated blood levels of ANP in women who have pre-eclampsia [87]. Partial upper airway obstruction (eg, as occurs in high upper airways resistance syndrome) is characterized by long periods of sleep during which there are continuous strong inspiratory efforts against a partially occluded upper airway. Each inspiratory effort is associated with increasingly negative intrathoracic pressures. This prolonged stimulation of the atria and atrial dilatation may lead to even greater release of ANP than in the "traditional" apneic patient who has intermittent obstruction followed by arousal. Such an increase in ANP could lead to reduced intravascular volume and reduced cardiac preload.

Thus, by reversing some of the factors involved of the cascade of events, specifically those associated with SDB, nasal CPAP treatment can directly impact many of the wide array of clinical and pathologic features of the disease.

Gestational diabetes and sleep-disordered breathing

Another important outcome of SDB in pregnancy may be the development of gestational diabetes mellitus. Although there currently is no evidence to link SDB in pregnancy to the development of gestational diabetes, there is a link between SDB and both hyperinsulinemia and type II diabetes mellitus (reviewed in Ref. [88]), independent of other risk factors, including obesity and hypercholesterolemia. Furthermore, studies in which blood glucose control is enhanced following successful treatment with nasal CPAP suggest a causal link [89]. Gestational diabetes mellitus and type II diabetes have similar origins; indeed, women who have gestational diabetes are known to be at a much greater risk of developing type II diabetes later in life [90–93]. Clearly, the pathophysiology of these two diseases is closely related. Given the clinical impact of gestational diabetes, it is imperative that this potential link between SDB and gestational diabetes mellitus be investigated.

Fetal effects of sleep-disordered breathing in pregnancy

Although sleep disorders in pregnancy clearly have important adverse maternal implications, the effects on the fetus have the potential to be much less transient and to have a greater impact on the long-term well-being of the neonate, child, and subsequent adult. A number of pathophysiologic outcomes that result from maternal SDB, including maternal hypoxemia, repetitive hypertensive peaks associated with maternal apneic cycles, reductions in maternal cardiac output, and increased maternal peripheral vascular resistance, have the potential to impact the well-being of the developing fetus both acutely and chronically. The first study showing the impact that SDB has on the developing fetus was published in 1978 [94], demonstrating that marked decelerations in fetal heart rate (an indication of fetal distress) and significant fetal acidosis (as indicated by a reduced pH in fetal scalp vein samples during maternal labor) were associated with episodes of maternal obstructive apnea during sleep. (Two of the participants in this study had been admitted for ruptured membranes, allowing the authors to access fetal scalp veins to sample fetal venous blood.) Since then, several studies have confirmed that maternal SDB has a marked impact on fetal outcome, leading to fetal growth restriction [41,94–97] and, in an extreme case, fetal death [96].

The authors recently have completed a series of studies investigating the impact of maternal SDB on the nocturnal fetal movement profile in both normal and pre-eclamptic pregnancy. In both instances, they found significant impairment in fetal movement indices. The number of fetal movements per hour of maternal non-REM sleep in women who had SDB was reduced to half that in non-REM sleep of women who had normal sleep breathing indices. Crucially, this effect was potentiated in maternal REM sleep in which the number of fetal movements per hour of maternal REM sleep was reduced by 65% in women who had SDB [98]. Furthermore, the normal variation in fetal movements also was compromised in pregnancy-complicated SDB, with the number of fetal movements per hour of maternal sleep decreasing throughout the maternal sleep period. This finding is in marked contrast to normal pregnancy, in which fetal movements increased throughout the maternal sleep period [98]. When SDB is reversed with the use of nocturnal nasal CPAP, the number of fetal movements per hour of sleep increased significantly (Fig. 3). The mechanism of reduced fetal movement in maternal SDB almost certainly is related to impaired maternal cardiac output and increased total peripheral vascular resistance, both leading to uteroplacental hypoperfusion and fetal hypoxemia. The placenta plays a critical role in maintaining normal fetal development, and it is evident that research directed at determining the effects of SDB on placental function is needed.

Maternal sleep-disordered breathing and fetal programming

Fetal and neonatal compromise is evident in pregnancy complicated by SDB, and the long-term

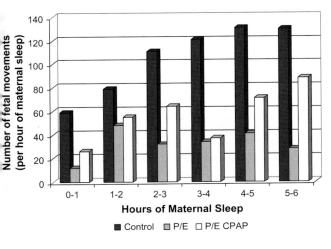

Fig. 3. The number of fetal movements per hour of maternal sleep in normal pregnancy (control, n = 10) and in pre-eclamptic pregnancy with SBD (n = 10), both before (P/E) and during treatment with nasal CPAP (P/E CPAP). The number of movements per hour of sleep was suppressed in pre-eclamptic patients. In contrast to the increase in the number of movements over the sleep period in normal pregnancy, there was a trend toward a reduction in the number of movements in pre-eclampsia. The absolute number of movements and the normal pattern were partially restored during maternal treatment with nasal CPAP. (*Data from* Edwards N, Blyton DM, Sullivan CE. Fetal movement is suppressed during maternal sleep in preeclampsia. Paper presented at the Associated Professional Sleep Societies. Minneapolis, MN, June 9–14, 2007.)

impact of this compromise must be considered. It is now recognized that fetal programming may have profound influences on adult disease. According to the Barker hypothesis, fetal growth restriction, particularly asymmetric growth restriction, indicative of impaired placental function, is associated with a significantly increased risk of adult cardiovascular disease [99]. In a recent study from Norway, women who themselves were small for gestational age at birth (less than the fifth percentile) were two to three times more likely than women who were in the twenty-fifth to seventy-fifth percentile for birth weight to develop hypertension during pregnancy [100]. One intriguing possibility is that reduced fetal movements [98], and specifically reduced respiratory movements in the fetal upper airway, may lead to the development of a relatively small upper airway, thereby "programming" the fetus for the development of SDB in later life. Thus, it is imperative that SDB duringpregnancy be recognized early and treated promptly to ensure normal fetal growth and development.

Treatment of sleep-disordered breathing in pregnancy

Relatively few studies have described the treatment of SDB during pregnancy. One study described the use of tracheostomy, which resolved the SDB [101]. Nasal CPAP has been found to provide a safe and effective means of treating maternal SDB until delivery [80,91]. An important consideration regarding the use of nasal CPAP is the impact on maternal cardiac output. Results from the authors' studies suggest that cardiac output is increased during nasal CPAP treatment in pre-eclamptic pregnancy associated with SDB [85]; the

mechanism almost certainly is reduced total peripheral resistance leading to reduced afterload. In the authors' studies of nasal CPAP treatment in non–pre-eclamptic pregnancy, cardiac output remained normal during treatment. A recent study in which SDB in hypertensive pregnancy was treated with nasal CPAP early in pregnancy showed a beneficial effect on both blood pressure and pregnancy outcomes [102].

Although there is clear evidence that there is a beneficial effect of treating pre-eclampsia once it has developed [53], the evidence regarding initiating treatment before development of pre-eclampsia is less clear. Guilleminault and colleagues [103] treated 12 women who had risk factors for the development of pre-eclampsia and flow limitation during sleep and showed that introducing nasal CPAP treatment early had no beneficial effect.

No studies have investigated other treatment modalities. Although in the general population weight loss often is a very effective treatment option [104], it is less of an option for this population. There has been no investigation of the efficacy of mandibular advancement splints in treating SDB in pregnancy; however, this area would need to be approached with caution because of the musculoskeletal changes (including ligament laxity) that are associated with pregnancy.

Identifying the pregnant patient who has obstructive sleep apnea

In women, presenting symptoms of OSA may include insomnia and depression [7], and because both daytime fatigue and excessive daytime sleepiness are highly prevalent in pregnancy [42], suspicion for OSA should be high when there are reports of snoring, especially in the presence of hypertension.

Both maternal prepregnancy BMI and neck circumference are strong indicators that should alert clinicians to the possibility of the presence of SDB during pregnancy. Oral examination and the Mallampati score also may be clinically useful. Of the few studies that have investigated clinical features that are suggestive of SDB, there seems to be some association with neck circumference [34], although BMI does seem to be somewhat predictive of SDB in pregnancy [49].

Summary

SDB seems to be prevalent in pregnancy, in contrast to traditional dogma that pregnancy is protective against developing SDB. The strong link between SDB and adverse outcomes in men and nonpregnant women seems to be even stronger in pregnancy, particularly for hypertension. Adverse outcomes not only affect the mother but also have a marked impact on fetal well-being, with the potential to increase the risk of lifelong cardiovascular and metabolic morbidities. In this group, treatment of SDB with nasal CPAP is associated with clear improvement in both maternal and fetal well-being and should be implemented immediately to maximize maternal, fetal, and neonatal well-being.

References

[1] Vickers MH, Breier BH, Cutfield WS, et al. Fetal origins of hyperphagia, obesity, and hypertension and postnatal amplification by hypercaloric nutrition. Am J Physiol Endocrinol Metab 2000; 279(1):E83–7.

[2] Oken E, Gillman MW. Fetal origins of obesity. Obes Res 2003;11(4):496–506.

[3] Ismail-Beigi F, Catalano PM, Hanson RW. Metabolic programming: fetal origins of obesity and metabolic syndrome in the adult. Am J Physiol Endocrinol Metab 2006;291(3):E439–40.

[4] Drager LF, Pereira AC, Barreto-Filho JA, et al. Phenotypic characteristics associated with hypertension in patients with obstructive sleep apnea. J Hum Hypertens 2006;20(7):523–8.

[5] Mooe T, Franklin KA, Holmstrom K, et al. Sleep-disordered breathing and coronary artery disease: long-term prognosis. Am J Respir Crit Care Med 2001;164(10 Pt 1):1910–3.

[6] Lugaresi E, Cirignotta F, Coccagna G, et al. Some epidemiological data on snoring and cardiocirculatory disturbances. Sleep 1980;3(3–4):221–4.

[7] Shepertycky MR, Banno K, Kryger MH. Differences between men and women in the clinical presentation of patients diagnosed with obstructive sleep apnea syndrome. Sleep 2005; 28(3):309–14.

[8] Guilleminault C, Stoohs R, Clerk A, et al. A cause of excessive daytime sleepiness. The upper airway resistance syndrome. Chest 1993;104(3) 781–7.

[9] Bearpark H, Elliott L, Grunstein R, et al. Occurrence and correlates of sleep disordered breathing in the Australian town of Busselton a preliminary analysis. Sleep 1993;16(Suppl 8) S3–5.

[10] Young T, Palta M, Dempsey J, et al. The occurrence of sleep-disordered breathing among middle-aged adults. N Engl J Med 1993 328(17):1230–5.

[11] Bixler EO, Vgontzas AN, Lin HM, et al. Prevalence of sleep-disordered breathing in women effects of gender. Am J Respir Crit Care Med 2001;163(3 Pt 1):608–13.

[12] Richman RM, Elliott LM, Burns CM, et al. The prevalence of obstructive sleep apnoea in an obese female population. Int J Obes Rela Metab Disord 1994;18(3):173–7.

[13] Dempsey J, Olson EB, Skatrud J. In: Hormone and neurochemicals in the regulation of breathing. vol. 2. Washington, DC: American Physiological Society; 1986.

[14] Bayliss DA, Millhorn DE. Central neural mechanisms of progesterone action: application to the respiratory system [review]. J Appl Physiol 1992;73(2):393–404.

[15] Feinsilver SH, Hertz G. Respiration during sleep in pregnancy [review]. Clin Chest Med 1992 13:637–44.

[16] Brownell LG, West P, Kryger MH. Breathing during sleep in normal pregnant women. Am Rev Respir Dis 1986;133(1):38–41.

[17] Edwards N, Wilcox I, Sullivan C. Haemodynamic responses to obstructive sleep apnoea in premenopausal women. J Hypertens 1999 17(5):603–10.

[18] Driver HS, McLean H, Kumar DV, et al. The influence of the menstrual cycle on upper airway resistance and breathing during sleep. Sleep 2005;28(4):449–56.

[19] Skatrud JB, Dempsey JA. Interaction of sleep state and chemical stimuli in sustaining rhythmic ventilation. J Appl Physiol 1983;55:813–22.

[20] Popovic RM, White DP. Upper airway muscle activity in normal women: influence of hormonal status. J Appl Physiol 1998;84(3) 1055–62.

[21] Jordan AS, Catcheside PG, O'Donoghue FJ, et al. Long-term facilitation of ventilation is not present during wakefulness in healthy men or women. J Appl Physiol 2002;93(6):2129–36.

[22] Bayliss DA, Millhorn DE, Gallman EA, et al. Progesterone stimulates respiration through a central nervous system steroid receptor mediated mechanism in cat. Proc Natl Acad Sci U S A 1987;84(21):7788–92.

[23] Stachenfeld NS, Taylor HS. Effects of estrogen and progesterone administration on extracellular fluid. J Appl Physiol 2004;96(3):1011–8.

[24] Mabry RL. Rhinitis of pregnancy. South Med J 1986;79:965–71.

[25] Hisaw F. Experimental relaxation of the pubic ligament of the guinea pig. Proc Soc Exp Biol Med 1926;23:661–3.

[26] Sherwood OD. Relaxin's physiological roles and other diverse actions. Endocr Rev 2004; 25(2):205–34.

[27] Craig DB, Toole MA. Airway closure in pregnancy. Can Aneasth Soc J 1975;22(6):665–72.

[28] Series F, Cormier Y, Desmeules M. Influence of passive changes of lung volume on upper airways. J Appl Physiol 1990;68(5):2159–64.

[29] Mallampati SR, Gatt SP, Gugino LD, et al. A clinical sign to predict difficult tracheal intubation: a prospective study. Can Anaesth Soc J 1985;32(4):429–34.

[30] Friedman M, Tanyeri H, La Rosa M, et al. Clinical predictors of obstructive sleep apnea. Laryngoscope 1999;109(12):1901–7.

[31] Pilkington S, Carli F, Dakin MJ, et al. Increase in Mallampati score during pregnancy. Br J Anaesth 1995;74(6):638–42.

[32] Izci B, Riha RL, Martin SE, et al. The upper airway in pregnancy and pre-eclampsia. Am J Respir Crit Care Med 2003;167(2):137–40.

[33] Davey DA, MacGillivray I. The classification and definition of the hypertensive disorders of pregnancy. Am J Obstet Gynecol 1988;158(4):892–8.

[34] Izci B, Vennelle M, Liston WA, et al. Sleep-disordered breathing and upper airway size in pregnancy and post-partum. Eur Respir J 2006; 27(2):321–7.

[35] Bradley TD, Brown IG, Grossman RF, et al. Pharyngeal size in snorers, nonsnorers, and patients with obstructive sleep apnea. N Engl J Med 1986;315(21):1327–31.

[36] Martin SE, Marshall I, Douglas NJ. The effect of posture on airway caliber with the sleep-apnea/hypopnea syndrome. Am J Respir Crit Care Med 1995;152(2):721–4.

[37] Hoffstein V, Zamel N, Phillipson EA. Lung volume dependence of pharyngeal cross-sectional area in patients with obstructive sleep apnea. Am Rev Respir Dis 1984;130(2):175–8.

[38] Loube DI, Poceta JS, Morales MC, et al. Self-reported snoring in pregnancy. Association with fetal outcome. Chest 1996;109(4):885–9.

[39] Guilleminault C, Querra-Salva M, Chowdhuri S, et al. Normal pregnancy, daytime sleeping, snoring and blood pressure. Sleep Med 2000;1(4):289–97.

[40] Leung PL, Hui DS, Leung TN, et al. Sleep disturbances in Chinese pregnant women. BJOG 2005;112(11):1568–71.

[41] Franklin KA, Holmgren PA, Jonsson F, et al. Snoring, pregnancy-induced hypertension, and growth retardation of the fetus. Chest 2000; 117(1):137–41.

[42] Pien GW, Fife D, Pack AI, et al. Changes in symptoms of sleep-disordered breathing during pregnancy. Sleep 2005;28(10):1299–305.

[43] Edwards N, Blyton DM, Hennessy A, et al. Severity of sleep-disordered breathing improves following parturition. Sleep 2005;28(6):737–41.

[44] Kowall J, Clark G, Nino Murcia G, et al. Precipitation of obstructive sleep apnea during pregnancy. Obstet Gynecol 1989;74:453–5.

[45] Kim SY, Dietz PM, England L, et al. Trends in pre-pregnancy obesity in nine states, 1993–2003. Obesity (Silver Spring) 2007;15(4): 986–93.

[46] Callaway LK, Prins JB, Chang AM, et al. The prevalence and impact of overweight and obesity in an Australian obstetric population. Med J Aust 2006;184(2):56–9.

[47] Catalano PM. Management of obesity in pregnancy. Obstet Gynecol 2007;109(2 Pt 1): 419–33.

[48] Strobel RJ, Rosen RC. Obesity and weight loss in obstructive sleep apnea: a critical review. Sleep 1996;19(2):104–15.

[49] Maasilta P, Bachour A, Terama K, et al. Sleep-related disordered breathing during pregnancy in obese women. Chest 2001;120(5):1448–54.

[50] Ekholm EM, Polo OJ, Rauhala ER, et al. Sleep quality in pre-eclampsia. Am J Obstet Gynecol 1992;167:1262–6.

[51] Edwards N, Blyton DM, Kirjavainen TT, et al. Hemodynamic responses to obstructive respiratory events during sleep are augmented in women with preeclampsia. Am J Hypertens 2001;14(11):1090–5.

[52] Edwards N, Blyton DM, Kesby GJ, et al. Preeclampsia is associated with marked alterations in sleep architecture. Sleep 2000;23(5):619–25.

[53] Edwards N, Blyton DM, Kirjavainen T, et al. Nasal continuous positive airway pressure reduces sleep-induced blood pressure increments in preeclampsia. Am J Respir Crit Care Med 2000;162:252–7.

[54] Perez-Chada D, Videla AJ, O'Flaherty ME, et al. Snoring, witnessed sleep apnoeas and pregnancy-induced hypertension. Acta Obstet Gynecol Scand 2007;86(7):788–92.

[55] Connolly G, Razak AR, Hayanga A, et al. Inspiratory flow limitation during sleep in preeclampsia: comparison with normal pregnant and nonpregnant women. Eur Respir J 2001; 18(4):672–6.

[56] Coccagna G, Mantovani M, Brignani F, et al. Continuous recording of the pulmonary and systemic arterial pressure during sleep in syndromes of hypersomnia with periodic breathing. Bull Physiopathol Respir (Nancy) 1972; 8(5):1159–72.

[57] Hedner JA, Wilcox I, Laks L, et al. A specific and potent pressor effect of hypoxia in patients with sleep apnea. Am Rev Respir Dis 1992; 146(5 Pt 1):1240–5.

[58] Carlson JT, Rangemark C, Hedner JA. Attenuated endothelium-dependent vascular relaxation in patients with sleep apnoea. J Hypertens 1996; 14(5):577–84.

[59] Kato M, Roberts-Thomson P, Phillips BG, et al. Impairment of endothelium-dependent vasodilation of resistance vessels in patients with obstructive sleep apnea. Circulation 2000;102: 2607–10.

[60] Chung S, Yoon IY, Shin YK, et al. Endothelial dysfunction and C-reactive protein in relation with the severity of obstructive sleep apnea syndrome. Sleep 2007;30(8):997–1001.

[61] Kraiczi H, Caidahl K, Samuelsson A, et al. Impairment of vascular endothelial function and left ventricular filling: association with the severity of apnea-induced hypoxemia during sleep. Chest 2001;119(4):1085–91.

[62] Nacher M, Serrano-Mollar A, Farre R, et al. Recurrent obstructive apneas trigger early systemic inflammation in a rat model of sleep apnea. Respir Physiol Neurobiol 2007;155(1):93–6.

[63] Faulx MD, Larkin EK, Hoit BD, et al. Sex influences endothelial function in sleep-disordered breathing. Sleep 2004;27(6):1113–20.

[64] Narkiewicz K, Somers VK. Sympathetic nerve activity in obstructive sleep apnoea. Acta Physiol Scand 2003;177(3):385–90.

[65] Kuo CD, Chen GY, Yang MJ, et al. Biphasic changes in autonomic nervous activity during pregnancy. Br J Anaesth 2000;84(3):323–9.

[66] Gant NF, Daley GL, Chand S, et al. A study of angiotensin II pressor response throughout primigravid pregnancy. J Clin Invest 1973;52:2682–9.

[67] Lewinsky RM, Riskin-Mashiah S. Autonomic imbalance in preeclampsia: evidence for increased sympathetic tone in response to the supine-pressor test. Obstet Gynecol 1998;91(6):935–9.

[68] Peppard PE, Young TB, Palta M, et al. Prospective study of the association between sleep-disordered breathing and hypertension. N Engl J Med 2000;342(19):1378–84.

[69] Motta J, Guilleminault C, Schroeder JS, et al. Tracheostomy and hemodynamic changes in sleep-inducing apnea. Ann Intern Med 1978; 89(4):454–8.

[70] Wolk R, Shamsuzzaman AS, Somers VK. Obesity, sleep apnea, and hypertension. Hypertension 2003;42(6):1067–74.

[71] Lavie P, Hoffstein V. Sleep apnea syndrome: a possible contributing factor to resistant hypertension. Sleep 2001;24(6):721–5.

[72] Lefcourt LA, Rodis JF. Obstructive sleep apnea in pregnancy. Obstet Gynecol Surv 1996; 51(8):503–6.

[73] Champagne K, Schwartzman K, Morin L, et al. Association between obstructive sleep apnea and gestational hypertension. Proc Am Thorac Soc 2006;3:A515.

[74] Lie RT, Rasmussen S, Brunborg H, et al. Fetal and maternal contributions to risk of preeclampsia: population based study. BMJ 1998; 316(7141):1343–7.

[75] Zhou Y, Damsky CH, Fisher SJ. Preeclampsia is associated with failure of human cytotrophoblasts to mimic a vascular adhesion phenotype. One cause of defective endovascular invasion in this syndrome? J Clin Invest 1997;99(9): 2152–64.

[76] Conrad KP, Benyo DF. Placental cytokines and the pathogenesis of preeclampsia. Am J Reprod Immunol 1997;37(3):240–9.

[77] Redman CW, Beilin LJ, Bonnar J. Reversed diurnal blood pressure rhythm in hypertensive pregnancies. Clin Sci (Lond) 1976;3(Suppl): 687s–9s.

[78] Lavie L. Obstructive sleep apnoea syndrome–an oxidative stress disorder. Sleep Med Rev 2003; 7(1):35–51.

[79] Chiu KL, Ryan CM, Shiota S, et al. Fluid shift by lower body positive pressure increases pharyngeal resistance in healthy subjects. Am J Respir Crit Care Med 2006;174(12):1378–83.

[80] Voto LS, Illia R, Darbon Grosso HA, et al. Uric acid levels: a useful index of the severity of preeclampsia and perinatal prognosis. J Perinat Med 1988;16(2):123–6.

[81] El Solh AA, Akinnusi ME, Baddoura FH, et al. Endothelial cell apoptosis in obstructive sleep apnea: a link to endothelial dysfunction. Am J Respir Crit Care Med 2007;175(11):1186–91.

[82] Serin IS, Ozcelik B, Basbug M, et al. Predictive value of tumor necrosis factor alpha (TNF-alpha) in preeclampsia. Eur J Obstet Gynecol Reprod Biol 2002;100(2):143–5.

[83] LaMarca BB, Cockrell K, Sullivan E, et al. Role of endothelin in mediating tumor necrosis factor-induced hypertension in pregnant rats. Hypertension 2005;46(1):82–6.

[84] Gallery ED, Hunyor SN, Gyory AZ. Plasma volume contraction: a significant factor in both pregnancy-associated hypertension (preeclampsia) and chronic hypertension in pregnancy. Q J Med 1979;48(192):593–602.

[85] Blyton DM, Sullivan CE, Edwards N. Reduced nocturnal cardiac output associated with preeclampsia is minimized with the use of nocturnal nasal CPAP. Sleep 2004;27(1):79–84.

[86] Krieger J, Laks L, Wilcox I, et al. Atrial natriuretic peptide release during sleep in patients with obstructive sleep apnoea before and during treatment with nasal continuous positive airway pressure. Clin Sci 1989;77(4):407–11.

[87] Irons DW, Baylis PH, Butler TJ, et al. Atrial natriuretic peptide in preeclampsia: metabolic clearance, sodium excretion and renal hemodynamics. Am J Physiol 1997;273(3 Pt 2):F483–7.

[88] Strohl KP. Diabetes and sleep apnea [review]. Sleep 1996;19(Suppl 10):225–8.

[89] Babu AR, Herdegen J, Fogelfeld L, et al. Type 2 diabetes, glycemic control, and continuous positive airway pressure in obstructive sleep apnea. Arch Intern Med 2005;165(4):447–52.

[90] Catalano PM, Kirwan JP, Haugel-de Mouzon S, et al. Gestational diabetes and insulin resistance: role in short- and long-term implications for mother and fetus. J Nutr 2003;133(5 Suppl 2): 1674S–83S.

[91] Herbison P, Wilson D. Implications of gestational diabetes for the future health of the mother. BJOG 1995;102(5):427–8.

[92] Dornhorst A. Implications of gestational diabetes for the health of the mother. BJOG 1994; 101(4):286–90.

[93] Henry OA, Beischer NA. Long-term implications of gestational diabetes for the mother. Baillieres Clin Obstet Gynaecol 1991;5(2):461–83.

[94] Joel-Cohen SJ, Schoenfeld A. Fetal response to periodic sleep apnea: a new syndrome in obstetrics. Eur J Obstet Gynecol Reprod Biol 1978;8(2):77–81.

[95] Charbonneau M, Falcone T, Cosio MG, et al. Obstructive sleep apnea during pregnancy. Therapy and implications for fetal health. Am Rev Respir Dis 1991;144:461–3.

[96] Brain KA, Thornton JG, Sarkar A, et al. Obstructive sleep apnoea and fetal death: successful treatment with continuous positive airway pressure. BJOG 2001;108(5):543–4.

[97] Schoenfeld A, Ovadia Y, Neri A, et al. Obstructive sleep apnea (OSA)-implications in maternal-fetal medicine. A hypothesis. Med Hypotheses 1989;30(1):51–4.

[98] Edwards N, Blyton DM, Sullivan CE. Fetal movement is suppressed during maternal sleep in preeclampsia. Paper presented at the Associated Professional Sleep Societies. Minneapolis, MN, June 9–14, 2007.

[99] Barker DJ. The fetal and infant origins of adult disease. BMJ 1990;301(6761):1111.

[100] Rasmussen S, Irgens LM. Pregnancy-induced hypertension in women who were born small. Hypertension 2007;49(4):806–12.

[101] Hastie SJ, Prowse K, Perks WH, et al. Obstructive sleep apnoea during pregnancy requiring tracheostomy. Aust N Z J Obstet Gynaecol 1989;29(3 Pt 2):365–7.

[102] Poyares D, Guilleminault C, Hachul H, et al. Pre-eclampsia and nasal CPAP. Part II: hypertension during pregnancy, chronic snoring, and early nasal CPAP intervention. Sleep Med 2008;9:15–24.

[103] Guilleminault C, Palombini L, Poyares D, et al. Pre-eclampsia and nasal CPAP. Part I: early intervention with nasal CPAP in pregnant women with risk-factors for pre-eclampsia: preliminary findings. Sleep Med, in press.

[104] Peppard PE, Young TB, Palta M, et al. Longitudinal study of moderate weight change and sleep-disordered breathing. JAMA 2000; 284(23):3015–21.

SLEEP
MEDICINE
CLINICS

Sleep Med Clin 3 (2008) 97–107

ELSEVIER
SAUNDERS

Socio-Cultural Considerations and Sleep Practices in the Pediatric Population

Judith A. Owens, MD, MPH[a,b,*]

Culture is the entire non-biological inheritance of human beings. Everything *that is socially developed and learned is a part of culture* [1].

Sleep behaviors and sleep practices in infants and children can serve as a reflection of cultural differences in human behavior in general and in parenting practices, beliefs, and values, in particular. Many of the host of variables that affect sleep patterns, habits, and even the definition of sleep problems within individual family units are highly culturally based. Sleep-related behaviors are ultimately the result of a complex amalgam of biologic, psychologic, developmental, environmental, and social influences, the relative contributions of which often vary across cultures. Although biologic determinants of sleep, including mechanisms of sleep regulation and chronobiologic (circadian) principles [2,3], form the universal infrastructure on which sleep behaviors are formed, the ways in which culture and biology interact play a major role in the establishment of sleep patterns and the development of sleep practices in a given cultural environment [4].

The evolution of sleep practices and behaviors across childhood is particularly sensitive to the important interplay between culture and the normal trajectory of child development. Culture and biology, as well as parental expectations regarding children's sleep, help define behavioral and developmental norms. Thus, both culture and biology must be considered in examining sleep behaviors and in defining what constitutes problematic sleep behavior. Furthermore, because sleep practices in

[a] Division of Pediatric Ambulatory Medicine, Rhode Island Hospital, Potter Bldg., Suite 200, 593 Eddy St., Providence, RI 02903, USA
[b] Warren Alpert School of Medicine at Brown University Box G, Providence, RI, USA
* Division of Pediatric Ambulatory Medicine, Rhode Island Hospital, Potter Bldg., Suite 200, 593 Eddy St., Providence, RI 02903.
E-mail address: owensleep@gmail.com

doi:10.1016/j.jsmc.2007.10.005

young children, in particular, are necessarily embedded in the socio-emotional context of the child–caregiver relationship, the influence of key developmental concepts such as attachment and temperament also must be considered within this same cultural perspective.

When seen through this cultural lens, it is clear that sleep, and its attendant spectrum of problems and behaviors, are grounded both in the physical, psychologic, and social microecology of human sleep (eg, sleeping arrangements, sleep space, bedding, and other factors) and in the macroecology that incorporates the structure and organization of daily life in different cultures (Fig. 1) [5]. It therefore would follow that, notwithstanding the basic and immutable biology of sleep architecture and regulation, there is unlikely to be one universally acceptable right way (or time or place) to sleep. How we sleep, where we sleep, and with whom and for how long we sleep are molded by culture and customs. Ultimately, cross-cultural comparisons of infant and childhood sleep practices across societies of different political, economic, ideological, and historical backgrounds are invaluable in providing the opportunity to understand better the ways in which adult sleep practices evolve. The following article attempts to illustrate how cultural variables impact the development of sleep patterns, behaviors, and problems in children by examining important cultural differences (and similarities) in a number of critical sleep behaviors, including co-sleeping/bed sharing, bedtime practices, napping, sleep needs, and lifestyle factors affecting sleep hygiene.

Ontogeny of sleep

To appreciate fully how culture influences the normal trajectory of sleep development in infants, children, and adolescents, some basic understanding of normal sleep behaviors and patterns in different age groups is extremely helpful. Although sleep in neonates and infants is quite different from that in adults, the structure of children's sleep and sleep-wake patterns begin to resemble that of adults as children mature [6]. In sleep architecture, there is a dramatic decrease in the proportion of both slow-wave and rapid-eye-movement sleep from birth through childhood to adulthood. In addition, several general trends in the maturation of sleep patterns over time may be identified. First, there is a decrease in the 24-hour average total sleep duration from infancy through adolescence, with a less marked and more gradual continued decrease in nocturnal sleep amounts into late adolescence [7]. This decline includes a decrease in nocturnal sleep throughout childhood as well as a significant decline in daytime sleep (scheduled napping) between 18 months and 5 years of age. There is also a gradual but marked circadian-mediated shift to a later bedtime and sleep-onset time that begins in middle childhood and accelerates in early to mid-adolescence. Finally, sleep/wake patterns on school nights and nonschool nights become

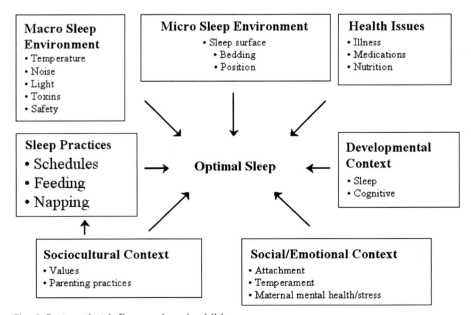

Fig. 1. Factors that influence sleep in children.

increasingly irregular from middle childhood through adolescence.

Infancy: sleep consolidation and regulation

In infancy, two important developmental sleep milestones normally are achieved during the first 9 months of life, both of which are highly influenced by homeostatic and circadian mechanisms and by the socio-cultural context in which they occur. These milestones are sleep consolidation and sleep regulation [8].

Sleep consolidation generally is described as an infant's ability to sleep for a continuous period of time that is concentrated during the nocturnal hours, augmented by shorter periods of daytime sleep (naps). Infants develop the ability to consolidate sleep between 6 weeks and 3 months, and approximately 70% to 80% of infants achieve sleep consolidation (ie, "sleeping through the night") by 9 months.

Sleep regulation refers to the infant's ability to control internal states of arousal both to fall asleep at bedtime without parental intervention or assistance and to fall back asleep following normal brief arousals during the night. The capacity to self-soothe begins to develop in the first 12 weeks of life and is a reflection of both neurodevelopmental maturation and learning. Not all cultures or families, however, share the developmental goal of independent self-soothing in infants at bedtime and after night wakings; voluntary or lifestyle bed and/or room sharing of infants and parents is a common and accepted practice in many cultures and ethnic groups.

Toddlers

During the toddler stage (12–36 months), both developmental and environmental issues begin to have more impact on sleep. Examples include an increase in separation anxiety, which may lead to bedtime resistance and problematic night wakings, the development of imagination, which may result in increased nighttime fears, increased understanding by toddlers of the symbolic meaning of objects, which can lead to increased interest in and reliance on transitional objects to allay normal developmental and separation fears, and an increased drive for autonomy and independence, which may result in increased bedtime resistance.

Preschool

In preschool-aged children, developmental and cultural issues that particularly affect sleep include expanded language and cognitive skills, which may lead to increased bedtime resistance. As children become more articulate about their needs, they may engage in more limit-testing behavior. A developing capacity to delay gratification and anticipate consequences enables preschoolers to respond to positive reinforcement for appropriate bedtime behavior, and increasing interest in developing literacy skills reinforces the importance of reading aloud at bedtime as an integral part of the bedtime routine. Bedtime routines and rituals, the use of transitional objects, and sleep/wake schedules are all important sleep-related issues at this developmental stage.

Most children give up napping by 5 years, although approximately 25% of children continue to nap at age 5 years, and, as discussed later, there is some evidence that napping patterns and the preservation of daytime sleep periods into later childhood may be influenced by cultural and ethnic differences [9].

Middle childhood

Middle childhood is a critical time for the development of healthy sleep habits. Increasing independence from parental supervision and a shift in responsibility for health habits as children approach adolescence may result in less enforcement of appropriate bedtimes and inadequate sleep duration. Parents also may be less aware of their children's sleep patterns and sleep problems, if problems do exist.

Adolescence

Finally, adolescence is a period of significant upheaval and change in sleep patterns and behaviors, including the biologically based alterations in circadian rhythm occurring in conjunction with the onset of puberty that result in a significant phase delay relative to the sleep-wake cycles of middle childhood [10,11]. This phase delay results in adolescents not feeling sleepy at their scheduled bedtimes.

Environmental factors and lifestyle/social demands, such as homework, activities, and after-school jobs, also have a significant impact on sleep amounts in adolescents, and the early starting times of many high schools may contribute to insufficient sleep. There also is significant weekday/weekend variability in sleep/wake patterns in adolescents, often accompanied by weekend oversleeping in an attempt to address the chronic sleep debt accumulated during the week. This oversleeping contributes further to circadian disruption and associated decreased levels of daytime alertness. Nonetheless, adolescents' sleep needs do not seem to differ dramatically from the sleep needs of preadolescents, and optimal sleep amounts remain at about 9 to 9.25 hours per night.

Sleep problems in childhood: cross-cultural perspectives

A number of important culturally determined child, parental, and environmental variables affect the type, relative prevalence, chronicity, and severity of sleep problems in childhood. Child-related factors that may affect children's sleep significantly include temperament and behavioral style [12], individual variations in circadian preference, cognitive and language delays [13], and the presence of comorbid medical and psychiatric conditions [14,15]. Parental factors include parenting and discipline styles, parents' education level and knowledge of child development, mental health issues such as maternal depression [16], family stress [17], and the quality and quantity of parents' sleep [18]. Environmental factors include the physical environment [19] (space, noise, perceived environmental threats to safety, room and bed sharing), family composition (number, ages, and health status of siblings and extended family members), and lifestyle issues (parental work status, competing priorities for time).

Despite these obvious cross-cultural differences, sleep problems in childhood are both common and universal. The prevalence of sleep problems in childhood reported in studies from diverse cultures is remarkably similar and consistent, with an overall prevalence of 25%. For example, international studies have shown that 23.5% of children aged 2 to 6 years in Beijing, China had sleep problems reported by parents, and 20% of Swiss 3-year-olds awaken every night. Community- and school-based studies conducted in Europe, Asia, and America suggest that a similar percentage of adolescents across cultures report difficulties in one or more of the following behavioral dimensions of sleep quality: going to bed [20,21], falling asleep [22–24], maintaining undisturbed sleep [25], reinitiating sleep after nocturnal awakenings [24], and returning to wakefulness in the morning [23]. In other studies, however, the prevalence of sleep problems varies more widely. For example, according to a recent international study published by the US Department of Health and Human Services, a greater percentage of 15-year-olds in the United States (40%) were likely to report feeling tired in the morning compared with students in other countries (less than 15% in the lowest ranked countries) [26]. A common disorder in adolescence, delayed sleep phase syndrome, in which circadian rhythms for sleep onset and offset are substantially later than the normal bedtime, also seems to vary in prevalence across populations [27].

These discrepancies in the scope and frequency of childhood sleep problems may result from actual differences across cultures, but they also may reflect differences in methodology and measurement of sleep problems across studies, making it difficult to compare results reliably. Furthermore, not only is the range of sleep behaviors that may be considered normal or pathologic wide, but the very

definition of what constitutes a problem often is quite subjective and highly dependent on culturally determined factors. These factors include parental awareness of, expectations for, and tolerance of sleep behaviors. For example, culturally based interpretations of the cause, meaning, and significance of parasomnias such as nightmares, night terrors, sleep walking, and sleep talking affect the parental interpretation of these sleep-related phenomena. Definitions of sleep problems also may be influenced by the perceived societal impact of sleep problems and insufficient sleep time on children's health, behavior, learning, and general well being. In addition, other cultural determinants not directly related to sleep, such as gender role expectations and work ethic, may play a role in defining acceptable sleep/wake behaviors.

Vulnerable populations, such as children who are at high risk for developmental and behavioral problems because of poverty, parental substance abuse and mental illness, or violence in the home, may be even more likely to experience double jeopardy as a result of sleep problems. In other words, these children are at higher risk for developing sleep problems as a result of such conditions as chaotic home environments, chronic medical issues, and neglect and also are less likely to be diagnosed as having sleep problems because of limited access to health care services. Finally, they are less likely to receive adequate treatment and are more likely to suffer serious consequences from those sleep problems than their less vulnerable peers [28].

Cultural issues in sleep practices: differences and similarities

Drawing on the concept of the developmental niche, sleep may be viewed as occurring within an organized framework of physical and social settings, customs and practices of care, and caretaker cultural beliefs or "ethnotheories" [29]. As such, sleep is affected by such variables as cultural beliefs about the perceived function and meaning of sleep, the relative value and importance of sleep as a health behavior, cultural norms for sleep practices, and social interactions, networks, and relationships, to name a few. For example, in some societies and cultural settings (tribal, kibbutz), sleep is a communal phenomenon, whereas solitary sleep is the cultural ideal in many Anglo-European societies [5]. In a number of tribal societies across the globe sleep patterns are polyphasic rather than monophasic. These patterns are characterized by lengthy daytime sleep in social groups including children, and periods of both daytime and nighttime sleep with frequent arousals which may include intervals of conversation, play, or other social interaction [5,30].

Cosleeping

A baby must not sleep in an empty room alone, and an adult must keep watch next to it. (Korean proverb)

"Cosleeping" is an umbrella term that generally is considered to include the practices of bed sharing with a caretaker(s) or other family members, proximate sleeping arrangements, and room sharing during sleep. Cosleeping also may be defined further as occurring as an isolated (occurring only under extraordinary circumstances, such as illness) or occasional phenomenon or on a regular nightly basis (habitual cosleeping); a distinction sometimes is made between all-night and part-night cosleeping as well.

By any definition, cosleeping of infants and parents is a common and accepted practice in the majority of cultures around the world [4]. A recent study of school-aged children in urban mainland China, for example, reported that the prevalence of regular bed sharing was 18.2% and as high as 55.8% in 7-year-olds [31]. In a study of bed sharing in Korean children, Yang and Hahn [32] found that 73.5% of mothers approved of bed sharing between 3 and 6 years of age; there was no association between cosleeping and socio-economic status, parent education, or number of household members. In that study, mothers also determined at what age the transition to a solitary sleeping arrangement was made. In another study, rates of cosleeping in Japan (59%) were reported to be much higher than in their American counterparts (15%), although in this study, the cosleeping occurred largely with the maternal caretaker, and fathers slept separately in 23% of the families surveyed [33].

Cosleeping also is common in some Western European cultures, although the age and demographic patterns of cosleepers may be quite different. One recent Italian study found a 3.5% prevalence of cosleeping among 10- to 11-year-old children living in Rome [34]. Other Italian survey studies have shown the highest rate of cosleeping in children aged 4 to 6 years (17%) compared with 2% at 6 to 12 months, 10% at 12 to 24 months [35], and 5% in 6- to 12- year-olds, with a mean duration of cosleeping of 6.4 years. Cosleeping in the latter study, and in some others (eg, in the United States [36]) was associated with child sleep problems, low socio-economic status, single-parent status, parent shift work, and a family history of cosleeping. A longitudinal study of sleep habits in Swiss children found the greatest prevalence of bed sharing between the ages of 1 month and 10 years was in

4-year-old children at 38% [37]. In contrast, a recent national survey conducted in the United States between 1993 and 2000 indicated that 9.2% of infants usually shared a bed with parents [38]. Even in the United States, however, certain ethnic groups, including African Americans, Hispanics, and South-east Asians, have high rates of cosleeping [39–41]. In the United States, cosleeping often is associated with lower socio-economic status, limited parental education, increased family stress, and a more ambivalent maternal attitude toward child-rearing in white families [36], although these factors do not seem to apply in black families (in which it has been reported as many as 50% to 70% habitually cosleep). In Hispanic families, cosleeping seems to be related to single parenting and status of the child, with the oldest child or only child cosleeping more commonly [40].

These differences in cosleeping patterns are likely to be intimately related to what different cultures define as appropriate developmental goals for children. In many Asian cultures, for example, the emphasis is on cultivating mutual dependence, not independence [42]. Therefore, not all families may share the developmental goal of independent self-soothing in infants at bedtime and after night wakings. As noted previously, in many traditional societies, sleep is heavily embedded in social practices, and both the sleeping environment and the positioning of sleep periods within the context of other activities is much less solitary and less rigid than in more Westernized cultures. Morelli and colleagues [43] point out that a Mayan mother would be shocked at the American habit of placing babies in a separate room and would view this practice as an indicator of Westerners shirking their parental responsibility for creating closeness with their children.

The results of an 18-year longitudinal study by Okami and colleagues [44] may be interpreted as supportive evidence for the contention that cosleeping as a lifestyle choice, at least in selected populations, is unlikely to result in either delayed attainment of developmental goals or in long-term psychologic harm. (By the same token, cosleeping in this study did not seem to confer any long-term advantages over solitary sleeping.) On the other hand, a distinction needs to be made between lifestyle cosleeping and the institution of cosleeping by parents as an attempt to address an underlying sleep problem, usually bedtime resistance or night wakings, so-called "reactive cosleeping." This practice, which is the more common scenario for the initiation of cosleeping after the first year of life, is likely to yield only a temporary respite from the sleep problem and may set the stage for more significant sleep issues later on [45].

Thus, cosleeping may have very different short and long-term effects, depending on the population, the context, and the specific circumstances under which it occurs.

One of the most serious potential consequences of cosleeping, which has garnered considerable attention in the past several years, is an increase in the risk of sudden infant death syndrome. The results of a number of large-scale epidemiologic studies have indicated that cosleeping, most specifically in the context of certain high-risk situations that are likely to be particularly prevalent in urban poor families (maternal obesity, smoking, alcohol, and drug use, overcrowding, use of "non-bed" sleeping surfaces such as couches or chairs), may increase the risk of accidental suffocation. These findings have prompted the American Academy of Pediatrics to issue a recommendation against bed sharing in the first year of life [46]. As tragic as these sporadic instances of infant death are, the widespread prevalence of cosleeping practices around the world suggests that in the vast majority of cases it is both safe and well accepted. The ability to identify and address differential vulnerabilities of child, parent, and the parent–child dyad to potential risks and benefits of cosleeping and to understand the cultural context of the practice in the individual family may help professionals guide parents more effectively in making informed choices that are in their family's best interest.

Bedtime rituals

In Anglo-European cultures, the presleep bedtime ritual centers on the private space of a separate bedroom and involves a patterned set of activities that often includes bathing, putting on special clothing, songs, story-telling, and use of a transitional or "security" object [47]. The bedtime routine is meant both to increase the child's readiness for sleep by leading to a gradual diminution of stimulation in the environment and to provide reassurances of safety to the child from the caregiver before the child is left alone in the room. More recently, the bedtime ritual has become an integral part of the "quality time" that many working parents in Anglo-European societies devote to their children and has been promoted as a way to increase literacy skills in young children (eg, the Reach Out and Read, and Read To Me programs).

Alternatively, bedtime rituals may be viewed as representing the conflict between the need to respond sensitively to the child's need for comfort and closeness and the need to adjust the child to the family routine. When infant care practices in families from the greater Boston, Massachusetts area, for example, were compared with those of families from a small town north of Rome in Italy,

the authors found that American children were much more likely to have a bedtime ritual and were required to go to bed regardless of their resistance. Italian children, in contrast, typically were allowed to participate in the family's late evening life and to fall asleep in the company of adults [48]. Bedtime routines are also not observed in the Guatemalan Mayan community [43], in which infants and children simply fall asleep when sleepy, do not wear specific sleep clothes or use traditional transitional objects, room share and cosleep with parents or siblings, and nurse on demand during the night. The benefits for the child of these less structured practices are considered to include increased intimacy and an enhanced opportunity to observe and learn from adults. In other cultures such as the Balinese society, children typically do not have bedtime rituals because babies are encouraged to acquire quickly the capacity to sleep under any circumstances, including situations of high stimulation, musical performances, and other noisy observances which reflect their more complete integration into adult social activities [5].

Sleeping environment

Sleeping rooms and sleeping surfaces also differ across cultures. A number of reviews are available regarding sleeping arrangements in different societies [49,50]. For example Japanese children and parents often sleep in the same room on futons that are separate but in close proximity to one another. This arrangement allows the parent to reach out easily to calm or comfort a child during the night. A recent Japanese study of *yonaki* (sleep-related night crying) suggested that the phenomenon may be closely linked to this particular sleeping arrangement because parents sleeping in close proximity to their infant are more likely to be aware of (and respond to) any (even brief) night wakings [51]. In India, particularly in rural areas, infants typically sleep either carried in close physical proximity to their mothers in a pouch-like arrangement or in a traditional cloth- cradle sling suspended from bamboo poles. Older infants may sleep in wooden cradles, cotton beds, or bamboo mats, all of which are placed in a communal living space rather than a separate bedroom. Mosquito nets and coils as well as fans are an integral part of the sleeping environment. In a recent study, Italian parents also reported it customary and preferable to have infants sleep in their rooms with them, irrespective of the availability of separate rooms for children and parents, and considered the American norm of putting children to bed in separate rooms to be unkind [52]. In comparison with non-Western societies, the sleeping space regarded as optimal in Western settings is much more likely to be free of or to provid minimal sensory stimulation (noise, light, odors, temperature extremes) [5].

Daytime sleep (Napping)

Cultural preferences also may play an important role in regulating napping behavior [53,54]. Although a biphasic sleep pattern is still predominant in countries around the Mediterranean Sea and in South America, Africa, and Asia, in the era of globalization and "24/7" economies, daytime napping behavior (ie, "siesta cultures") as a cultural standard seems to be slowly disappearing [55]. For example, most Icelandic children [56] stop napping by the age of 3 years, whereas the majority of American children typically drop their naps between the ages of 4 and 5 years [54]. Napping practices also may have substantial inter- and intracultural variations, however. For example, in a recent study of 2- to 5-year-old children sampled from pediatric patient populations in a major Midwestern center in the United States, Lavigne and colleagues [57] found that minority children (African American, Hispanic, and "other") were reported to take substantially more and longer daytime naps and to sleep less at night than non-Hispanic white children. A recent study also showed marked ethnic differences in napping tendencies in an examination of white and African American 2- to 8-year-old children from a tri-county area in southern Mississippi [58]. Black children napped significantly more days per week, had shorter average nocturnal sleep durations, and slept significantly less on weeknights than on weekends compared with white children. Despite these differences in the distribution of sleep, however, the total sleep duration was nearly identical for the two ethnic groups.

Ethnic and racial variability in napping may result from a number of factors, including differences in daytime schedules and activities that are more or less likely to permit napping, cultural differences in attitudes about the acceptability of daytime sleep periods, and cultural beliefs regarding the relative value of nocturnal sleep and regular bedtimes and sleep-wake schedules. For example, the social acceptability in Japan of the unique form of napping called *inemuri* (literally, "to be present and sleep"), in which the sleeper is in a situation not ordinarily meant for sleep such as at work or at a social event, demonstrates the influence of cultural values on sleep patterns [30]. The recent emergence of policies eliminating napping in some preschool and kindergarten settings in the United States in the interest of increasing time devoted to more academic pursuits seems to reflect an increasing societal focus on academic achievement and performance on standardized tests (eg, "No Child Left Behind"), potentially to the decrement of the substantial percentage of 4- and 5-year-olds who still require a daytime nap. Finally, there may be fundamental racial and ethnic differences either in sleep need or in the functioning of the chronobiologic and/or homeostatic mechanisms regulating sleep patterns.

Sleep amounts

Despite basic biologic dictates regarding the amount of sleep needed for optimal functioning, normative values for sleep duration in infants and children also seem to vary somewhat across cultures [7]. In a study of cultural differences in sleep habits and complaints of 40,303 children aged 11 to 16 years from 11 European countries [59], sleep habits varied significantly between countries, with Israeli children sleeping the shortest and Swiss children sleeping the longest amounts. Super and colleagues [60] compared sleep patterns between American and Dutch children using parental reports. Whereas American infants in the 1990s slept 13 hours per day at age 3 months, Dutch babies slept 15 hours per day at the same age. Up to 8 years of age, Dutch children went to bed significantly earlier than American children, which the authors attribute to the influence of the "three R's"—*rust, regelmaat eet reinheid* (rest, regularity, and cleanliness)—fundamental cultural principles for Dutch parents. In contrast, in another Western European study, Italian preschool children in the 1990s were reported to go to bed later and to wake up earlier, resulting in shorter sleep duration [35], than children in other countries, presumably because Italian children regularly participated in the evening social activities of adults [48].

As with napping, there may be racial differences in sleep amounts. For example, in one study minority children in the United States were almost five times more likely to have a bedtime later than 11 PM than white children and were thus more likely to get less sleep; older minority boys obtained the least sleep [61]. In another American study of 2- to 7-year-olds, African American children had later bedtimes and slept fewer hours than their white counterparts, independent of socio-economic status [62].

Studies of this nature have almost universally used parental reports of "average" sleep amounts, which then often are interpreted to be equivalent to sleep needs. From a historical perspective, the normative values for sleep duration at different ages also have tended to reflect somewhat arbitrary cultural standards rather than any empirically based observations of sleep needs based on documentation of the daytime consequences of inadequate sleep. As with other sleep behaviors, the family environment also plays a key role in determining when children are put to bed and how long they are encouraged or allowed to sleep. For instance, a recent study found that the presence of marital conflict adversely affected both the quantity and quality of children's sleep [63], and in one of the few longitudinal studies of sleep behavior in a single cohort, Iglowstein and coworkers [7] demonstrated a decrease in sleep duration and a delay in bedtime between cohorts in Switzerland in the 1970s and the 1990s. These shifts were accompanied by a decrease in bedtime resistance, leading the authors to speculate that parents were increasingly adjusting (delaying) their child's bedtime to reflect the child's preferred sleep-onset time, irrespective of the children's potential sleep needs.

Lifestyle issues and sleep

Lifestyle issues with a potential impact on children's sleep, such as television viewing habits, video and computer games, and an increasing number of evening activity demands, seem to be increasingly common across cultures. In addition, school-related factors such as school starting times and pressures on students to excel academically increasingly transcend cultural differences. For example, sleep habits in adolescents in such diverse countries as India, Italy, Korea, China, and Japan [64,65] reflect the fact that school starting times are early (usually before 7:30 AM), there are homework demands, and late nights are common. Thus average sleep time in grades 10 through 12 is considerably reduced by homework and pressures at school, and sleep problems are common. This finding may indicate some degree of homogenization across cultures, especially in urban areas (which tend to look quite different from the more rural and thus less "Westernized" areas in terms of sleep problems).

Electronic devices

The use of a variety of electronic devices affects sleep habits in both children and adolescents. In one study in the United States, 76% of households surveyed reported that television was part of the "bedtime routine" for 4- to 10-year-olds, 20% of parents reported arguing about bedtime television, and 26% of these children had a television set in the bedroom. Subsequent surveys have reported even higher numbers, and the most recent 2006 National Sleep Foundation poll on sleep in adolescents found that almost 100% of the teenagers surveyed had at least one electronic device (ie, computer, DVD player, television) in the bedroom. More importantly, a number of studies also have demonstrated an association between television-viewing habits and sleep problems (difficulty initiating sleep, shortened sleep duration). In one

qualitative study of inner city middle school students, the students themselves cited television viewing as the primary reason for inadequate sleep [66].

Caffeine

Caffeine is the most widely consumed drug in the world and is the only psychoactive drug that is legally available to children and adolescents. The variety of caffeinated beverages and other caffeine vehicles (eg, candy, gum, pills) now available on supermarket shelves worldwide, from food and beverage vendors, in school vending machines, and over the Internet is astounding and is increasing every year; more than 500 new "energy drinks" reached the international market in 2006 alone. The 2006 National Sleep Foundation poll showed that 75% of adolescents drink at least one caffeinated beverage per day and that almost a third consume two or more. Twenty-six percent of students in grades 6 through 8 (age 10–14 years) drink at least two cans or cups of a caffeinated beverage per day.

Although caffeine has short-term effects in reversing some performance decrements associated with sleep deprivation (eg, decreased in vigilance, increased reaction time), any potential beneficial effects of this stimulant on performance must be balanced against potential health effects. The adverse effects of caffeine range from acute direct effects on mood and anxiety, somatic symptoms (eg, headache and gastrointestinal disturbance) and increased sleep disruption to possible long-term cardiovascular and carcinogenic effects and issues related to dependency, tolerance, and withdrawal and caffeine's potential role as a "gateway drug." A particularly disturbing recent trend is the increased purposeful use of caffeinated beverages by adolescents as a "performance enhancer," attempting both to counteract the effects of voluntary sleep restriction and to mitigate or eliminate the effect of alcohol consumption on performance and alertness and allow the user to consume greater amounts of alcohol. One interesting study of 12- to 24-month-old Guatemalan children, for whom coffee intake is very common, examined the effect of randomized discontinuation of caffeine in daily coffee drinkers. Sleep amounts were increased by an average of 30 minutes per night [67].

Summary

Cultural issues shape how, where, and when children and families sleep (see Fig. 1) and the types of sleep problems they experience. Cultural background therefore must be a key consideration in determining future research directions in pediatric sleep, education of both health care professionals and the public, and pediatric clinical practice ncreased cross-cultural pediatric sleep research is critically needed to improve the standard of care across nations and ethnic groups and to enhance basic knowledge about the causes and impact of pediatric sleep disorders. Unfortunately, the current state of pediatric sleep research in many countries is, at best, rudimentary. A key component of cross-cultural research also involves the development and testing of culturally sensitive epidemiologic tools such as surveys that also are comparable across cultures.

There is also a critical need for educational materials for parents regarding normal sleep, healthy sleep patterns and behaviors, and signs of sleep problems that are appropriately tailored for differences in literacy level, language, cultural values, and knowledge level of the target audience. Finally, the availability of clinical sleep diagnostic and treatment services for children, especially subspecialty expertise, varies but generally is inadequate in most countries, even in urban centers. Therefore, there is an urgent need to share clinical resources regarding the diagnosis and treatment of sleep problems in children (eg, educational materials, sleep questionnaires, behavioral treatment strategies). Although treatment should be evidence-based whenever possible, there is also a need to share clinical experiences, because many of the treatments available in clinical practice have little empiric data to support their use.

Ultimately, culturally competent health care involves awareness of one's own cultural sensitivities and biases, requires an adequate knowledge base regarding culturally based patient beliefs and practices, and necessitates an appreciation of both the beneficial effects and negative impact that culture and related issues such as health literacy have on health care. It also includes the acquisition of cultural skills such as the use of culturally appropriate language and the consideration of culture in assessment and treatment of patients and requires exposure to and encounters with cultural issues in clinical practice. International nonprofit organizations, such as Sleeping Children Around the World (www.scaw.org), which provides culturally appropriate bedkits to needy children in developing countries around the world, are examples of culturally competent care that is mindful of and responsive to the experience of health and illness from the patient's and family's perspective and should be the model to which sleep medicine professionals should aspire.

References

[1] Hufford D. Cultural and social perspectives on alternative medicine: background and assumptions. Altern Ther Health Med 1995;1(1):53–61.

[2] Borbely AA. A two process model of sleep regulation. Hum Neurobiol 1982;1(3):195–204.

[3] Borbely A, Achermann P. Sleep homeostasis and models of sleep regulation. In: Kryger M, Roth T, Dement W, editors. Principles and practice of sleep medicine. 4th edition. Philadelphia: Elsevier/Saunders; 2005. p. 405–17.

[4] Jenni OG, O'Connor BB. Children's sleep: an interplay between culture and biology. Pediatrics 2005;115(1 Suppl):204–16.

[5] Worthman C, Melby M. Toward a comparative developmental ecology of human sleep. In: Carskadon M, editor. Adolescent sleep patterns: biological, social, and psychological influences. Cambridge (UK): Cambridge University Press; 2002. p. 69–117.

[6] Mindell JA, Carskadon MA, Owens JA. Developmental features of sleep. Child Adolesc Psychiatr Clin N Am 1999;8(4):695–725.

[7] Iglowstein I, Jenni OG, Molinari L, et al. Sleep duration from infancy to adolescence: reference values and generational trends. Pediatrics 2003; 111(2):302–7.

[8] Goodlin-Jones BL, Burnham MM, Gaylor EE, et al. Night waking, sleep-wake organization, and self-soothing in the first year of life. J Dev Behav Pediatr 2001;22(4):226–33.

[9] LeBourgeois MK, Giannotti F, Cortesi F, et al. The relationship between reported sleep quality and sleep hygiene in Italian and American adolescents. Pediatrics 2005;115(1 Suppl):257–65.

[10] Carskadon MA, Wolfson AR, Acebo C, et al. Adolescent sleep patterns, circadian timing, and sleepiness at a transition to early school days. Sleep 1998;21(8):871–81.

[11] Carskadon MA, Vieira C, Acebo C. Association between puberty and delayed phase preference. Sleep 1993;16(3):258–62.

[12] Owens-Stively J, Frank N, Smith A, et al. Child temperament, parenting discipline style, and daytime behavior in childhood sleep disorders. J Dev Behav Pediatr 1997;18(5):314–21.

[13] Wiggs L. Sleep problems in children with developmental disorders. J R Soc Med 2001;94(4):177–9.

[14] Dahl RE, Ryan ND, Matty MK, et al. Sleep onset abnormalities in depressed adolescents. Biol Psychiatry 1996;39(6):400–10.

[15] Sachs H, McGuire J, Sadeh A, et al. Cognitive and behavioural correlates of mother reported sleep problems in psychiatrically hospitalized children. Sleep Research 1994;23:207–13.

[16] Hiscock H, Wake M. Infant sleep problems and postnatal depression: a community-based study. Pediatrics 2001;107(6):1317–22.

[17] Gallagher K, Tobia A, Wolfson A. Sleep and waking behaviours in kindergarten: impact of stressful life events. J Sleep Res 1995;24:96–107.

[18] Owens J, Boergers J, Streisand R, et al. Relationship between maternal and child sleep disturbances. Presented at the 13th annual meeting of the Association of Professional Sleep Societies. Orlando, June 1999.

[19] Sadeh A. Stress, trauma and sleep in children. Child Adolesc Psychiatr Clin N Am 1996;5(3): 685–700.

[20] Liu X, Uchiyama M, Okawa M, et al. Prevalence and correlates of self-reported sleep problems among Chinese adolescents. Sleep 2000;23(1): 27–34.

[21] Tynjala J, Kannas L, Levalahti E, et al. Perceived sleep quality and its precursors in adolescents. Health Promot Int 1999;14:155–66.

[22] Gau SF, Soong WT. Sleep problems of junior high school students in Taipei. Sleep 1995; 18(8):667–73.

[23] Morrison DN, McGee R, Stanton WR. Sleep problems in adolescence. J Am Acad Child Adolesc Psychiatry 1992;31(1):94–9.

[24] Roberts RE, Roberts CR, Chen IG. Impact of insomnia on future functioning of adolescents. J Psychosom Res 2002;53(1):561–9.

[25] Giannotti F, Cortesi F. Sleep patterns and daytime functions in adolescents: an epidemiological survey of Italian high-school student population. In: Carskadon MA, editor. Adolescent sleep patterns: biological, social and psychological influences. New York: Cambridge University Press; 2002.

[26] U.S. Department of Health and Human Services HRaSA. U.S. teens in our world. Rockville (MD): U.S. Department of Health and Human Services; 2003.

[27] Pelayo R, Thorpy M, Glovinsky P. Prevalence of delayed sleep phase syndrome among adolescents. J Sleep Res 1988;17:392.

[28] Owens JA, Witmans M. Sleep problems. Curr Probl Pediatr Adolesc Health Care 2004;34(4): 154–79.

[29] Harkness S, Super CM. The developmental niche: a theoretical framework for analyzing the household production of health. Soc Sci Med 1994;38(2):217–26.

[30] Steger B, Brunt L. Introduction: into the night and the world of sleep. In: Steger B, Brunt L, editors. Night-time and sleep in Asia and the West: exploring the dark side of life. London: Routledge Curzon; 2003.

[31] Claudill W, Plath D. Who sleeps by whom? Parent-child involvement in urban Japanese families. Psychiatry 1966;29:344–66.

[32] Yang CK, Hahn HM. Cosleeping in young Korean children. J Dev Behav Pediatr 2002; 23(3):151–7.

[33] Latz S, Wolf AW, Lozoff B. Cosleeping in context: sleep practices and problems in young children in Japan and the United States. Arch Pediatr Adolesc Med 1999;153(4):339–46.

[34] Cortesi F, Giannotti F, Sebastiani T, et al. Cosleeping and sleep behavior in Italian school-aged children. J Dev Behav Pediatr 2004;25(1):28–33.

[35] Ottaviano S, Giannotti F, Cortesi F, et al. Sleep characteristics in healthy children from birth to 6 years of age in the urban area of Rome. Sleep 1996;19(1):1–3.

[36] Lozoff B, Wolf A, Davis N. Cosleeping in urban families with young children in the United States. Pediatrics 1984;74(2):171–82.

[37] Jenni OG, Fuhrer HZ, Iglowstein I, et al. A longitudinal study of bed sharing and sleep problems among Swiss children in the first 10 years of life. Pediatrics 2005;115(1 Suppl):233–40.

[38] Willinger M, Ko CW, Hoffman HJ, et al. Trends in infant bed sharing in the United States, 1993–2000: the National Infant Sleep Position study. Arch Pediatr Adolesc Med 2003;157(1):43–9.

[39] Lozoff B, Askew GL, Wolf AW. Cosleeping and early childhood sleep problems: effects of ethnicity and socioeconomic status. J Dev Behav Pediatr 1996;17(1):9–15.

[40] Schachter FF, Fuchs ML, Bijur PE, et al. Cosleeping and sleep problems in Hispanic-American urban young children. Pediatrics 1989;84(3): 522–30.

[41] Stein MT, Colarusso CA, McKenna JT, et al. Cosleeping (bedsharing) among infants and toddlers. J Dev Behav Pediatr 1997;18(6):408–12.

[42] Claudill W, Weinstein H. Maternal care and infant behavior in Japan and America. Psychiatry 1969;32:12–43.

[43] Morelli G, Rogoff B, Oppenheim D, et al. Cultural variation in infants' sleeping arrangements: questions of independence. Dev Psychol 1992; 28:604–13.

[44] Okami P, Weisner T, Olmstead R. Outcome correlates of parent-child bedsharing: an eighteen year longitudinal study. J Dev Behav Pediatr 2002;23(4):244–53.

[45] Owens JA. Cosleeping. J Dev Behav Pediatr 2002; 23(4):254–5.

[46] American Academy of Pediatrics. The changing concept of sudden infant death syndrome: diagnostic coding shifts, controversies regarding the sleeping environment, and new variables to consider in reducing risk. Pediatrics 2005;116(5): 1245–55.

[47] Burnham MM, Goodlin-Jones BL, Gaylor EE, et al. Use of sleep aids during the first year of life. Pediatrics 2002;109(4):594–601.

[48] New R, Richman A. Maternal beliefs and infant care practices in Italy and the United States. In: Harkness S, Super C, editors. Parents' cultural belief systems: their origins, expressions, and consequences. New York: Guilford Press; 1996.

[49] Stearns P, Rowland P. Children's sleep: sketching historical change. J Soc Hist 1996;30:345–67.

[50] McKenna JJ, Thoman EB, Anders TF, et al. Infant-parent co-sleeping in an evolutionary perspective: implications for understanding infant sleep development and the sudden infant death syndrome. Sleep 1993;16(3):263–82.

[51] Fukumizu M, Kaga M, Kohyama J, et al. Sleep-related nighttime crying (yonaki) in Japan: a community-based study. Pediatrics 2005; 115(1 Suppl):217–24.

[52] Wolf A, Lozoff B, Latz S, et al. Parental theories in the management of young children's sleep

in Japan, Italy, and the United States. In: Harkness S, Super C, editors. Parents' cultural belief systems: their origins, expressions, and consequences. New York: Guilford Press; 1996.

[53] Webb W, Dinges D. Development of human napping. In: Dinges D, Broughton R, editors. Sleep and alertness: chronobiological, behavioral, and medical aspects of napping. New York: Raven Press; 1989. p. 31–51.

[54] Weissbluth M. Naps in children: 6 months–7 years. Sleep 1995;18(2):82–7.

[55] Yi L. Discourse of mid-day napping: a political windsock in contemporary China. In: Steger B, Brunt L, editors. Night-time and sleep in Asia and the West: exploring the dark side of life. London: Routledge Curzon; 2003. p. 45–64.

[56] Thorleifsdottir B, Bjornsson JK, Benediktsdottir B, et al. Sleep and sleep habits from childhood to young adulthood over a 10-year period. J Psychosom Res 2002;53(1):529–37.

[57] Lavigne JV, Arend R, Rosenbaum D, et al. Sleep and behavior problems among preschoolers. J Dev Behav Pediatr 1999;20(3):164–9.

[58] Crosby B, LeBourgeois MK, Harsh J. Racial differences in reported napping and nocturnal sleep in 2- to 8-year-old children. Pediatrics 2005;115(1 Suppl):225–32.

[59] Tynjala J, Kannas L, Valimaa R. How young Europeans sleep. Health Educ Res 1993;8(1):69–80.

[60] Super C, Harkness S, Van Tijen N, et al. The three R's of Dutch childrearing and the socialization of infant arousal. In: Super C, Harkness S, editors. Parents' cultural belief systems: their origins, expressions, and consequences. New York: Guilford Press; 1996.

[61] Spilsbury JC, Storfer-Isser A, Drotar D, et al. Sleep behavior in an urban US sample of school-aged children. Arch Pediatr Adolesc Med 2004;158(10):988–94.

[62] McLaughlin Crabtree V, Beal Korhonen J, Montgomery-Downs HE, et al. Cultural influences on the bedtime behaviors of young children. Sleep Med 2005;6(4):319–24.

[63] El-Sheikh M, Buckhalt JA, Mize J, et al. Marital conflict and disruption of children's sleep. Child Dev 2006;77(1):31–43.

[64] Tagaya H, Uchiyama M, Ohida T, et al. Sleep habits and factors associated with short sleep duration among Japanese high-school students: a community study. Sleep Biol Rhythms 2004; 2(1):57–64.

[65] Ohida T, Osaki Y, Doi Y, et al. An epidemiologic study of self-reported sleep problems among Japanese adolescents. Sleep 2004;27(5):978–85.

[66] Owens JA, Stahl J, Patton A, et al. Sleep practices, attitudes, and beliefs in inner city middle school children: a mixed-methods study. Behav Sleep Med 2006;4(2):114–34.

[67] Engle PL, VasDias T, Howard I, et al. Effects of discontinuing coffee intake on iron deficient Guatemalan toddlers' cognitive development and sleep. Early Hum Dev 1999;53(3):251–69.

SLEEP
MEDICINE
CLINICS

Sleep Med Clin 3 (2008) 109–119

ELSEVIER
SAUNDERS

Insomnia: Therapeutic Options for Women

Judith R. Davidson, PhD[a,b,c,*]

- Predisposing factors
- Precipitating factors
- Perpetuating factors
- Therapeutic options
- Pharmacotherapy
  Benzodiazepines
  Nonbenzodiazepines
  Melatonin
  Ramelteon
  Sedating antidepressants
  Antihistamines as hypnotics
  Herbal therapies
- Nonpharmacologic interventions

Stimulus control therapy
Sleep restriction therapy
Relaxation-based interventions
Cognitive therapy
Sleep hygiene education
Treatment format
Evidence base for nonpharmacologic interventions
- Choice of treatment
- Clinical considerations
- Summary
- Acknowledgments
- References

Recognition of the special circumstances in which women develop insomnia is important for understanding, supporting, and treating women when they seek help for sleep difficulty. Insomnia, by definition, is difficulty falling asleep or staying asleep, waking up too early, or nonrestorative sleep, with associated fatigue, distress, or impairment in functioning [1–3]. Insomnia may be situational, intermittent, or persistent. It can also be a symptom of, or be concurrent with, another sleep disorder, a medical condition, a psychiatric disorder, emotional distress, or substance use. It is especially important to treat persistent insomnia because it tends not to resolve on its own and can have a significant effect on quality of life [4,5]. Persistent insomnia increases the risk of subsequent psychiatric conditions, especially depression [6–9]. It also predicts a rise in health care use, including number of

physician visits [10–12]. Fortunately, several effective pharmacologic and nonpharmacologic interventions are available for improving sleep in the short term and for reversing persistent insomnia.

Any given case of insomnia is likely to involve a diathesis for sleep difficulty combined with circumstances or events that trigger a bout of poor sleep, followed by phenomena that maintain the poor sleep. The factors associated with these phases in the development of insomnia have been termed, respectively, predisposing, precipitating and perpetuating factors [13].

Predisposing factors

Women are 1.4 to 2.0 times more likely to report insomnia than are men [14–18]. Depending on how insomnia is defined in a survey, the prevalence in

[a] Department of Psychology, Queen's University, 62 Arch Street, Kingston, ON, Canada K7L 3N6
[b] Department of Oncology, Queen's University, Kingston, ON, Canada
[c] Kingston Family Health Team, Kingston, ON, Canada
* Department of Psychology, Queen's University, 62 Arch Street, Kingston, ON, Canada K7L 3N6.
E-mail address: davidsnj@queensu.ca

women can range from 2% (stringently-defined disorder of initiating or maintaining sleep) [19] to 61% (report of regular insomnia or trouble sleeping during the past 12 months) [14]. In a telephone survey with detailed questions to establish an insomnia designation consistent with psychiatric (*Diagnostic and Statistical Manual of Mental Disorders, 4th Edition* [DSM-IV]) [2] and World Health Organization (*International Classification of Diseases and Related Health Problems, 10th Revision* [ICD-10]) [3] criteria—including sleep difficulty at least 3 nights per week for a minimum of 1 month with associated impairment or distress—the estimated prevalence of insomnia syndrome in Quebec women was 11% [18]. Many more women than this are dissatisfied with their sleep but their symptoms do not meet clinical definitions of insomnia [18,20]. The higher rates in women as compared with men may be due to greater symptom awareness in women, socialization that encourages women more than men to acknowledge and report distress, biological differences (eg, reproductive hormones, pregnancy, menstruation, menopause), possible greater involvement in nighttime child care and elder care, and the greater prevalence of anxiety and depression in women [21,22].

A family history of insomnia appears to increase the likelihood of developing insomnia, especially if one's mother had insomnia [23]. The extent to which this represents genetic predisposition and/or the environment in which one grows up is unknown. The prevalence of insomnia increases with age and, in women, there appears to be a steep rise at midlife [20,24]. Being prone to cognitive and emotional hyperarousal [25] and overactivation of the hypothalamic–pituitary–adrenal axis [26] are believed to increase vulnerability to insomnia.

Precipitating factors

Commonly reported precipitants of insomnia include stressful life events, such as death of a loved one or other personal loss; illness; work or school stress; family concerns; and interpersonal conflict [24,27,28]. It appears that arousal and distress, rather than the stressful events themselves, are associated with insomnia [29,30]. Japanese women reported that aging, living with a child under age 6, undergoing medical treatment, experiencing major life events, following irregular bedtimes, having sleep apnea–type symptoms, and living near heavy traffic were associated with insomnia [31]. Pregnancy, childbirth, and caring for an infant are times when a woman's sleep is bound to be disturbed. Women who develop chronic insomnia sometimes identify childbirth as the initial precipitant of their poor sleep. At insomnia clinics, mothers of infants frequently describe the reciprocal influence of infant and maternal sleep—wake patterns. Surprisingly however, there is very little research on the interaction of child and parent sleep. Surprisingly, however, there is little research on the interaction of child and parent sleep. Meijer and van der Wittenboer [32] found that a mother's insomnia was worse than the father's before childbirth and it remained worse over the first year. A mother is often nocturnally vigilant for her baby's crying and responsive to nighttime feeding needs. The sleep quality of young children influences the mother's sleep and daytime functioning. Meltzer and Mindell [33] found, for example, that the quality of children's sleep predicted the quality of maternal sleep, and that poor sleep in the child and mother was associated with maternal stress, mood disturbance, and fatigue. When children reach adolescence, parents may stay awake until their son or daughter returns home late at night. During perimenopause and menopause, women's sleep may be disrupted by nocturnal hot flashes [34,35]. During the menopausal transition, and at midlife in general, psychological distress is associated with sleep difficulty [30,36]. A high proportion of postmenopausal women have some level of sleep-disordered breathing [37]. Snoring bed partners are another potential precipitant of sleep difficulty. Caring for aging parents or an aging spouse, or caring for anyone with a disordered sleep schedule (eg, a person with Alzheimer's disease) will disrupt the caregiver's sleep. One's own illness or pain syndrome can precipitate a bout of poor sleep.

Perpetuating factors

Insomnia can be maintained by a variety of physiological, behavioral, emotional, and cognitive factors. Sometimes a precipitant of poor sleep, such as pain or ongoing worries about life circumstances, will persist, leading to chronic insomnia. However, in addition to ongoing precipitants, several perpetuating factors tend to develop over time, often independent of the initial precipitant. Typical perpetuating factors are (1) maladaptive sleep–wake habits, especially sleep scheduling; (2) learned associations of the bed with sleeplessness; and (3) dysfunctional cognitions that prevent sufficient presleep reduction in arousal.

Maladaptive sleep–wake habits include a tendency to go to bed early or stay in bed later in the morning in an attempt to make up for poor sleep. This strategy tends to backfire, leading to increased sleep disruption and more nights of poor sleep. Similarly, sleep tends to remain poor for those who have inconsistent sleep times and wake times (for example, those who rise at different times each day or hose who nap at various times during the day). In hese cases the homeostatic and circadian processes hat regulate sleep [38] are constantly being reset. This ongoing desynchronization between sleep need (homeostatic) and the time of day (circadian) prevents sleep from improving.

Learned associations of the bed with sleeplessness develop when a person stays in bed when she is not sleeping. After several nights of not sleeping well in one's bed, there is an association of the bed and bedroom with being awake, and sometimes with frustration and dread. In classical conditioning terms, the bed and the bedroom are stimuli that elicit a conditioned arousal response that is incompatible with sleep. This phenomenon, although commonly accepted, has been the subject of very little research. A recent study found supportive but nonspecific evidence for insomnia-associated classical conditioning [39]. In such cases, the person sometimes discovers that she can fall asleep on the sofa, in another bed, or when away from home. Thus, the difficulty with sleeping in her own bed and bedroom persists.

Dysfunctional cognitions that perpetuate poor sleep tend to be troubling thoughts about the feared consequences of not sleeping. Some typical worries are:

Here I go again, why can't I sleep? There must be something wrong with me.
I won't be able to function tomorrow.
My health will deteriorate. I am making myself prone to cancer.

Naturally these troubling thoughts are associated with cognitive and emotional arousal, preventing the reduction in arousal that allows sleep to come.

Therapeutic options

Women make up the majority of participants in insomnia trials (eg, Refs. [40,41]) and are more likely than men to be using prescribed hypnotics [42]. Subsequently, much of the outcome data for insomnia treatments of all kinds are based on the experiences of women. A variety of pharmacologic and nonpharmacologic interventions have been shown to be efficacious for improving sleep [43]. The choice of intervention is influenced by many factors, including the nature of the insomnia, especially whether it is acute or chronic; age; the presence of medical or psychiatric comorbidity; condition of pregnancy or nursing; concurrent medications and substances; availability of treatments; time; cost; and personal preference.

Pharmacotherapy

Pharmacotherapy is a treatment option for acute, situational insomnia. The most commonly prescribed hypnotic medications are the broad class of benzodiazepine receptor agonists. These agents bind to the benzodiazapine site of the γ-aminobutyric acid A ($GABA_A$) receptor complex. In doing so, they enhance GABA-induced neuronal inhibition. The benzodiazepine receptor agonists include the traditional benzodiazepines (eg, flurazepam, estazolam, temazepam, and triazolam) and the newer nonbenzodiazepine agents (eg, zolpidem, zaleplon, zopiclone, and eszopiclone), hereafter referred to as the nonbenzodiazepines. Nonbenzodiazepines may bind selectively to the α1 subunit of the $GABA_A$ receptor complex [44] or have a totally separate binding site on the benzodiazepine receptor complex [45]. Whereas the traditional benzodiazepines have sedative and hypnotic properties, the nonbenzodiazepines have more specific hypnotic properties.

Benzodiazepines

The benzodiazepines are effective at increasing sleep duration and in reducing patient-reported time to sleep onset [46]. However, they also have some less desirable effects, including altered sleep stage composition (usually an increase in stages 1 and 2 and a reduction in slow-wave sleep); tolerance after 1 to 3 weeks; potential for dependence; rebound insomnia after discontinuation; next-day hangover; effects on vigilance, concentration, and memory; and respiratory depression [47]. The benzodiazepines, especially alprazolam, should be avoided during pregnancy and nursing because of risks to the fetus, including congenital defects [48]. Temazepam is contraindicated in pregnancy according to the US Food and Drug Administration [49]. Benzodiazepines and the nonbenzodiazepines (described below) should be used with caution by women 60 years old or older. Although the benzodiazepine receptor agonists improve sleep in this age group, they are associated with dangerous cognitive and psychomotor side effects, including memory problems, confusion, disorientation, dizziness, loss of balance, and falls [50].

Nonbenzodiazepines

Zolpidem and zaleplon show efficacy for reducing sleep latency. Zopiclone and eszopiclone (an isomer of racemic zopiclone) show efficacy for reducing sleep latency, number of awakenings, and wake time after sleep onset, and for increasing sleep duration and depth of sleep [45,51,52]. Dorsey and colleagues [53] found zolpidem to be useful in the treatment of perimenopausal insomnia. Tolerance and rebound insomnia are unlikely with the nonbenzodiazepines [45,52,54–56]. The nonbenzodiazepines are generally better tolerated than the benzodiazpenines. Potential side effects for zolpidem include headache, dizziness, drowsiness, and nausea [52]. Zopiclone and eszopiclone may have a bitter taste [54,57] and patients taking eszopiclone are more likely than placebo-taking patients to experience somnolence and myalgia [58]. The literature is mixed about whether the nonbenzodiazepines are safer than benzodiazepines for older patients [40,50].

As discussed by Sloan in this issue, caution should be exercised in taking nonbenzodiazapines during pregnancy and nursing [45,47]. In the labelling of drugs for use in pregnancy, the US Food and Drug Administration gives better ratings to zolpidem and zaleplon than to the benzodiazepines. Also, Diav-Citrin and colleagues [59] found that zopiclone taken during the first trimester was not associated with an increase in the rate of malformations. However, because the safety information is very limited, current recommendations for the use of nonbenzodiazepines during pregnancy and nursing are that they be used only if the potential benefits to the mother justify the potential risks to the fetus [45].

Melatonin

Although there are very few studies, the available research indicates that exogenous melatonin is not useful for insomnia. It appears to help sleep only for naps or sleep that is taken at times other than during the usual nocturnal sleep period, such as during the daytime or in the period just before normal bedtime called the "wake maintenance zone" [60,61]. Melatonin can be useful for preventing eastbound jet lag and for night-shift work [62,63] but only if taken at a very specific time with respect to the circadian rhythm of sleep-wakefulness. It should be used with caution unless the timing of administration with respect to circadian phase is carefully planned.

Ramelteon

Ramelteon is a melatonin receptor agonist that reduces sleep latency and sometimes increases sleep duration. It is generally well tolerated by patients, including those aged 65 and older [64]. Patients do not show signs of cognitive impairment, rebound insomnia, or withdrawal effects [64,65]. Potential side effects include headache, dizziness, somnolence, fatigue, and nausea. Patients with severe hepatic impairment should avoid ramelteon [66]. In pregnancy, it should be used only if the benefits clearly outweigh the risks to the fetus [67].

Sedating antidepressants

There have been few trials of sedating antidepressants in people with insomnia who are not depressed [68]. Walsh and colleagues [69] found trazodone to be somewhat useful, but less so than zolpidem, in the treatment of primary insomnia as measured by patient self-report. There has been a surge of prescription of trazodone as a hypnotic [70]. Although this antidepressant increases sleep duration in people with major depressive disorder, there appears to be no efficacy or tolerance data for trazodone as a hypnotic in nondepressed individuals [71]. Potential side effects include dizziness, arrhythmias, sedation, and psychomotor impairment [68]. Concern about safety, especially in elderly patients, is higher with trazodone than with the conventional hypnotics [71].

Antihistamines as hypnotics

Most over-the-counter sleep remedies contain the antihistamine diphenhydramine. These remedies cause daytime sleepiness but there is little evidence that they are useful for people with chronic insomnia [44]. Placebo-controlled trials of diphenhydramine have shown some efficacy for self-reported or physician-reported measures of insomnia symptoms in the short term (1–2 weeks) [72–74]. With polysomnographic measures, Morin and colleagues [74] found that diphenhydramine improved sleep efficiency over placebo in patients with mild insomnia during the first 2 weeks of treatment. Diphenhydramine can cause some psychomotor performance deficits [44] and may also have abuse potential [75]. Although the negative effects on performance may recede after 3 days, diphenhydramine's effects on sleepiness also appear to decline within the same period [76]. Diphenhydramine may offer help for those with mild insomnia but its effects seem short-lived.

Herbal therapies

Fifteen percent of a Canadian community sample reported the use of herbal or dietary products for insomnia within the previous year [18]. Data from the US National Health Interview indicated that 82% of people with sleep trouble who had tried herbal therapies found them to be helpful [14]. Various herbal preparations are purported to help with sleep, including valerian root, lavender, hops, kava kava, and chamomile [77,78]. The efficacy of these therapies has been difficult to evaluate because of their unstandardized formulation and the paucity of sound clinical research [77,78]. A recent review of valerian as a sleep aid concluded that there is, as yet, no evidence of clinical efficacy [79]. Currently, there is insufficient or absent evidence of efficacy for the vast majority of herbal products for insomnia. See Meoli and colleagues [78] for a review. Although some herbal therapies appear to be generally well tolerated (eg, valerian [79]), others are associated with adverse effects (eg, risk of hepato-toxicity with kava kava [78]).

Nonpharmacologic interventions

Insomnia-specific cognitive and behavioral treatments are the interventions of choice for insomnia that lasts for 1 month or longer. These treatments are not only efficacious, they are also safer than medication. They are associated with a higher degree of acceptance and satisfaction by patients as compared with hypnotic medication [80,81].

The efficacy of these insomnia-specific therapies is believed to be due specifically to their ability to alter the main factors that perpetuate poor sleep. Perpetuating factors, as described above, include maladaptive sleep–wake habits, especially sleep scheduling; learned associations of the bed with sleeplessness; and dysfunctional cognitions that prevent sufficient presleep reduction in arousal.

Interventions are designed to adjust sleep–wake scheduling to achieve rapid sleep onset and uninterrupted sleep, or to maximize the association of bedtime with reduced arousal and increased sleep tendency. Some of the interventions improve the conditions for the homeostatic and circadian processes that regulate sleep propensity. In doing so, they increase the likelihood of sleep and wakefulness occurring at desired hours. Insomnia-specific therapies generally fall into five categories: stimulus control therapy, sleep restriction, relaxation training, cognitive therapy, and sleep hygiene education.

Stimulus control therapy

As previously described, people with insomnia often come to associate their bed and bedroom with sleeplessness rather than with sleep. Stimulus control therapy is a brief set of instructions for going to and getting up from bed, designed to maximize the association of the bed with sleepiness and sleep. It also emphasizes a consistent rise time, which helps support the circadian component of the rhythm of sleep tendency. The standard stimulus control instructions are:

- Go to bed only when sleepy.
- Use the bed only for sleeping. Sexual activity is the only exception.
- Leave the bed and the bedroom if you can't fall asleep within 15 to 20 minutes. Return when sleepy. Repeat this step as often as necessary during the night.

- Maintain a regular rising time in the morning.
- Do not nap, or limit naps to the midafternoon.[1]

Sleep restriction therapy

Sleep restriction therapy is the prescription of a specific amount of time in bed that is as close as possible to the actual sleep time. This procedure is designed to curtail the time in bed that is spent awake. Restriction of sleep builds up the homeostatic component of the sleep drive, and is therefore conducive to a rapid sleep onset and reduced time awake during the night. With this technique, time in bed is gradually increased as sleep becomes more consolidated. Sleep diaries are used to guide the prescription of time in bed. The steps for sleep restriction are:

- Calculate mean daily subjective total sleep time from sleep diaries kept for at least 1 week.
- Prescribe time in bed as the mean total sleep time or 5 hours, whichever is greater.
- The patient chooses a rise time that is sustainable.
- Work backward (rise time minus time in bed) to establish the bedtime.
- For one week, the patient goes to bed no earlier than the prescribed bedtime and rises no later than the prescribed rise time. This interval is the "sleep window."
- At the end of the week, adjust the sleep window based on that week's mean sleep efficiency (time asleep divided by time in bed times 100%) as follows: (1) If sleep efficiency is 90% or more, then increase time in bed by 15 minutes; (2) if sleep efficiency is between 85% and 90%, then keep time in bed constant; (3) if sleep efficiency is less than 85%, then decrease time in bed by 15 minutes. Adjustments to the window are usually made by altering the bedtime rather than the rise time.
- Make weekly adjustments until optimal sleep efficiency and duration are reached with minimal daytime sleepiness.

Relaxation-based interventions

Relaxation techniques for insomnia include a variety of approaches to release somatic and mental tension, thereby reducing physiological, cognitive, and emotional arousal that interferes with sleep onset. Several relaxation techniques have been shown to be effective in treating insomnia. These include progressive muscle relaxation, imagery, meditation,

---

This is a variation of the original instruction to avoid napping altogether. An afternoon nap, no longer than 1 hour, starting before 3 PM, can be taken if sleepiness is overwhelming. A brief midafternoon nap is unlikely to interfere with nighttime sleep [82,83].

and autogenic training [84]. Relaxing music has shown some potential for assisting sleep in older adults [85,86], but more research is required.

Cognitive therapy

The goal of cognitive therapy in the context of insomnia is to identify and alter maladaptive thinking patterns associated with arousal and the maintenance of sleep difficulty. For example, patients sometimes believe that they must get 8 hours of sleep per night; or that, if they do not sleep well, they will be unable to function the next day. Such thoughts lead to increased worry and arousal, thereby perpetuating the sleep disturbance. The Dysfunctional Beliefs and Attitudes Scale [87] is useful to help patients identify their own particular sleep-related worries. The aim of insomnia-specific cognitive therapy is for the patient to replace the maladaptive sleep-related cognitions with ones that are realistic but less worrisome and arousing. This decatastrophization works well with empathy and education about the particular sleep-related fears. For example, it may be helpful to discuss interindividual variation in sleep need or changes in sleep with aging. Patients whose fears arise from an expectation of their inability to function after a sleepless night often benefit from knowing that fatigue, mood effects, and increased perceived exertion may occur but that objective measures of performance generally show only subtle deficits with sleep loss (eg, Ref. [88]). Paradoxical intention can be useful for some people who try too hard to fall asleep, believing that they "must sleep." This technique involves instructing the patient to try to stay awake, rather than try to sleep, thereby reducing performance anxiety.

Sleep hygiene education

Sleep hygiene education involves provision of information about sleeping conditions and lifestyle habits that promote sleep or minimize sleep interference. A typical set of sleep hygiene recommendations follows:

- **Avoid stimulants, including caffeine and nicotine, several hours before bed. Caffeine and nicotine can impede sleep onset and reduce sleep quality.**
- **Do not drink alcohol 4 to 6 hours before bedtime. Alcohol can lead to fragmented sleep and early morning awakenings.**
- **Avoid heavy meals within 2 hours of bedtime. These can interfere with sleep. A light snack, however, may be sleep inducing.**
- **Regular exercise in the late afternoon or early evening may deepen sleep. However,** **exercising too close to bedtime may have a stimulating effect and delay sleep onset.**
- **Keep the bedroom environment quiet, dark, and comfortable.**

Treatment format

Insomnia-specific cognitive and behavioral interventions can be offered as part of individual therapy or group programs. In individual therapy, interventions are tailored to the set of factors believed to perpetuate that person's insomnia based on the assessment. The various interventions are not incompatible and they can easily be introduced sequentially. The patient continues to track her progress with the use of sleep diaries. Typically, group programs involve a combination of sleep hygiene education, stimulus control therapy and/or sleep restriction, relaxation techniques, and cognitive therapy. There may be four to seven patients and one or two therapists per group. Group programs have the advantages of lower costs in therapist time and the mutual support provided by group members.

Evidence base for nonpharmacologic interventions

The benefits of insomnia-specific cognitive and behavioral treatments for insomnia are well established from research with people who have primary insomnia, who are from the community at large, who are predominantly women (approximately 60%) with mean age in the early 40s, and who are healthy, nonusers of hypnotics, with mean duration of insomnia of 11 years [41,89]. There is sound empirical support for the efficacy of stimulus control therapy, relaxation training, paradoxical intention, sleep restriction, biofeedback, and multicomponent cognitive-behavioral therapy in the treatment of insomnia [84,90]. Sleep hygiene education, on its own, appears to have limited therapeutic value for people with insomnia [90–92]. The relation between sleep hygiene practices by midlife women and sleep variables is low [93], suggesting that good sleep hygiene plays a fairly small role in predicting the quality of sleep.

On average, with insomnia-specific cognitive and behavioral interventions, patients with chronic insomnia see a reduction of about 30 minutes in sleep latency and/or 30 minutes in time awake after sleep onset [41]. Sleep duration is increased, on average, by approximately 30 minutes. Patients' ratings of sleep quality and satisfaction with sleep are significantly enhanced. Improvements in sleep are well maintained and sometimes further improved at follow-up six to eight months after treatment. There is evidence of maintenance of gains even at 24 months [81] post-treatment. The limited data on the effect of these interventions on daytime functioning suggest that depressive and anxiety symptoms are reduced [94] but more research is required on other aspects of functioning, including fatigue, cognitive performance, and quality of life. Patients who participate in group programs achieve results broadly comparable to those of patients who participate in individual sleep therapy [95]. Self-help programs are associated with significant but modest improvements in sleep [96,97].

There is abundant evidence that older adults benefit from insomnia-specific cognitive and behavioral techniques [90,98]. Patients who use hypnotic medications also see improvements to their sleep with the use of these techniques [84,90]. It is becoming clear that these interventions are helpful for patients whose insomnia is associated with medical or psychiatric illness [90,99]. In the past, insomnia in patients with comorbid conditions was often called "secondary" insomnia, and clinicians sometimes hesitated to treat the insomnia, focusing instead on the "underlying" problem. However, the temporal and causal relations between illness and insomnia are usually quite difficult to discern, and there is a move to favor the term "comorbid insomnia" for insomnia with another condition [100]. For medical conditions, the efficacy of insomnia-specific cognitive and behavioral treatments has been demonstrated for people with chronic pain [101] and for people with cancer [102]. For psychiatric conditions, the scant literature suggests that patients with depressive disorders can benefit from insomnia-specific cognitive and behavioral interventions for insomnia [103,104], both in terms of sleep improvement and mood improvement. Patients with subclinical anxiety or depressive symptoms appear to benefit from insomnia-specific cognitive and behavioral interventions [94]. Therefore, for several medical and mental-health problems, there seems little reason to delay insomnia treatment if the patient wishes to improve her sleep. However, patients with bipolar disorder or seizures should avoid sleep restriction because of the possibility of triggering mania or a seizure [99].

Choice of treatment

Insomnia-specific pharmacologic and psychological interventions are both efficacious [43]. However, the timing of their benefits differs. Whereas medications (eg, benzodiazepine receptor agonists) work immediately to improve sleep, and are useful in the short to medium term (generally 1 day to 4 weeks, although some newer agents have potential for use over longer terms), the cognitive and behavioral approaches are useful in the medium to long term (1–2 weeks to at least 2 years).

Nonpharmacologic interventions are not without side effects. Patients using sleep restriction or stimulus control therapy may experience daytime sleepiness in the first few days or weeks of treatment. Patients should be warned about the dangers of driving or operating dangerous equipment while sleepy. The nonpharmacologic interventions are initially more time-consuming and expensive than hypnotic medication (because of clinician's time), but they have longer-term benefits. Unfortunately, few psychologists or other clinicians have training in the nonpharmacologic treatments, so the availability of these interventions is currently limited in many communities.

Clinical considerations

For patients with severe depression, anxiety disorders, or substance abuse problems, the need to receive treatment for those disorders is a priority. Sleep disorders other than insomnia—such as sleep apnea, hypopneas, restless legs syndrome and periodic limb movement disorder—should be screened for and treated if present. Circadian rhythm disorders need to be kept in mind. For example, occasionally a complaint of chronic sleep initiation problems arises from delayed sleep phase syndrome. When sleep is disturbed by nocturnal hot flashes (see article by Polo-Kantola in this issue), treatment directed at the hot flashes themselves can be considered [105]. If the disturbance persists, cognitive and behavioral techniques aimed at reducing the duration of awakenings may be helpful. Insomnia often occurs with medical conditions [106] and, if the direct cause of the problem is treatable (eg, hyperthyroidism, acute pain due to injury), then medical treatment is the first course of action. Of course, sleep difficulty associated with stimulants, such as amphetamines and caffeine, or medications (eg, certain antihypertensives, levothyroxin) needs to be ruled out.

When the patient works on rotating shifts, designing an insomnia treatment protocol can be especially challenging because of the instability of the circadian rhythm of sleep and wakefulness. Circadian rhythms, sleep, and countermeasures to optimize sleep for women working shifts are discussed in the article by Shechter and colleagues in this issue. Also, for individuals who are using such techniques as stimulus control therapy and sleep restriction, vacations and travel to other time zones can complicate and prolong the treatment process. For users of hypnotics, decisions need to be made about whether, when, and how to withdraw from the medication. If the decision is to withdraw, it is preferable to do so in parallel with insomnia-specific cognitive and behavioral treatment. The withdrawal program should be systematic and medically supervised. A withdrawal protocol is outlined by Morin and Espie [87].

Useful areas of future clinical research are the prevention of insomnia; the cotreatment of mothers, infants, and children; the treatment of insomnia with comorbid mental health issues; raising awareness of nonpharmacologic treatments; and making nonpharmacologic treatments available through the health care system [107,108].

Summary

Women are at greater risk of developing insomnia than are men, and the circumstances of pregnancy, childbirth, midlife, and menopause are key times of sleep disturbance. These are opportunities to prevent sleep disruption from transforming into chronic insomnia. For immediate relief of acute insomnia, short-term use of nonbenzodiazepine hypnotics can be helpful. To restore and maintain healthy sleep patterns, several insomnia-specific cognitive and behavioral interventions are recommended. The choice of a specific treatment depends on the nature and duration of insomnia, the presence of medical or mental-health problems, the stage of a woman's life, the availability of the treatments, and personal preference.

Acknowledgments

The author thanks Richard J. Beninger and Brenda Bass for their helpful comments on earlier versions of this manuscript.

References

[1] American Sleep Disorders Association. The International classification of sleep disorders, revised: diagnostic and coding manual. Rochester (MN): American Sleep Disorders Association; 1997.

[2] American Psychiatric Association. Diagnostic and statistical manual of mental disorders. 4th edition. Washington, D.C.: American Psychiatric Association; 1994.

[3] World Health Organization. International statistical classification of diseases and related health problems 10th revision. Version for 2007.

[4] Zammit GK, Weiner J, Damato N, et al. Quality of life in people with insomnia. Sleep 1999;22: S379–85.

[5] Roth T, Ancoli-Israel S. Daytime consequences and correlates of insomnia in the United States: results of the 1991 National Sleep Foundation Survey II. Sleep 1999;22:S354–8.

[6] Ford DE, Kamerow DB. Epidemiologic study of sleep disturbances and psychiatric disorders. J Am Med Assoc 1989;262:1479–84.

[7] Breslau N, Roth T, Rosenthal L, et al. Sleep disturbance and psychiatric disorders: a longitudinal epidemiological study of young adults. Biol Psychiatry 1996;39:411–8.

[8] Roberts RE, Shema SJ, Kaplan G, et al. Sleep complaints and depression in an aging cohort: a prospective perspective. Am J Psychiatry 2000;157:81–8.

[9] Perlis ML, Giles DE, Buysse DJ, et al. Self-reported sleep disturbance as a prodromal symptom in recurrent depression. J Affect Disord 1997;42:209–12.

[10] Simon GE, VonKorff M. Prevalance, burden, and treatment of insomnia in primary care. Am J Psychiatry 1997;154:1417–23.

[11] Weissman MM, Greenwald S, Nino-Murcia G, et al. The morbidity of insomnia uncomplicated by psychiatric disorders. Gen Hosp Psychiatry 1997;19:245–50.

[12] Weyerer S, Dilling H. Prevalence and treatment of insomnia in the community: results from the Upper Bavarian field study. Sleep 1991;14:392–8.

[13] Spielman AJ, Glovinsky PB. Introduction: the varied nature of insomnia. In: Hauri PJ, editor. Case studies in insomnia. New York: Plenum; 1991. p. 1–15.

[14] Pearson NJ, Johnson LL, Nahin RL. Insomnia, trouble sleeping, and complementary and alternative medicine. Arch Intern Med 2006;166: 1775–82.

[15] Leger D, Guilleminault C, Dreyfus JP, et al. Prevalence of insomnia in a survey of 12,778 adults in France. J Sleep Res 2000;9:35–42.

[16] Stewart R, Besset A, Bebbington P, et al. Insomnia comorbidity and impact and hypnotic use by age group in a national survey population aged 16 to 74 years. Sleep 2006;29: 1391–7.

[17] Ohayon MM, Caulet M, Guilleminault C. How a general population perceives its sleep and how this relates to the complaint of insomnia. Sleep 1997;20:715–23.

[18] Morin CM, Leblanc M, Daley M, et al. Epidemiology of insomnia: Prevalence, self-help treatments, consultations, and determinants of help-seeking behaviors. Sleep Med 2006;7: 123–30.

[19] Liljenberg B, Almqvist M, Hetta J, et al. The prevalence of insomnia: the importance of operationally defined criteria. Ann Clin Res 1988;20:393–8.

[20] Ohayon MM. Epidemiology of insomnia: what we know and what we still need to learn. Sleep Med Rev 2002;6:97–111.

[21] Barsky AJ, Peekna HM, Borus JF. Somatic symptom reporting in women and men. J Gen Intern Med 2001;16:266–75.

[22] Soares CN. Insomnia in women: an overlooked epidemic? Arch Womens Ment Health 2005;8: 205–13.

[23] Bastien C, Morin CM. Familial incidence of insomnia. J Sleep Res 2000;9:49–54.

[24] Tjepkema M. Insomnia. Health Reports, Statistics Canada, Catalogue 82-003. 2005;17:9–25.

[25] Espie CA. Insomnia: conceptual issues in the development, maintenance and treatment of sleep disorder in adults. Annu Rev Psychol 2002;53:1–44.

[26] Vgontzas AN, Chrousos GP. Sleep, the hypothalamic-pituitary-adrenal axis, and cytokines: multiple interactions and disturbances in sleep disorders. Endocrinol Metab Clin North Am 2002;31:15–36.

[27] Bastien CH, Vallieres A, Morin CM. Precipitating factors of insomnia. Behav Sleep Med 2004;2:50–62.

[28] Healey ES, Kales A, Monroe LJ, et al. Onset of insomnia: role of life-stress events. Psychosom Med 1981;43(5):439–51.

[29] Morin CM, Rodrigue S, Ivers H. Role of stress, arousal, and coping skills in primary insomnia. Psychosom Med 2003;65:259–67.

[30] Shaver JLF, Johnston SK, Lentz MJ, et al. Stress exposure, psychological distress, and physiological stress activation in midlife women with insomnia. Psychosom Med 2002;64:793–802.

[31] Kageyama T, Kabuto M, Nitta H, et al. A population study on risk factors for insomnia among adult Japanese women: a possible effect of road traffic volume. Sleep 1997;20:963–71.

[32] Meijer AM, van den Wittenboer GLH. Contribution of infants' sleep and crying to marital relationship of first-time parent couples in the 1st year after childbirth. J Fam Psychol 2007;21:49–57.

[33] Meltzer LJ, Mindell JA. Relationship between child sleep disturbances and maternal sleep, mood, and parenting stress: a pilot study. J Fam Psychol 2007;21:67–73.

[34] Shaver JLF, Zenk SN. Sleep disturbance and menopause. J Womens Health Gend Based Med 2000;9:109–18.

[35] Savard J, Davidson JR, Ivers H, et al. The association between nocturnal hot flashes and sleep in breast cancer survivors. J Pain Symptom Manage 2004;27:513–22.

[36] Kloss JD, Tweedy K, Gilrain K. Psychological factors associated with sleep disturbance among perimenopausal women. Behav Sleep Med 2004;2:177–90.

[37] Guilleminault C, Palombini L, Poyares D, et al. Chronic insomnia, postmenopausal women, and sleep disrordered breathing: part 1. Frequency of sleep disordered breathing in a cohort. J Psychosom Res 2002;53:611–5.

[38] Borbely AA. Sleep mechanisms. Sleep Biol Rhythms 2004;2:S67–8.

[39] Robertson JA, Broomfield NM, Espie CA. Prospective comparison of subjective arousal during the pre-sleep period in primary sleep-onset insomnia and normal sleepers. J Sleep Res 2007;16:230–8.

[40] Dolder C, Nelson M, McKinsey J. Use of non-benzodiazepine hypnotics in the elderly. Are all agents the same? CNS Drugs 2007;21:389–405.

[41] Morin CM, Culbert JP, Schwartz SM. Nonpharmacological interventions for insomnia: a meta-analysis of treatment efficacy. Am J Psychiatry 1994;151:1172–80.

[42] Kassam A, Patten SB. Hypnotic use in a population-based sample of over thirty-five thousand interviewed Canadians. Popul Health Metr 2006;4:doi:10.1186/1478-7954-4-15.

[43] Smith MT, Perlis ML, Park A, et al. Comparative meta-analysis of pharmacotherapy and behaviour therapy for persistent insomnia. Am J Psychiatry 2002;159:5–11.

[44] Mendelson WB, Roth T, Cassella J, et al. The treatment of chronic insomnia: drug indications, chronic use and abuse liability. Sleep Med Rev 2004;8:7–17.

[45] Najib J. Eszopiclone, a nonbenzodiazepine sedative-hypnotic agent for the treatment of transient and chronic insomnia. Clin Ther 2006;28:491–516.

[46] Holbrook AM, Crowther R, Lotter A, et al. Meta-analysis of benzodiazephine use in the treatment of insomnia. Can Med Assoc J 2000;162:225–33.

[47] Montplaisir J, Hawa R, Moller H, et al. Zopiclone and zaleplon vs benzodiazepines in the treatment of insomnia: Canadian consensus statement. Hum Psychopharmacol 2003;18:29–38.

[48] Iqbal MM, Sobhan T, Ryals T. Effects of commonly used benzodiazepines on the fetus, the neonate, and the nursing infant. Psychiatr Serv 2002;53:39–49.

[49] Santiago JR, Nolledo MS, Kinzler W, et al. Sleep and sleep disorders in pregnancy. Ann Intern Med 2001;134:396–408.

[50] Glass J, Lanctot KL, Herrmann N, et al. Sedative hypnotics in older people with insomnia: meta-analysis of risks and benefits. Br Med J 2005;331:1169.

[51] Benca R. Diagnosis and treatment of chronic insomnia: a review. Psychiatr Serv 2005;56:332–43.

[52] Swainston Harrison T, Keating GM. Zolpidem: a review of its use in the management of insomnia. CNS Drugs 2005;19:65–89.

[53] Dorsey CM, Lee KA, Scharf MB. Effect of zolpidem on sleep in women with perimenopausal and postmenopausal insomnia: a 4-week, randomized, multicenter, double-blind, placebo-controlled study. Clin Ther 2004;26:1578–86.

[54] Melton ST, Wood JM, Kirkwood CK. Eszopiclone for insomnia. Ann Pharmacother 2005;39:1659–65.

[55] Krystal AD, Walsh JK, Laska E, et al. Sustained efficacy of eszopiclone over 6 months of nightly treatment: results of a randomized, double-blind, placebo-controlled study in

adults with chronic insomnia. Sleep 2003;26: 793–9.

[56] Roth T, Walsh JK, Krystal AD, et al. An evaluation of the efficacy and safety of eszopiclone over 12 months in patients with chronic primary insomnia. Sleep Med 2005;6:487–95.

[57] Hajak G. A comparative assessment of the risks and benefits of zopiclone. A review of 15 years' clinical experience. Drug Saf 1999;21:457–69.

[58] Walsh JK, Krystal AD, Amato DA, et al. Nightly treatment of primary insomnia with eszopiclone for six months: effect on sleep, quality of life, and work limitations. Sleep 2007;30: 959–68.

[59] Diav-Citrin O, Okotore B, Lucarelli K, et al. Pregnancy outcome following first-trimester exposure to zopiclone: a prospective controlled cohort study. Am J Perinatol 1999;16: 157–60.

[60] Wyatt JK, Dijk D-J, Ritz-de Cecco A, et al. Sleep-facilitating effect of exogenous melatonin in healthy young men and women is circadian-phase dependent. Sleep 2006;29:609–18.

[61] Scheer FAJL, Czeisler CA. Melatonin, sleep, and circadian rhythms. Sleep Med Rev 2005;9:5–9.

[62] Burgess HJ, Sharkey KM, Eastman CI. Bright light, dark and melatonin can promote circadian adaptation in night shift workers. Sleep Med Rev 2002;6:407–20.

[63] Revell VL, Eastman CI. How to trick mother nature into letting you fly around or stay up all night. J Biol Rhythms 2005;20:353–65.

[64] Roth T, Seiden D, Sainati S, et al. Effects of ramelteon on patient-reported sleep latency in older adults with chronic insomnia. Sleep Med 2006;7:312–8.

[65] Erman M, Seiden D, Zammit G, et al. An efficacy, safety, and dose-response study of ramelteon in patients with chronic primary insomnia. Sleep Med 2006;7:17–24.

[66] Borja NL, Daniel KL. Ramelteon for the treatment of insomnia. Clin Ther 2006;28:1540–55.

[67] Rozerem (ramelteon) prescribing information. Available at: www.rozerem.com/index.aspx/PI. pdf. Accessed September 9, 2007.

[68] Mendelson WB. A review of the evidence for the efficacy and safety of trazodone in insomnia. J Clin Psychiatry 2005;66:469–76.

[69] Walsh JK, Erman M, Erwin CW, et al. Subjective hypnotic efficacy of trazodone and zolpidem. Hum Psychopharmacol 1998;13:191–8.

[70] Walsh JK, Schweitzer PK. Ten-year trends in the pharmacological treatment of insomnia. Sleep 1999;22:371–5.

[71] James SP, Mendelson WB. The use of trazodone as a hypnotic: a critical review. J Clin Psychiatry 2004;65:752–5.

[72] Kudo Y, Kurihara M. Clinical evaluation of diphenhydramine hydrochloride for the treatment of insomnia in psychiatric patients: a double-blind study. J Clin Pharmacol 1990; 30:1041–8.

[73] Rickels K, Morris RJ, Newman H, et al. Diphenhydramine in insomniac family practice patients: a double-blind study. J Clin Psychiatry 1983;23:235–42.

[74] Morin CM, Koetter U, Bastien C, et al. Valerian hops combination and diphenhydramine for treating insomnia: a randomized placebo-controlled clinical trial. Sleep 2005;28:1465–71.

[75] Halpert AG, Olmstead MC, Beninger RJ. Mechanisms and abuse liability of the anti-histamine dimenhydrinate. Neurosci Biobehav Rev 2002; 26:61–7.

[76] Richardson GS, Roehrs TA, Rosenthal L, et al. Tolerance to daytime sedative effects of H antihistamines. J Clin Pharmacol 2002;22: 511–5.

[77] Wheatley D. Medicinal plants for insomnia: a review of their pharmacology, efficacy and tolerability. J Psychopharmacol 2005;19:414–21.

[78] Meoli AL, Rosen C, Kristo D, et al. Oral nonprescription treatment for insomnia: an evaluation of products with limited evidence. J Clin Sleep Med 2005;1:173–87.

[79] Taibi DM, Landis CA, Petry H, et al. A systematic review of valerian as a sleep aid: safe but not effective. Sleep Med Rev 2007;11:209–30.

[80] Morin CM, Gaulier B, Barry T, et al. Patients' acceptance of psychological and pharmacological therapies for insomnia. Sleep 1992;15:302–5.

[81] Morin CM, Colecchi C, Stone J, et al. Behavioral and pharmacological therapies for late-life insomnia. A randomized controlled trial. J Am Med Assoc 1999;281:991–9.

[82] Aber R, Webb WB. Effects of a limited nap on night sleep in older subjects. Psychol Aging 1986;1:300–2.

[83] Aschoff J. Naps as integral parts of the wake time within the human sleep-wake cycle. J Biol Rhythms 1994;9:145–55.

[84] Morin CM, Bootzin RR, Buysse DJ, et al. Psychological and behavioral treatment of insomnia: update of the recent evidence (1998–2004). Sleep 2006;29:1398–414.

[85] Lai H-L, Good M. Music improves sleep quality in older adults. J Adv Nurs 2005;49:234–44.

[86] Johnson JE. The use of music to promote sleep in older women. J Community Health Nurs 2003;20:27–35.

[87] Morin CM, Espie CA. Insomnia: a clinical guide to assessment and treatment. New York: Kluwer Academic / Plenum Publishers; 2003.

[88] Riedel BW, Lichstein KL. Insomnia and daytime functioning. Sleep Med Rev 2000;4:277–98.

[89] Murtagh DRR, Greenwood KM. Identifying effective psychological treatments for insomnia: a meta-analysis. J Consult Clin Psychol 1995; 63:79–89.

[90] Morgenthaler T, Kramer M, Alessi C, et al. Practice parameters for the psychological and behavioural treatment of insomnia: an update. An American Academy of Sleep Medicine report. Sleep 2006;29:1415–9.

[91] Schoicket SL, Bertelson AD, Lacks P. Is sleep hygiene a sufficient treatment for sleep-maintenance insomnia? Behav Ther 1988;19: 183–90.

[92] Engle-Friedman M, Bootzin RR, Hazlewood L, et al. An evaluation of behavioral treatments for insomnia in the older adult. J Clin Psychol 1992;48:77–90.

[93] Cheek RE, Shaver JL, Lentz MJ. Lifestyle practices and nocturnal sleep in midlife women with and without insomnia. Biol Res Nurs 2004;6:46–58.

[94] Vallieres A, Bastien CH, Ouellet M, et al. Cognitive-behaviour therapy for insomnia associated with anxiety or depression [abstract]. Sleep 2000;23(Suppl 2):A311.

[95] Bastien C, Morin C, Ouellet M-C, et al. Cognitive-behavioral therapy for insomnia: comparison of individual therapy, group therapy, and telephone consultations. J Consult Clin Psychol 2004;72:653–9.

[96] Strom L, Pettersson R, Andersson G. Internet-based treatment for insomnia: A controlled evaluation. J Consult Clin Psychol 2004;72:113–20.

[97] Morin CM, Beaulieu-Bonneau S, Leblanc M, et al. Self-help treatment for insomnia: A randomized controlled trial. Sleep 2005;28:1319–27.

[98] Irwin MR, Cole JC, Nicassio PM. Comparative meta-analysis of behavioral interventions for insomnia and their efficacy in middle-aged adults and in older adults 55+ years of age. Health Psychol 2006;25:3–14.

[99] Smith MT, Huang MI, Manber R. Cognitive behavior therapy for chronic insomnia occurring within the context of medical and psychiatric disorders. Clin Psychol Rev 2005; 25:559–92.

[100] National Institute of Health State of the Science Conference statement; manifestations and management of chronic insomnia in adults. Sleep 2005;28:1049–57.

[101] Currie SR, Wilson KG, Pontefract AJ, et al. Cognitive-behavioral treatment of insomnia secondary to chronic pain. J Consult Clin Psychol 2000;68:407–16.

[102] Savard J, Simard S, Ivers H, et al. Randomized study of the efficacy of cognitive-behavioural therapy for insomnia secondary to breast cancer, Part I: sleep and psychological effects. Am J Clin Oncol 2005;23:6083–96.

[103] Morawetz D. Insomnia and depression: Which comes first? Sleep Res Online 2003;5:77–81.

[104] Dashevsky B, Kramer M. Behavioral treatment of chronic insomnia in psychiatrically ill patients. J Clin Psychiatry 1998;59:693–9.

[105] Hickey M, Davis SR, Sturdee DW. Treatment of menopausal symptoms: What shall we do now? Lancet 2005;366:409–21.

[106] Taylor DJ, Mallory LJ, Lichstein KL, et al. Comorbidity of chronic insomnia with medical problems. Sleep 2007;30:213–8.

[107] Espie CA, Inglis SJ, Tessier S, et al. The clinical effectiveness of cognitive behaviour therapy for chronic insomnia: implementation and evaluation of a sleep clinic in general medical practice. Behav Res Ther 2001;39:45–60.

[108] Davidson JR, Feldman-Stewart D, Brennenstuhl S, et al. How to provide insomnia interventions to people with cancer: insights from patients. Psychooncology 2007;16(11):1028–38.

ELSEVIER
SAUNDERS

SLEEP
MEDICINE
CLINICS

Sleep Med Clin 3 (2008) 121–131

Dealing with Menopausal Sleep Disturbances

Päivi Polo-Kantola, MD, PhD[a,b,*]

- Characteristics of the climacterium
- Female sex hormones and the brain
- Menopause and sleep disturbance
  Vasomotor symptoms
- The effect of hormone therapy on sleep
- Treatment of sleep disturbances during menopause

- Sleep-disordered breathing
- Other sleep disorders during menopause
- Summary
- References

During the climacterium, or menopausal transition, women are at increased susceptibility for several symptoms that significantly reduce their quality of life. Among these are sleep problems, including insomnia and/or nocturnal breathing disturbances. The symptoms of menopausal insomnia are often identical to those of general insomnia, with trouble falling asleep, frequent awakenings, or awakening too early in the morning [1,2]. However, the most typical symptoms of menopausal insomnia are nocturnal awakenings. Because menopausal insomnia may result from climacteric symptoms, it is normally considered secondary insomnia. However, a direct hormonal effect in the brain is also plausible. Treatment with hormone therapy normally eliminates, or at least alleviates, the symptoms. The situation is more complicated for women with insomnia before menopause. For these women, the climacterium causes the quality of sleep to further deteriorate. This co-occurrence presents a challenge for the clinician and, although hormone therapy often gives benefit, other treatment options have to be considered.

After menopause, nocturnal breathing problems also increase. Although sleep apnea occurs more often in men than in women, women are prone to partial upper-airway obstruction, a frequently undiagnosed condition. The adverse consequences of sleep-related breathing disturbances, such as fatigue, sleepiness, irritability, mood disorders, memory impairment, lack of concentration, and reduced daytime functioning, may lead to social impairment, work-related difficulties, and significantly decreased overall quality of life [3]. These symptoms are often the reason a woman eventually seeks clinical assistance.

This review illustrates the effects of the climacterium on sleep and related events and evaluates different treatment options. Aging is briefly discussed with a focus on the menopausal transition and related changes in biological functions.

Characteristics of the climacterium

Menopause, the time when menstruation ceases naturally or surgically, results in a variety of

[a] Department of Obstetrics and Gynecology, University Central Hospital of Turku, Kiinamyllykatu 4-8, SF-20520 Turku, Finland
[b] Sleep Research Center Dentalia, University of Turku, FIN-20520 Turku, Finland
* Department of Obstetrics and Gynecology, University Central Hospital of Turku, Kiinamyllykatu 4-8, SF-20520 Turku, Finland.
E-mail address: paivi.polo-kantola@tyks.fi

doi:10.1016/j.jsmc.2007.10.006

physiologic changes due to altered hormonal status [4,5]. The age range for natural menopause is from 45 to 55 years with an average age of 51 to 52 years [6]. Perimenopause is the period of time from the first signs of approaching menopause until 12 months of permanent amenorrhea, when the exact time of menopause can be determined. Postmenopause starts when menopause is diagnosed [7]. The climacterium covers the perimenopause through to the postmenopausal period when climacteric symptoms occur.

Hallmark symptoms during the climacterium comprise hot flashes and sweating, globally termed "vasomotor symptoms" [8]. Hot flashes are described as short transient and recurrent episodes of flushing and redness, and sensations of warmth or even intense heat, typically on the upper body, neck, and face. They vary from mild to severe in intensity and low to high in frequency in individual women. An increase in peripheral vasodilatation, skin temperature, and moisture can be demonstrated by measurements of skin conductance, thermograms, or plethysmography [9–11]. Hot flashes often couple with sweating and are followed by evaporative skin cooling and shivering. When present during the night, these symptoms often disturb sleep and may result in somatic, mental, or cognitive problems [12–14]. Approximately 75% of postmenopausal women and 40% of perimenopausal women suffer from vasomotor symptoms [13,15]. As with symptom severity, the duration of symptoms varies among individuals. Generally the occurrence of vasomotor symptoms is 1 to 2 years, but about 25% of women report them for 5 years and 9% experience them practically all their lifetime after menopause [16,17].

During the climacterium, other symptoms, both physical and mental, may appear. Palpitations, closely related to vasomotor symptoms as additional signs of autonomic nervous system dysfunction, are disturbing both during the daytime and at night [18]. During this period, many women also experience headaches, dizziness, deterioration in postural balance, numbness, muscle and joint pain, dry eyes and mouth, and reduced skin elasticity. These symptoms are often related to menopause, but do not necessarily correlate to the absolute estrogen levels [18]. Vaginal dryness, nocturia, and other urinary tract symptoms are female sex-hormone dependent and clearly get worse after menopause, typically with a latency of some years [18]. Mental symptoms, such as anxiety, depression, a decline in libido, lack of concentration, and memory impairment occur, and these symptoms may even surpass the severity of vasomotor symptoms. Furthermore, sleep problems are common, arising as distinct symptoms or more typically in addition to other climacteric symptoms [14]. Mental symptoms are reported in 50% to 80% of menopausal women. Similarly, 50% to 80% of menopausal women have sleep problems [13,19].

Female sex hormones and the brain

Menopause is associated with decreased plasma concentration of the endogenous female sex steroids, estrogen, and progesterone [4,5]. These hormones are mainly secreted by ovaries under hypothalamic-pituitary regulation predominately through the actions of follicle-stimulating hormone and luteinizing hormone [4]. At menopause, secretion of androgens also declines. Because female sex hormones, especially estrogen, have complex effects in the central nervous system (CNS), changes during menopause may cause, or at least contribute to, dysfunction in numerous brain functions, including sleep, mood, and cognitive performance [20–22].

In the brain, estrogen has fast-acting and short-duration "nongenomic" as well as slow-acting and long-lasting "genomic" actions [23,24]. Nongenomic mechanisms include an increase in excitability of neurons, activation of intracellular signaling pathways, modulation of proteins, and protection against neuronal damage [23]. At least two estrogen receptors (ER) that belong to the nuclear hormone receptor family are involved. ERα is the dominant receptor in the uterus, while ERβ is expressed at high levels in other estrogen target tissues, such as the ovary, testis, prostate, and vascular endothelium [24]. These ovarian steroid receptors are found in numerous brain areas, such as the cortex, hippocampus, hypothalamus, amygdala, basal forebrain, midbrain raphe nuclei, pituitary gland, locus coeruleus, and cerebellum [23–25], which are areas involved in sleep regulation [26].

Sex steroids have an affect on several neurotransmitter systems. In climacteric symptomatology, cholinergic, serotonergic, dopaminergic, and noradrenergic systems are crucial [27]. An imbalance, particularly in levels of serotonin and noradrenalin in the hypothalamic thermoregulatory centers, followed by a reduction in circulating estrogen has been suggested to result in hot flashes [11,28]. Also, glutamate, γ-aminobutric acid, opiate, and vasopressin systems, as well as insulinlike growth factor 1, transforming growth factor alpha, cyclic adenosine monophosphate, protein kinase activators, and various other neurotransmitters presumably are involved [29]. These neurotransmitters are also important for sleep [26]. Thus, the disturbance in their secretion or actions associated with menopausal changes may contribute to sleep problems.

Although changes in CNS-related circadian hormones, such as growth hormone, prolactin, cortisol, or melatonin, are age-dependent, menopause and decreased estrogen levels may add to the alterations [29]. These hormones are also involved in sleep regulation. After menopause, diurnal growth hormone and prolactin levels decrease [30,31], while cortisol levels increase [32]. Unopposed estrogen therapy induces an increase in growth hormone [33,34]. However, studies on the effects of estrogen therapy with combined hormone therapy have produced conflicting results [30,35,36]. The diurnal secretion of prolactin is higher in younger women than in postmenopausal women [37] and estrogen therapy with or without progestagen has been suggested to elevate serum prolactin [38]. Studies on the effect of hormone therapy on cortisol levels are inconclusive, showing a reduction [39,40], an increase [41,42], or no effect [39,40].

Menopause and sleep disturbance

In sleep surveys, women of all age groups report noticeably more sleep problems than men do [43–45]. After 50 years of age, around menopause, moderate insomnia is reported by 25% of women and severe insomnia by 15% [44]. The task of determining whether sleep problems are of menopausal origin or just coincident with the menopausal period is complex because several changes that are often age-related and that affect sleep also take place at the same time. Among these are respiratory disorders and cardiovascular, neurological, and endocrinological diseases. Further, pain, mood disorders, psychosocial factors, and medications may contribute or even cause sleep disorders. However, regardless of origin, menopause and the associated climacteric symptoms may essentially worsen these sleep problems.

The gradual cessation of hormonal secretion by the ovaries is heralded by irregularities in menstruation and the onset of climacteric symptoms. Sleep may be affected during this perimenopausal period. Sometimes sleep problems are the first symptoms of approaching menopause. Compared with premenopausal women, perimenopausal women report more frequent and longer arousals resulting in significantly less sleep. Several studies have confirmed the increase of sleep problems in the menopausal transition. In a study with 1000 women, the odds ratio for sleep problems, after controlling for age, was 1.5 in postmenopausal women compared with menstruating women [46]. Kuh and colleagues [47] found that the risk for sleep disturbance was 1.5 in perimenopausal women and 3.4 in postmenopausal women compared with premenopausal women in a population of over 1200

responders. In the multicenter Survey of Women's Health Across the Nation (SWAN) [48], odds ratios for sleep problems were 1.6 for postmenopausal and 1.3 for perimenopausal women compared with premenopausal women. According to an early study of 100 climacteric women recruited from a menopausal clinic, almost 80% suffered from insomnia and 90% experienced fatigue. Typical complaints were waking too early in the morning and intermittent sleep [49].

Vasomotor symptoms

Climacterically symptomatic women often report sleep problems, especially insomnia, which is typically evident in vasomotorically symptomatic but also mentally symptomatic women [13,48–52]. A study including over 5000 women showed a relationship between insomnia and vasomotor symptoms [13]. In the SWAN study with 12,600 women, an odds ratio for sleep problems in women with climacteric symptoms was 2.0 compared with asymptomatic women [48]. Baker and colleagues [51] reported an association between sleep disturbance and climacteric mood changes.

The evidence from clinical practice has confirmed the association between climacteric vasomotor symptoms and sleep problems. Symptomatic women describe their nocturnal activities as follows: Falling asleep is aggravated because of perspiration or palpitation; sleep is interrupted by frequent awakenings caused by sweating followed by shivering, necessitating a change in bedclothes. Despite these clear clinical observations, studies with objective measurements do not entirely support these associations. Thurston and colleagues [53] conducted a study involving symptomatic peri- and postmenopausal women. Hot flashes were measured with skin conductance, and women kept a sleep diary to subjectively track vasomotor symptoms and sleep quality. Although subjective hot flashes and sleep problems were connected, no association between measured hot flashes during sleep and sleep problems were found. Findings about the relationship between objectively measured sleep quality (with polysomnography, actigraphy, or quantitative analysis of electroencephalogram) and climacteric symptoms are also controversial. Most of the studies evaluated the effects of vasomotor symptoms on objective sleep quality measured by polysomnography while relying on subjective sensations of symptoms [50,52,54–56]. Apparently, because of the different research techniques and variety in severity of vasomotor symptoms, the results have been equivocal. Shaver and colleagues [50] reported more time in bed and longer rapid eye movement (REM) latency in symptomatic women compared with asymptomatic women. Erlik and colleagues [54] showed that hot flashes caused arousals. Three other studies could not distinguish any specific abnormalities in polysomnography in connection with climacteric symptoms [52,55,56].

Some polysomnography studies have included objective measures of vasomotor symptoms. Freedman and colleagues [57–60] conducted a series of studies to evaluate the effect of objectively measured hot flashes (by skin conductance or core body temperature) on objectively measured sleep quality. One of their first studies showed that vasomotor symptoms disrupted sleep by causing nocturnal awakenings, increasing sleep stage changes, and lowering sleep efficiency [57]. Subsequently, when comparing symptomatic postmenopausal women with asymptomatic or premenopausal women, no correlation between symptoms and objective sleep quality was found [58]. More recent studies by the same research group concluded that hot flashes presumably interfere with sleep quality in the first half but not in the second half of the night, when REM sleep predominates and hot flashes and associated arousals and awakenings are suppressed [59,60].

The effect of hormone therapy on sleep

The concept of hormone therapy[1] was first explored in the late nineteenth century [61]. The main indication for taking hormone therapy today is to relieve climacteric symptoms, especially vasomotor symptoms [8,19,61,62]. Epidemiological as well as clinical studies have demonstrated the protective effect of hormone therapy against osteoporosis and bone fractures [63]. Although controversial, data also suggest a cardio-protective effect of hormone therapy if initiated at menopause [64]. Because of the side effects, fear of adverse events, and an increased risk of breast cancer, compliance with hormone therapy is low and over 50% of women stop therapy after 1 year [61]. Because complications associated with hormone therapy are mainly connected with high doses, long duration of treatment, and use in older women [8,65], recommendations for therapy call for treatment for as short a time period as possible with the lowest effective dose.

Controlled studies evaluating the effect of hormone therapy on climacteric symptoms have usually also assessed the effect on subjective sleep quality [13,19,62,65–68]. Six months of estrogen therapy alleviated sleep problems in 95% of symptomatic women in a study with over 200 postmenopausal women [19]. In another study with over 220 postmenopausal women, 12 weeks of hormone substitution resulted in a significant reduction of sleep disturbance [66]. Low-dose hormone therapy has been shown to be effective as well [68]. In a study with 50 postmenopausal women, sleep problems for women treated with low-dose hormone therapy were alleviated after 6 weeks and improved further after 12 weeks compared with sleep problems of women in a control group.

Sixty-three postmenopausal women, both vasomotorically symptomatic and asymptomatic, where recruited for a 7-month study to evaluate the effect of hormone therapy on various sleep problems [67]. Compared to placebo, estrogen facilitated falling asleep and decreased nocturnal restlessness and awakenings, as well as decreased tiredness in the morning and during the daytime. The degree of improvement in vasomotor symptoms was an important predictor for the degree of improvement in sleep disturbance. Nevertheless, the vasomotorically asymptomatic women who experienced at least some degree of insomnia also reported improved sleep quality with estrogen therapy. A recent large study, the Women's Health Initiative, assessed the long-term effects of hormone therapy on the quality of life in asymptomatic or low symptomatic women and confirmed the beneficial effect of hormone therapy on sleep quality [65].

Researchers say the improved sleep quality after hormone therapy in vasomotorically symptomatic women stems from the elimination of vasomotor symptoms [62,67]. For asymptomatic women, the improvement in sleep may be explained by one of two reasons. One explanation is that these women may not be asymptomatic at all. Rather they may underestimate, or poorly perceive, their vasomotor symptoms. The hormone therapy eliminates these poorly perceived symptoms, resulting in improved sleep. The other explanation is that female sex hormones introduced with hormone therapy have potent direct CNS effects that may improve sleep [27].

Although studies of the effect of hormone therapy on subjective sleep quality are consistent, the findings using objective measurements are less so. Hormone therapy has been found to increase REM sleep [69–71], to reduce awakening [54,69,72,73], and to decrease nocturnal wakefulness during the entire night [69,74] or in the first sleep cycle [71]. In addition, a shortening of sleep latency [70,75], an improvement in sleep efficiency [72,74], and a reduction of the rate of cyclic

---

[1]Because sleep studies have been conducted with various drug compounds, hormone therapy here means estrogen and progesterone therapy or estrogen therapy alone unless otherwise specified.

alternating patterns of sleep [72] have also been shown. Other studies have found no effect of hormone therapy on polysomnography sleep measures [76–78]. Furthermore, in an observational study without a placebo group, postmenopausal hormone-therapy users, compared with nonusers, had less slow-wave sleep, more stage 1 sleep, and more fragmented sleep [55]. Thus, postmenopausal hormone-therapy users had worse sleep quality compared with nonusers.

Because of disparities in design, subject recruitment, and treatment administration (form, dose, and duration) in previous studies relating hormone therapy with sleep, conclusions on the effect of hormone therapy on objectively measured sleep quality are difficult to determine. Some studies have enrolled both peri- and postmenopausal women without hormone level measurements [69] or both naturally and surgically menopausal women [70]. Thus bias may result because of a wide age range or differences in biological changes and clinical symptoms in natural and surgical menopause [79]. Also, the follow-up in prospective studies has been short, from 4 weeks to 7 months, and investigations into the possible long-term effects of hormone therapy are lacking. Self-selected use of hormone therapy in observational studies [55,75] might also have influenced the inconclusive outcomes. The ambiguity among findings in objective sleep studies calls into question the value of the techniques employed in hormone therapy studies. In clinical practice, assessment of subjective sleep quality by questionnaires is more suitable and cost-effective. However, sleep laboratory studies may be needed to ascertain possible underlying sleep disorders, such as sleep apnea and narcolepsy, or sleep movement disorders as a contributing factors to, or root causes of, patients' insomnia.

Treatment of sleep disturbances during menopause

Because climacteric insomnia is complex, amelioration or alleviation of the symptoms is challenging. In women with climacteric vasomotor symptoms, the cornerstone of management is hormone therapy. Hormone therapy is generally acknowledged as the most effective therapy for reducing climacteric vasomotor symptoms and related secondary insomnia [13,19,62,65–68]. Moreover, women whose insomnia is apparently related to mood symptoms benefit from hormone therapy as do some women with insomnia but without vasomotor symptoms [67]. The window for initiation of hormone therapy is critical. Treatment should be started when entering menopause, not after a delay of a year or more. Lowest effective doses should be employed and

the need for treatment reevaluated annually [8]. As an additional precaution, breast mammography with at least two dimensions should be performed every second year and women should be reminded to self-screen by palpating the breast. If after a few months of hormone therapy there has been no symptom relief, or if symptoms and signs suggest other underlying causes, further medical examinations are necessary. In women over 60 years old, the vascular side effects of hormone therapy must be considered [65] and thus, for these women, the treatment is not recommended.

In women who seek treatment but prefer to avoid hormone therapy or for whom hormone therapy is contraindicated, treatments that directly target the thermoregulatory mechanism may be an option. A large body of literature has indicated that noradrenalin and serotonin have a central role in the pathophysiology of hot flashes [28]. Thus clonidine, an α_2 adrenergic agonist [28,80], or serotonin-reuptake inhibitors (SSRIs) [28] have been found to alleviate climacteric symptoms and, accordingly, related sleep problems. As discussed below, an improvement of nocturnal breathing has been reported as well. However, the most important side effect, weight gain, may restrict the use of SSRIs. Also, the antiepileptic drug gabapentin has been shown to have a benefit [28], although adverse events, such as dizziness, rash, or weight gain, often result in the discontinuation of the treatment.

Estrogens in plants, the phytoestrogens, have varying degrees of selectivity for ERα and ERβ [24] and there is evidence that diets rich in unrefined grains, vegetables, and fruits are associated with lower risk of diabetes, inflammatory diseases, and cardiovascular diseases [81]. Although controversial, dietary isofavones, a type of phytoestrogen found in soy and red clover, may alleviate vasomotor symptoms [82]. Dietary isofavones can be tested individually, taking into account the safeness of these treatments, though caution is advised in women at high risk for breast cancer. Some women evidently require hypnotic therapy, which should be used for short periods, and is discussed in more detail in the article by Davidson in this issue.

Essential for good sleep quality is good sleep hygiene as noted in the article by Davidson in this issue. A dark, quiet room with a comfortable bed is important. If a woman has vasomotor symptoms, low ambient temperature is often helpful, and lightweight bedclothes may be more comfortable. Daytime napping as well as irregular bedtimes should be avoided. Beverages (tea, coffee, some soft drinks and herbal drinks), smoking, and alcohol intake before bedtime may interfere with, or cause, sleep disruption [83] and thus should be restricted, at least in the evening. Relaxation therapies or cognitive sleep therapy help to improve sleep.

Sleep-disordered breathing

Nocturnal breathing disorders increase around menopause because of several contributing factors, mostly structural but also physiological. After menopause, body fat composition changes, leading in particular to increases in the waist/hip ratio and neck circumference [84], either of which may impair breathing. Further, the decrease in female sex hormones, particularly progesterone, may partly be responsible for nocturnal breathing disorders [85] because progesterone has respiratory stimulant properties [86,87] and affects genioglossus muscle tone [88]. The lack of estrogen has indirect importance in breathing as well because progesterone receptors are estrogen-dependent. An overview on the effects of estrogen and progesterone on sleep-related breathing is provided in the article by Edwards and Sullivan in this issue.

The obstructive sleep apnea syndrome (OSAS) is distinguished by repeated episodes of upper-airway narrowing or closure, increased breathing efforts, snoring, and arousals. The symptoms of OSAS include snoring, witnessed apneas, daytime sleepiness, and morning headaches, which are typical symptoms in men, whereas women have more symptoms of morning headaches and depression as reviewed by Banno and Kryger in this issue. Previously, OSAS has been considered a male disease. However, based on more recent literature, prevalence in men ranges 3% to 7.5% and in women 2% to 3% [89]. When lower criteria of obstructive sleep apnea are considered, 28% of the adult population may be affected [90]. The large data set of the Wisconsin Sleep Cohort study [84] showed that the male/female ratio in OSAS was 3:1 and that the prevalence of sleep-disordered breathing in women aged 30 to 60 years was 9%. In a study of a group of women aged 40 to 59 years, both pre- and postmenopausal, OSAS occurred in 2.5% [91] and among 1000 postmenopausal women enrolled from general population, 3.9% had OSAS [92].

In late menopause, partial upper-airway obstruction—characterized as hypoventilation and carbon dioxide retention—seems to be a more common nocturnal breathing disorder than sleep apnea in women [93]. Symptoms in nocturnal upper-airway obstruction are similar to those of sleep apnea, including heavy snoring, daytime sleepiness, sweating, morning headache, nocturia, lack of energy, cognitive difficulties, and mental symptoms. Sometimes differentiation from climacteric symptoms is also difficult, which may delay diagnosis.

In a study with 63 postmenopausal women from the general population, significant partial upper-airway obstruction was found in 17% but OSAS only in 1.5% [94].

The most effective therapy for OSAS or partial upper-airway obstruction is continuous positive airway pressure [95]. However, compliance with using the device varies from 40% to 80% [96]. While surgical options in OSAS have decreased, various drugs have been investigated [97]. Serotoninergic drugs, SSRIs, and 5-hydroxytryptamine receptor antagonists have been shown to play roles in the neurochemical control of the upper airway. For instance, a reduction of the apnea/hypopnea index (AHI) by up to 50% has been reported with mirtatzapine [98].

The therapeutic action of hormone therapy after menopause has also been considered, with conflicting outcomes. Improvement of nocturnal breathing, especially reduced AHI, with hormone therapy has been found in some [76,92,99] but not all studies [100]. A placebo-controlled crossover study with unopposed estrogen found only little improvement in nocturnal breathing problems in a general population [93], while in a pilot study with hormone therapy but no placebo group a decrease in AHI was seen in OSAS patients [101].

Progestin (medroxyprogesterone acetate [MPA]) has been used in studies evaluating the effect of progestin on breathing. The dosages of MPA in these trials have been higher than those in conventional menopausal hormone therapy treatment. A decrease in duration of apneas [102] as well as an improvement in ventilation [103] has been shown. However, because the studies using hormone therapy or progesterone alone are limited and were conducted mainly without placebo groups, and because the results of those studies conflict somewhat, no definite recommendation of hormone therapy as an option for sleep-disordered breathing can be made.

Other sleep disorders during menopause

Although sleep problems significantly increase around menopause, the causal connection is not always evident. Several factors, such as depressed mood, stress, behavioral or cognitive factors, systemic diseases, and medications, as well as restless legs syndrome (RLS) and periodic limb movement syndrome (PLMS), may explain the symptoms while the menopausal state is only coincident and possibly causes further decreases in sleep quality.

Affective symptoms and mood disorders typically cause sleep disturbances. According to a United States survey, 24% of patients with insomnia and 28% with hypersomnia have a diagnosis of anxiety disorders [104]. The relationship with depression s even more obvious because 69% of depressed patients complain about sleep difficulties [105]. Women report mood symptoms, especially depression, anxiety, and lack of initiative, more frequently than men do [106,107]. The influence of hormonal fluctuations is conceivable because mood symptoms have been connected to the female reproductive lifespan, including the premenstrual, as reviewed by Baker and colleagues in this issue, postpartum, as reviewed in the article by Sloan in this issue, and climacterium periods. In menopausal clinics, 70% to 90% of women report depressive symptoms [49]. Several studies have reported a relationship between mood symptoms and sleep disturbance in peri- and postmenopausal women [51,52,108]. However, detrimental factors totally unconnected to hormonal state may influence mood during menopause. Depressive symptoms may stem from an unsatisfying social life, unemployment, or health problems, or from being separated, divorced, or widowed [109]. As sleep quality is sensitive to mood disturbances, sleep problems may be the first sign of low affect. Although early morning awakening typically originates from depressive mood, difficulties in falling asleep or sleep disruption may occur.

Several systemic diseases increase during the menopausal transition [110]. Although they are mainly due to aging or other existing risk factors, lack of endogenous female sex hormones may play a role. Furthermore, a decrease takes place not only in sex hormones, but also in the secretion of other endogenous hormones, such as thyrotropin. About 25% of postmenopausal women show clinical or subclinical thyroid disease, which often causes symptoms similar to those of the climacteric [111]. Among postmenopausal women, fibromyalgia, which almost always causes insomnia, is common, as discussed in the article by Shaver in this issue. Pulmonary diseases, especially asthma; heart disease; gastrointestinal disease, such as gastroesophageal reflux; renal failure; rheumatic diseases; and muscular and joint pains; as well as neurological diseases, such as Parkinson's and Alzheimer's diseases, may be involved. Several medications may cause insomnia. These include stimulating antidepressants, CNS stimulants, antiepileptic drugs, antihypertensives, diuretics, bronchodilators, corticosteroids, and thyroid hormones. The response is individual and may depend on the dose or time of administration [110].

RLS and PLMS are considered as parallel movement disorders with disparity in timing. RLS occurs during wakefulness, intensifying in the evening, whereas PLMS takes place while asleep. Characteristics of RLS are unpleasant sensations, typically in the limbs, which provokes an overwhelming urge to move them. In PLMS, rapid movements recur with short intervals (about every 20 seconds). Prevalence rates of these movement disorders slightly increase with age [112] and, according to recent studies, a female predominance is suggested [113]. RLS occurs in 5% to 15% of the adult population and PLMS in 30% to 45% [26]. RLS and PLMS are idiopathic with a high genetic predisposition or secondary, for example, to iron metabolism, magnesium decency, renal failure, peripheral neuropathies, or the use of drugs, especially CNS stimulants and dopamine antagonists. As estrogen has been suggested to have dopaminergic actions, an effect of estrogen on these syndromes is probable. Further, RLS and PLMS are more frequent during pregnancy [114], as described in the article by Sloan in this issue, and even in multiple pregnancies [115] with high estrogen levels. However, studies in this field are few. One study with 62 postmenopausal women on estrogen therapy showed no effect on the frequency of PLMS [116]. Aging, rather than menopause or a decrease in female sex hormones, seems to be responsible on these nocturnal movement disorders.

Summary

Menopause and related climacteric symptoms often cause, or exacerbate, sleep disturbances. Subjective symptoms have not been systematically corroborated with objective findings, possibly because the measurement tools have not been refined to detect what may be subtle changes. According to subjective reports, hormone therapy considerably improves sleep quality. However, the reports are ambiguous about the effect of hormone therapy on the quality of sleep when measured objectively. Hormone therapy is thus the first-line therapy for menopausal sleep problems, especially if other climacteric symptoms are also present. Initiating effective treatment around the menopausal transition leads to the best therapeutic result. In addition, hormone therapy prevents osteoporosis and probably also cardiovascular diseases when started in menopause.

Postmenopausal sleep disturbances may be part of an aging process and have no specific root cause related to steroid hormones. In aging, breathing or movement disorders (RLS, PLMS) increase. Whether hormone therapy may improve these conditions is unclear. However, using hormone therapy simultaneously does not appear to worsen the disorders. To conclude, women in general report significant improvement in sleep quality with hormone therapy. However, if such therapy does not bring relief within a few months, further medical assessments are warranted.

References

[1] American Sleep Disorders Association: Diagnostic Classification Steering Committee. International classification of sleep disorders. Diagnostic and coding manual. Rochester (MN); 1990.

[2] American Psychiatric Association. Diagnostic and statistical manual of mental disorders. 4th edition. Washington, DC, USA: APA; 1993.

[3] Moul DE, Nofzinger EA, Pilkonis PA, et al. Symptom reports in severe chronic insomnia. Sleep 2002;25:553–63.

[4] Speroff L. The menopause. A signal for the future. In: Lobo RA, editor. Treatment of the postmenopausal woman: basic and clinical aspects. New York: Raven Press Ltd; 1994. p. 1–8.

[5] Wise PM, Krajnak KM, Kashon ML. Menopause: the aging of multiple pacemakers. Science 1996; 273:67–70.

[6] McKinlay SM, Brambilla BJ, Posner JG. The normal menopausal transition. Maturitas 1992;14: 103–15.

[7] World Health Organization (WHO) Scientific Group. In: Research on the menopause in the 1990s. Geneva; 1996. p. 12–21.

[8] International Menopause Society. IMS updated recommendations on postmenopausal hormone therapy. Climacteric 2007;10:181–94.

[9] Sturdee DW, Reece BL. Thermography of menopausal hot flushes. Maturitas 1979;1:201–5.

[10] Freedman RR. Physiology of hot flashes. Am J Hum Biol 2001;13:453–64.

[11] Freedman RR. Pathophysiology and treatment of menopausal hot flashes. Semin Reprod Med 2005;23(2):117–25.

[12] Collins A, Landgren BM. Reproductive health, use of estrogen and experience of symptoms in perimenopausal women: a population based study. Maturitas 1994;20:101–11.

[13] Oldenhave A, Jaszmann LJ, Haspels AA, et al. Impact of climacteric on well-being. A survey based on 5213 women 39 to 60 years old. Am J Obstet Gynecol 1993;168:772–80.

[14] Moe KE. Hot flashes and sleep in women. Sleep Med Rev 2004;8:487–97.

[15] Guttuso T, Kurlan R, McDermott M, et al. Gabapentin's effects on hot flashes in postmenopausal women: a randomized controlled trial. Am J Obstet Gynecol 2003; 101(2):337–45.

[16] Belchetz PE. Drug therapy: hormonal treatment of postmenopausal women. N Engl J Med 1994;330:1062–71.

[17] Rodstrom K, Bengtsson C, Lissner L, et al. A longitudinal study of the treatment of hot flushes: the population study of women in Gothenburg during a quarter of the century. Menopause 2002;9:156–61.

[18] Milsom I. Menopause-related symptoms and their treatment. In: Erkkola R, editor. The menopause. Elsevier; 2006. p. 9–16.

[19] Erkkola R, Holma P, Järvi T, et al. Transdermal oestrogen replacement therapy in a Finnish population. Maturitas 1991;13:275–81.

[20] Toran-Allerand CD. Novel sites and mechanisms of oestrogen action in the brain. Novartis Found Symp 2000;230:56–69.

[21] Sherwin BB. Hormones, mood and cognitive functioning in postmenopausal women. Obstet Gynecol 1996;87(Suppl):20–6.

[22] Natale V, Albertazzi P, Zini M, et al. Exploration of cyclical changes in memory and mood in postmenopausal women taking sequential combined oestrogen and progestogen preparations. Int J Obstet Gynecol 2001;108:286–90.

[23] Moss RL, Gu Q, Wong M. Estrogen: nontranscriptional signalling pathway. Recent Prog Horm Res 1997;52:33–68.

[24] Koehler KF, Helguero LA, Haldosen L-A, et al. Reflections on the discovery and significance of estrogen receptor β. Endocr Rev 2005 26(3):465–78.

[25] McEwen BS, Alves SE. Estrogen actions in the central nervous system. Endocr Rev 1999;20 279–307.

[26] Shneerson JM, editor. Handbook of sleep medicine. 1st edition. Oxford (UK): Blackwell Science Ltd; 2000. p. 237.

[27] Barrett-Connor E. Rethinking estrogen and the brain. J Am Geriatr Soc 1998;46:90–2.

[28] Rapkin AJ. Vasomotor symptoms in menopause: physiologic condition and central nervous system approaches to treatment. Am J Obstet Gynecol 2007;196:97–106.

[29] Dzaja A, Arber S, Hislop J, et al. Women's sleep in health and disease. J Psychiatr Res 2005;39:55–76.

[30] Fonseca E, Ochoa R, Galván R, et al. Increased serum levels of growth hormone and insulin-like growth factor-I associated with simultaneous decrease of circulating insulin in postmenopausal women receiving hormone replacement therapy. Menopause 1999;6:56–60.

[31] Fernandez B, Malde JL, Montero A, et al. Relationship between adenohypophyseal and steroid hormones and variations in serum and urinary melatonin levels during the ovarian cycle, perimenopause and menopause in healthy women. J Steroid Biochem 1990;35:257–62.

[32] Woods NF, Carr MC, Tao EY, et al. Increased urinary cortisol levels during the menopausal transition. Menopause 2006;13:212–21.

[33] Moe KE, Prinz PN, Larsen LH, et al. Growth hormone in postmenopausal women after long term oral estrogen replacement therapy. J Gerontol A Biol Sci Med Sci 1998;53A:B117–24.

[34] Bellantoni MF, Vittone J, Campfield AT, et al. Effects of oral versus transdermal estrogen on the growth hormone/insulin-like growth factor I axis in younger and older postmenopausal women: a clinical research center study. J Clin Endocrinol Metab 1996;81:2848–53.

[35] Weissberger AJ, Ho KKY, Lazarus L. Contrasting effects of oral and transdermal routes of

estrogen replacement therapy on 24-hour growth hormone secretion, insulin-like growth factor I, and GH-binding protein in postmenopausal women. J Clin Endocrinol Metab 1991; 72:374–81.

[36] Cano A, Castelo-Branco C, Tarin JJ. Effect of menopause and different combined estradiol-progestin regimens on basal and growth hormone-releasing hormone-stimulated serum growth hormone, insulin-like growth factor-1, insulin-like growth factor binding protein (IGFBP)-1, and IGFBP-3 levels. Fertil Steril 1999;71:261–7.

[37] Katznelson L, Riskind PN, Saxe VC, et al. Prolactin pulsatile characteristics in postmenopausal women. J Clin Endocrinol Metab 1998; 83:761–4.

[38] Chang RJ, Davidson BJ, Carlson HE, et al. Circadian pattern of prolactin secretion in postmenopausal women receiving estrogen with or without progestin. Am J Obstet Gynecol 1982; 144:402–7.

[39] Bernardi F, Pieri M, Stomati M, et al. Effect of different hormonal replacement therapies on circulating allopregnanolone and dehydroepiandrosterone levels in postmenopausal women. Gynecol Endocrinol 2003;17:65–77.

[40] Pluchino N, Genazzani AD, Bernardi F, et al. Tibolone, transdermal estradiol or oral estrogen-progestin therapies: effects on circulating allopregnanolone, cortisol and dehydroepiandrosterone levels. Gynecol Endocrinol 2005; 20:144–9.

[41] Gudmundsson A, Goodman B, Lent S, et al. Effects of estrogen replacement therapy on the circadian rhythms of serum cortisol and body temperature in postmenopausal women. Exp Gerontol 1999;34:809–18.

[42] Fonseca E, Basurto L, Veláquez S, et al. Hormone replacement therapy increases ACTH/dehydroepiandrosterone sulfate in menopause. Maturitas 2001;39:57–62.

[43] Ohayon M. Epidemiological study on insomnia in the general population. Sleep 1996;19:7–15.

[44] Leger D, Guilleminault C, Dreyfus JP, et al. Prevalence of insomnia in a survey of 12,778 adults in France. J Sleep Res 2000;9:35–42.

[45] Zhang B, Wing YK. Sex differences in insomnia: a meta-analysis. Sleep 2006;29(1):85–93.

[46] Ledesert B, Ringa V, Breart G. Menopause and perceived health status among the women of the French GAZEL cohort. Maturitas 1994;20:113–20.

[47] Kuh DL, Wadsworth M, Hardy R. Women's health in midlife: the influence of the menopause, social factors and health in earlier life. Br J Obstet Gynaecol 1997;104:923–33.

[48] Kravitz HM, Ganz PA, Bromberger J, et al. Sleep difficulty in women at midlife. Menopause 2003;10:19–28.

[49] Anderson E, Hamburger S, Liu JH, et al. Characteristics of menopausal women seeking assistance. Am J Obstet Gynecol 1987;156:428–33.

[50] Shaver J, Giblin E, Lentz M, et al. Sleep patterns and stability in perimenopausal woman. Sleep 1988;11:556–61.

[51] Baker A, Simpson S, Dawson D. Sleep disruption and mood changes associated with menopause. J Psychosom Res 1997;43:359–69.

[52] Polo-Kantola P, Erkkola R, Irjala K, et al. Climacteric symptoms and sleep quality. Obstet Gynecol 1999;94:219–24.

[53] Thurston RC, Blumenthal JA, Babyak MA, et al. Association between hot flashes, sleep complaints, and psychological functioning among healthy menopausal women. Int J Behav Med 2006;13(2):163–72.

[54] Erlik Y, Tataryn IV, Meldrum DR, et al. Association of waking episodes with menopausal hot flushes. JAMA 1981;245:1741–4.

[55] Young T, Rabago D, Zgierska A, et al. Objective and subjective sleep quality in pre-, peri- and postmenopausal women in the Wisconsin sleep cohort study. Sleep 2003;26:667–72.

[56] Sharkey KM, Bearpark HM, Acebo C, et al. Effects of menopausal status on sleep in midlife women. Behav Sleep Med 2003;1:69–80.

[57] Woodward S, Freedman RR. The thermoregulatory effects of menopausal hot flashes on sleep. Sleep 1994;17(6):497–501.

[58] Freedman RR, Roehrs TA. Lack of sleep disturbance from menopausal hot flashes. Fertil Steril 2004;82:138–44.

[59] Freedman RR, Roehrs TA. Effects of REM sleep and ambient temperature on hot flash-induced sleep disturbance. Menopause 2006;13(4): 576–83.

[60] Freedman RR, Roehrs TA. Sleep disturbance in menopause. Menopause 2007;14(5):826–9.

[61] Rees M. The use of hormone replacement therapy in Europe and around the world. In: Erkkola R, editor. The menopause. Elsevier; 2006. p. 255–9.

[62] Wiklund I, Berg G, Hammar M, et al. Long-term effect of transdermal hormonal therapy on aspects of quality of life in postmenopausal women. Maturitas 1992;14:225–36.

[63] Rosen CJ. Postmenopausal osteoporosis. N Engl J Med 2005;353:595–603.

[64] Samsioe G. Current views on hormone replacement therapy and cardiovascular disease. In: Erkkola R, editor. The menopause. Elsevier; 2006. p. 63–80.

[65] Hays J, Ockene JK, Brunner RL, et al. Effects of estrogen plus progestin on health-related quality of life. N Engl J Med 2003;348:1839–54.

[66] Wiklund I, Karlberg J, Mattsson L-Å. Quality of life of menopausal women on a regimen of transdermal estradiol therapy: a double blind place-controlled study. Am J Obstet Gynecol 1993;168:824–30.

[67] Polo-Kantola P, Erkkola R, Helenius H, et al. When does estrogen replacement therapy improve sleep quality? Am J Obstet Gynecol 1998;178:1002–9.

[68] Gambacciani M, Ciaponi M, Cappagli B, et al. Effects of low-dose, continuous combined estradiol and noretisterone acetate on menopausal quality of life in early postmenopausal women. Maturitas 2003;44:157–63.

[69] Thomson J, Oswald I. Effect of oestrogen on the sleep, mood, and anxiety of menopausal women. BMJ 1977;2:1317–9.

[70] Schiff I, Regestein Q, Tulchinsky D, et al. Effects of estrogens on sleep and psychological state of hypogonadal women. JAMA 1979; 242:2405–7.

[71] Antonijevic IA, Stalla GK. Steiger A Modulation of the sleep electroencephalogram by estrogen replacement in postmenopausal women. Am J Obstet Gynecol 2000;182:277–82.

[72] Scharf MB, McDannold MD, Stover R, et al. Effects of estrogen replacement therapy on rates of cyclic alternating patterns and hot-flush events during sleep in postmenopausal women: a pilot study. Clin Ther 1997;19:304–11.

[73] Polo-Kantola P, Erkkola R, Irjala K, et al. Effect of short-term transdermal estrogen replacement therapy on sleep: a randomized, double-blind crossover trial in postmenopausal women. Fertil Steril 1999;71:873–80.

[74] Montplaisir J, Lorrain J, Denesle R, et al. Sleep in menopause: differential effects of two forms of hormone replacement therspy. Menopause 2001;8:10–6.

[75] Moe KE, Larsen LH, Vitiello MV, et al. Estrogen replacement therapy modulates the sleep disruption associated with nocturnal blood sampling. Sleep 2001;24:886–94.

[76] Pickett CK, Regensteiner JG, Woodard WD, et al. Progestin and estrogen reduce sleep-disordered breathing in postmenopausal women. J Appl Physiol 1989;66:1656–61.

[77] Purdie DW, Empson JAC, Crichton C, et al. Hormone replacement therapy, sleep quality and psychological wellbeing. Br J Obstet Gynaecol 1995;102:735–9.

[78] Saletu-Zyhlarz G, Anderer P, Gruber G, et al. Insomnia related to postmenopausal syndrome and hormone replacement therapy: sleep laboratory studies on baseline differences between patients and controls and double-blind, placebo-controlled investigations on the effects of a novel estrogen-progestogen combination versus estrogen alone. J Sleep Res 2003;12:239–54.

[79] Kronenberg F. Hot flashes: epidemiology and physiology. Ann NY Acad Sci 1990;592:52–86.

[80] Miller RG, Ashar BH. Managing menopause: current therapeutic options for vasomotor symptoms. Adv Stud Med 2004;4:484–92.

[81] Mazur W, Adlercreutz H. Overview of naturally occurring endocrine-active substances in the human diet in relation to human health. Nutrition 2000;16:654–8.

[82] Speroff L. Alternative therapies for postmenopausal women. Int J Fertil Womens Med 2005; 50(3):101–14.

[83] Ancoli-Israel S. Insomnia in the elderly: a review for the primary care practitioner. Sleep 2000 23(Suppl 1):S23–30.

[84] Young T, Palta M, Dempsey J, et al. The occurrence of sleep-disordered breathing among middle-aged adults. N Engl J Med 1993;328:1230–5

[85] Manber R, Armitage R. Sex, steroids, and sleep a review. Sleep 1999;22:540–55.

[86] Skatrud JB, Dempsey JA, Kaiser DG. Ventilator responses to medroxyprogesterone acetate in normal subjects: time course and mechanism J Appl Physiol 1978;44:939–44.

[87] Regensteiner JG, Woodard WD, Hagerman DD et al. Combined effects of female hormone and metabolic rate on ventilatory drives in women. J Appl Physiol 1989;66:808–13.

[88] Popovic RM, White DP. Upper airway muscl activity in normal women: influence of hormonal status. J Appl Physiol 1998;84 1055–62.

[89] Villaneuva AT, Buchanan PR, Yee BJ, et al. Ethnicity and obstructive sleep apnoea. Sleep Med Rev 2005;9(6):419–36.

[90] Young T, Peppard PE, Gottlieb DJ. Epidemiology of obstructive sleep apnea: a population health perspective. Am J Respir Crit Care Med 2002;165:1217–39.

[91] Gislason T, Benediktsdottir B, Bjornsson J et al. Snoring, hypertension, and the sleep apnea syndrome. An epidemiologic survey of middle-aged women. Chest 1993;103:1147–51.

[92] Bixler EO, Vgontzas AN, Lin H-M, et al. Prevalence of sleep-disordered breathing in women Effect of gender. Am J Respir Crit Care Med 2001;163:608–13.

[93] Anttalainen U, Saaresranta T, Kalleinen N, et al Gender differences in age and BMI distribution in partial upper airway obstruction during sleep. Respir Physiol Neurobiol 2007;159(2) 219–26.

[94] Polo-Kantola P, Rauhala E, Helenius H, et al Breathing during sleep in menopause: a randomized, controlled, crossover trial with estrogen therapy. Obstet Gynecol 2003;102:68–75.

[95] Anttalainen U, Saaresranta T, Kalleinen N, et al CPAP adherence and partial upper airway obstruction during sleep. Sleep Breath 2007 11:171–6.

[96] Grunstein RR. Continuous positive airway pressure treatment for obstructive sleep apnea-hypopnea syndrome. In: Kryger MH, Roth T Dement WC, editors. Principles and practice of sleep medicine. Philadelphia: Elsevier Saunders; 2005. p. 1066–80, Chapter 89.

[97] Buchanan PR, Grunstein RR. Neuropharmacology of obstructive sleep apnea and central apnea. In: Pandi-Perumal SR, Monti JM, editors Clinical pharmacology of sleep. Switzerland Birkhäuser Verlag; 2006. p. 21–41.

[98] Carley DW, Olopade C, Seink S, et al. Serotonin antagonist improves obstructive sleep apnea Sleep Med 2003;4(Suppl 1):S1–56.

[99] Shahar E, Redline S, Young T, et al. Hormone replacement therapy and sleep-disordered breathing. Am J Respir Crit Care Med 2003; 167:1186–92.

[100] Cistulli PA, Barnes DJ, Grunstein RR, et al. Effect of short-term hormone replacement in the treatment of obstructive sleep apnoea in postmenopausal women. Thorax 1994;49: 699–702.

[101] Keefe DL, Watson R, Naftolin F. Hormone replacement therapy may alleviate sleep apnea in menopausal women: a pilot study. Menopause 1999;6:196–200.

[102] Block AJ, Wynne JW, Boysen PG, et al. Menopause, medroxyprogesterone and breathing during sleep. Am J Med 1981;70:506–10.

[103] Saaresranta T, Polo-Kantola P, Irjala K, et al. Respiratory insufficiency in postmenopausal women: sustained improvement of gas exchange with short-term medroxyprogesterone acetate. Chest 1999;115:1581–7.

[104] Ford DE, Kamerow DB. Epidemiologic study of sleep disturbances and psychiatric disorders: an opportunity for prevention? JAMA 1989;262: 1479–84.

[105] Johnson EO, Roth T, Breslau N. The association of insomnia with anxiety disorders and depression: exploration of the direction of risk. J Psychiatr Res 2006;40(8):700–8.

[106] Kornstein SG. Gender differences in depression: implications for treatment. J Clin Psychiatry 1997;58:12–8.

[107] Pigott TA. Gender differences in the epidemiology and treatment of anxiety disorders. J Clin Psychiatry 1999;60:4–15.

[108] Avis NE, Stellato R, Crawford S, et al. Is there a menopausal syndrome? Menopausal status and symptoms across racial/ethnic groups. Soc Sci Med 2001;52:345–56.

[109] Sakkas P, Soldatos CR. Primary insomnia: diagnosis and treatment. In: Pandi-Perumal SR, Monti JM, editors. Clinical pharmacology of sleep. Switzerland: Birkhäuser Verlag; 2006. p. 11–9.

[110] Lichstein KL, Gellis LA, Stone KC, et al. Primary and secondary insomnia. In: Pandi-Perumal SR, Monti JM, editors. Clinical pharmacology of sleep. Switzerland: Birkhäuser Verlag; 2006. p. 1–9.

[111] Genazzani AR, Cambacciani M, Cappagli B, et al. Endocrinology of the menopause. In: Erkkola R, editor. The menopause. Elsevier; 2006. p. 1–8.

[112] Rothdach AJ, Trenkwalder C, Haberstock J, et al. Prevalence and risk factors of RLS in elderly population. The MEMO study. Neurology 2000;54:1064–8.

[113] Zucconi M, Ferini-Strambi L. Epidemiologic and clinical findings of restless legs syndrome. Sleep Med 2004;5:293–9.

[114] Manconi M, Covoni V, De Vito A, et al. Restless legs syndrome and pregnancy. Neurology 2004; 63:1065–9.

[115] Nikkola E, Ekblad U, Ekholm E, et al. Sleep in multiple pregnancy: breathing patterns, oxygenation, and periodic leg movements. Am J Obstet Gynecol 1996;174(5):1622–5.

[116] Polo-Kantola P, Rauhala E, Erkkola R, et al. Estrogen replacement therapy and nocturnal periodic limb movements: a randomized trial. Obstet Gynecol 2001;97:548–54.

SLEEP
MEDICINE
CLINICS

Sleep Med Clin 3 (2008) 133–140

ELSEVIER
SAUNDERS

The Circuitous Route to Diagnosing Sleep Disorders in Women: Health Care Utilization and Benefits of Improved Awareness for Sleep Disorders

Katsuhisa Banno, MD[a], Meir H. Kryger, MD, FRCPC[b],*

Sleep disorders that are common in women include insomnia [1], sleep breathing disorders [2], restless legs syndrome (RLS) [3,4], and sleep disturbance caused by mental conditions such as depression [5]. It has been shown that there may be a long interval between the onset of symptoms and the correct diagnosis of some sleep disorders [3,4,6]. The increasing demand for the diagnosis and treatment of sleep-related breathing disorders has led to long waiting lists for consultation and therapeutic services in clinics and hospitals [6]. In addition, sleep disorders may

be comorbid with medical problems; when finally evaluated for their sleep problems, many patients who have sleep disorders have been found to have psychiatric and medical conditions [1,7–11]. Gender differences in symptoms and clinical presentation [12–15] also may result in delayed diagnosis in women who have a sleep disorder. The circuitous route to correct diagnosis of a sleep disorder, or sleep disorders, consequently may lead to a negative impact on health care systems, because patients who have untreated sleep disorders may develop new psychiatric and medical

Supported in part by National Institutes of Health grant RO1 HL082672-01.
[a] Sleep Disorders Center, Kitatsushima Hospital, 307 Yomefuri, Heiwa-cho, Inazawa-city, Aichi, 490-1323, Japan
[b] Sleep Research and Education, Gaylord Hospital, 400 Gaylord Farm Road, Wallingford, CT 06492, USA
* Corresponding author.
E-mail address: mkryger@gaylord.org (M.H. Kryger).

comorbidities. This article reviews the impact of sleep disorders in women on health care utilization and the benefits of diagnosis and treatment.

Sleep disorders are classified into more than 80 diagnostic entities by the International Classification of Sleep Disorders published in 2005 [16]. Some sleep disorders such as obstructive sleep apnea syndrome (OSAS), insomnia, and RLS are prevalent in women and may lead to a negative impact on the patient's health and quality of life [1–5]. These disorders may play a role in the development of new medical comorbidities and mental conditions [2,5,8]. Thus untreated and delayed diagnosis of primary sleep disorders ultimately may increase health care utilization. Each sleep disorder may have an impact on health care systems; however, few cost analysis data have been reported for specific sleep disorders. Therefore this article reviews the impact of common sleep disorders in women, especially OSAS and insomnia, on health care utilization.

Obstructive sleep apnea syndrome

OSAS is a common disorder characterized by repetitive cessation of breathing during sleep caused by upper airway obstruction, with consequences of hypoxemia and fragmented sleep. OSAS has been reported to affect middle-aged people (4% of men and 2% of women) [17]. A systemic review reported by Young and colleagues [2] in 2002 showed that OSAS may affect up to 5% of adults. The prevalence of OSAS may be higher now, however, because of recent trends of increasing obesity [18] and the greater awareness of OSAS compared with a decade ago. Common causes of OSAS include obesity, craniofacial malformation (eg, retrognathia and micrognathia), and obstruction of upper airway by enlarged tonsils and adenoids [19]. The abnormal breathing in sleep consequently leads to daytime sleepiness and impaired cognitive function, resulting in impaired quality of life [20]. Depressive symptoms may be present in patients who have OSAS [21]. Hypoxemia and metabolic dysfunction caused by repetitive apneas have been reported to play a role in the development of hypertension, heart failure, stroke, and insulin resistance [22–26].

Health care use in obstructive sleep apnea syndrome

For several years before diagnosis, patients who have OSAS use health care resources at higher rates than those who do not have OSAS [27–31]. Increased health care expenditure in patients who have OSAS may be caused by comorbidities, because many have been diagnosed with medical or psychiatric comorbidities before the recognition of OSAS. Health care utilization was assessed using total expenditure from physician claims and number of hospital stays or clinic visits, which are surrogates of health care cost [27–31]. One of the problems in estimating health care expenditure in a particular patient group is the variability of payer systems for health care in each region; this variability may skew data significantly. Thus a one-payer system with complete health care data, which allows accurate tracking of long-term health care utilization, (eg, the Manitoba Canada health database) [32] is considered appropriate for evaluation of health care expenditure.

The first study to confirm that patients who have OSAS are heavy users of health care was reported by Kryger and colleagues [27] in 1996. They compared physician claims and number of hospital stays of 97 obese patients who had OSAS with those of 97 controls for the 2 years before the initial OSAS diagnosis. Total health care expenditures calculated from physician claims were $82,238 (Canadian dollars) for the OSAS group versus $41,018 for the control group (P<.01). The OSAS group had 251 nights in hospital, compared with 90 nights for the control group, and they spent between $100,000 and $200,000 more in services than the control group. Thus, there is an increased health care cost in the few years just before evaluation for OSAS. This result led to the question of how far back the increased health care cost in the OSAS group was seen.

The study reported by Ronald and colleagues [28] in 1999 looked at health care utilization 10 years before diagnosis using the number of hospital stays and physician claims in 181 patients who had OSAS compared with those of age- and gender-matched controls. Health care expenditure calculated from physician claims was $686,365 ($3972 per patient) for the OSAS group, compared with $356,376 ($1969 per patient) for the control group for the 10-year period before OSAS diagnosis. In addition, the OSAS group also had more hospital stays: 1118 nights (6.2 per patient), versus 676 nights (3.7 per patient) for the control group. The OSAS group used more health care resources than the control group in 7 of 10 years before OSAS diagnosis.

In North America most patients who have OSAS are overweight or obese. The mean body mass index (BMI) at time of referral to a sleep disorders center has been reported to be 32.2 ± 0.1 kg/m^2 (SD) (95% confidence interval [CI], 32.0–32.4) in men versus 34.5 ± 0.2 kg/m^2 (95% CI, 34.1–35.0) in women (P < .0001) [18], indicating a high prevalence of obesity in patients who have OSAS. Obesity also may play a role in the increased health care use in patients who have OSAS, because obesity, which s associated with metabolic syndrome, is a known isk factor of ischemic heart diseases, stroke, and diabetes mellitus [33,34]. These two reports on health care utilization in patients who have OSAS verified increased health care utilization before OSAS diagnosis. The factors determining the health care resource have remained unclear, however.

Factors affecting health care use in patients who have obstructive sleep apnea syndrome

The comorbidities affecting health care utilization have been reported by Smith and colleagues [10]. The group investigated health care resources and medical diagnoses made before the diagnosis of OSAS in 773 patients and found that patients who have OSAS are more likely to receive a diagnosis of hypertension before the OSAS diagnosis is made (odds ratio [OR], 2.5; 95% CI, 2.0 to 3.3) [10]. Otake and colleagues [35] reported that many patients who have OSAS are taking antihypertensive medications before their OSAS diagnosis is made: the OR of OSAS patients taking medications indicated for the treatment of systemic hypertension was 2.71 (95% CI, 1.96–3.77) compared with controls. The use of medications indicated for the treatment of systemic hypertension was predicted by age, BMI, and apnea-hypopnea index.

Patients who have OSAS also are at higher risk for congestive heart failure (OR, 3.9; 95% CI, 1.7–8.9), cardiac arrhythmias (OR, 2.2; 95% CI, 1.2–4.0), chronic obstructive airways disease (COPD) (OR, 1.6; 95% CI, 1.2–2.0), and depression (OR, 1.4; 95% CI, 1.0–1.9) [10]. Age and BMI significantly predicted diagnoses of cardiovascular diseases and arthropathy in patients who had OSAS. Male gender predicted ischemic heart disease (OR, 2.98; 95% CI, 1.36–6.54). In contrast, female gender was a significant predictor for COPD (OR, 2.63; 95% CI, 1.85–3.72) and depression (OR, 2.24; 95% CI, 1.45–3.44).

Tarasiuk and colleagues [36], in another single-payer system (Israel), reported increased health care utilization in the 2 years before OSAS diagnosis in patients who had OSAS compared with a control group. The increased expenses particularly resulted from hospital stays (*P*<.001), consultations (*P*<.001), and cost of drugs (*P*<.05), especially for cardiovascular diseases. They also concluded that women who had a diagnosis of OSAS consumed more health care resources than men. In addition, patients who had OSAS and were older than 65 years consumed 2.2-fold more health care resources than controls (*P*<.001). The same research group reported that older age, use of antipsychotic and anxiolytic drugs, and asthma contribute significantly to the higher health care cost in women who have OSAS [37]. Age and female gender may be

possible factors affecting health care utilization in patients who have OSAS.

Changes in health care use before treatment and after treatment

The first report on a change of health care utilization by treatment intervention for OSAS was by Bahammam and colleagues [29], who used the Manitoba health database. The group compared physician claims and hospital stays of 344 men who had OSAS with those of controls from the general population, matched for age and geographic location, 1 and 5 years before treatment and for 2 years after treatment. The effect of continuous positive airway pressure (CPAP) adherence on health care resources was examined also. The difference in health care expenditure between the entire OSAS group and the control group 2 years after diagnosis and treatment ($174 ± 32 per year) was less than the difference in the year before diagnosis ($260 ± 36 per year) (*P* = .038). There was a significant difference in physician claims between the 282 patients adhering to CPAP therapy and controls: $267 ± 37 1 year before diagnosis versus $181 ± 36 2 years after treatment (*P* = .05). In contrast, a significant difference in physician claims was not observed between the 62 patients not adhering CPAP treatment: $236 ± 104 1 year before treatment, versus $141 ± 72 2 years after treatment (*P* = .44). Interestingly, in the 5 years before OSAS diagnosis, patients not adhering to CPAP treatment spent more on physician claims than patients adhering to CPAP treatment for cardiovascular disorders ($75.76 ± 25.97 versus $31.54 ± 3.41 per year; *P* = .0019) and genitourinary disorders ($13.39± 3.91 versus $6.93 ± 1.28 per year; *P* = .05). The noncompliant patients also were older and had a lower apnea-hypopnea index, which might have made adherence to therapy more problematic for this group.

Albarrak and colleagues [30] assessed the effect of long-term use of CPAP on health care utilization. They compared physician claims and physician visits for 342 men who had OSAS with those of matched controls for whom there were utilization data for 5 years before initial OSAS diagnosis and for 5 years of CPAP treatment. In the patients who had OSAS, physician visits increased by 3.46 ± 0.2 (95% CI, 2.57–4.36) during the year immediately before diagnosis compared with the fifth year preceding diagnosis and then decreased for the 5 years of treatment by 1.03 ± 0.49 (95% CI, −1.99 to −0.07; *P*<00,001). Physician claims also increased by $148.65 ± 27.27 (95% CI, 95.12–202.10) in the 5 years leading up to diagnosis in the patient group and decreased over the next 5 years by $13.92 ± 27.94 (95% CI, −68.68 to 40.83; *P* = .0009).

Thus, these two reports emphasize that early diagnosis and treatment result in long-term as well as short-term cost benefits. Patients who have OSAS, however, may already have been diagnosed with a comorbid condition that could affect health care use before OSAS diagnosis and after treatment. Smith and colleagues [10] reported that cardiovascular diseases, especially hypertension and heart failure, were more frequently diagnosed in both men and women who had OSAS than in their controls during the 5 years before OSAS diagnosis. Pre-existing ischemic heart disease at the time of OSAS diagnosis has been reported to predict about a fivefold increase in health care expenditure between the second and fifth year of treatment [30].

Health care use in women who have obstructive sleep apnea syndrome

Increasing trends in health care utilization before diagnosis and decreasing trends in physician claims and ambulatory clinic visits after assessment and treatment of OSAS have been found in women who have OSAS [31]. There was an increase in fees of $123.43 ± 25.01 in the 2 years before diagnosis and a reduction in fees of $37.96 ± 21.35 in the 2 years after diagnosis of OSAS (*P*<.0001). The number of clinic visits by women who had OSAS also increased by 2.32 ± 0.43 visits in the 2 years before diagnosis and decreased by 1.48 ± 0.42 visits during the next 2 years (*P*<.0001). Thus early diagnosis and treatment recommendation help stem the consumption of health care resources in women who have OSAS. A change in health care utilization after long-term use of CPAP is not yet clear in women who have OSAS, however.

Gender differences in the clinical presentation of obstructive sleep apnea syndrome

Some differences in the clinical presentation of OSAS between men and women have resulted in a referral bias to sleep clinics in favor of men [13,38–44]. Young and colleagues [45] reported that more than 90% of women who had moderate to severe OSAS may be undiagnosed. Larsson and colleagues [46] estimated the referral rate for men:-women, after correction for population and prevalence of symptoms, may be 1.25:1 (*P* = .012). Men who have OSAS are more likely to have symptoms of snoring, observed apnea, or sleepiness, whereas women who have OSAS have more symptoms of depression or morning headache [10,38,39]. Women first diagnosed as having OSAS are more likely than men to have been diagnosed previously with depression or COPD [10]. Comparing the clinical presentations before OSAS diagnosis of women with those of men matched

for sleep apnea severity, subjective sleepiness, BMI and age, Shepertycky and colleagues [13] concluded that a history of depression and hypothyroid disease and a presenting complaint of insomnia were seen more frequently in women; men were more likely to have a history of witnessed apnea and greater caffeine and alcohol consumption. Another study also reported that women who have OSA are more likely than men who have OSA to be diagnosed with hypothyroidism (OR, 4.7; 95% CI, 2.3–10) or arthropathy (OR, 1.6; 95% CI, 1.1–2.2), but the women had a lower risk for comorbid cardiovascular disease (OR, 0.7; 95% CI, 0.5–0.91) [37].

Different clinical presentations may result in fewer referrals of women to a sleep clinic, resulting in more undiagnosed OSAS in women. Women diagnosed as having OSAS are more obese than men who have OSAS [47,48] and are more likely to have comorbid mental disorders such as depression [10,49]. The updated data published in 2007 by Greenberg-Dotan and colleagues [37] on gender differences in health care use among patients who have OSAS showed that women who had OSAS received more antidepressants, hypnotics, and anxiolytics before OSAS diagnosis than men who had OSAS matched for age, BMI, and apnea-hypopnea index. In addition, the investigators concluded that health care expenditure for drugs was 1.3 times higher in women who had OSAS than in men who had OSAS (*P*<.0001).

Thus it is possible that undiagnosed OSAS in women may impact health care systems more significantly than undiagnosed OSAS in men. The prevalence of OSAS in men has been reported to be about double that in women [17]; however, overall health care utilization between the genders may be similar or greater in women than in men because of more severe obesity and the greater prevalence of comorbid psychiatric conditions in women. Early treatment of OSAS may contribute to the reduced consumption of health care resources in men.

Insomnia

Insomnia is characterized by difficulty in sleep initiation, maintenance, duration, or quality that occurs despite adequate time and opportunity for sleep, along with daytime impairments such as fatigue, attention impairment, sleepiness, mood disturbance, and social dysfunction [1,16,50,51]. Insomnia is classified into two types: idiopathic insomnia and comorbid insomnia. The former has no identified specific cause; in contrast, the latter refers to insomnia symptoms that are related to comorbid medical and psychiatric conditions or drugs [1,16,51]. Insomnia often may accompany acute or chronic medical conditions; changes in the sleep-wake schedule, pain, dyspnea, urinary incontinence, and the use of certain medications may lead to insomnia symptoms. Stress, symptoms of depression, or anxiety in reaction to the medical conditions and primary sleep disorders such as OSAS and RLS also may cause sleep disturbances.

Impact of insomnia on health care cost

Insomnia is a major public health problem affecting millions of individuals, along with their families and communities, in European countries, North America, and Australia [52–58]. The cost of medications used to treat insomnia has been reported to total $1.97 billion in the United States in 1995 [52]. Epidemiologic data reported by Leger and colleagues [53] estimated the total cost of insomnia in France at $2 billion, which was spent for hypnotics and fees for physicians and sleep specialists for treatment in outpatient clinics. The National Institutes of Health, in their Science Conference statement in 2005, concluded that the direct and indirect annual cost for chronic insomnia in adults was estimated to be tens of billions of dollars [1]. Updated data on the cost analysis for untreated insomnia in the United States by Ozminkowski and colleagues [59] published in 2007 showed that the average direct and indirect costs for younger adults who had insomnia were about $924 greater than for patients who did not have insomnia: $4755 for patients treated for insomnia, versus $3831 for controls ($P < .01$); among the elderly, direct costs were about $1143 greater for patients who had insomnia: $5790 for patients treated for insomnia, versus $4648 for controls ($P < .01$). Thus insomnia is a costly medical condition that burdens health care systems.

Association of insomnia with psychiatric conditions

Psychiatric conditions may result in sleep disturbance in many women. Starting from puberty until menopause, women are at twice the lifetime risk of developing major depression than men [60,61]. Sleep disturbance is common in depression; the most common subjective complaint is insomnia, including difficulty falling asleep, frequent awakenings, and early morning awakenings [7,62,63]. Psychiatric disturbance such as depression is a risk factor for insomnia in women [64–66]. People who have insomnia have been reported to be 9.82 times more likely to have clinically significant depression than people who do not have insomnia [7]. The risk of insomnia has been reported to be higher in patients who have depression (mild insomnia: OR, 2.6; 95% CI, 1.9–3.5; $P<.001$; severe insomnia: OR, 8.2; 95% CI, 5.7–12.0; $P<.001$) [67]. Breslau and colleagues [8] concluded that the

relative risk for new-onset depression in people who had insomnia was 4.0 (95% CI, 2.2–7.0). There are lifetime associations of insomnia with anxiety disorder and with depression [68]. Among those who have comorbid disorders, anxiety disorders preceded insomnia 73% of the time, whereas insomnia occurred first in 69% of patients who had comorbid insomnia and depression [68]. Using the Hospital Anxiety and Depression scale, Lindberg and colleagues [69] concluded that anxiety affected women more frequently than men (32.8% for women, versus 18.9% for men; $P < .001$).

Thus these reports suggest that a causal link between insomnia and psychiatric conditions seems to be bi-directional. Medical conditions may lead to the development of insomnia [1,16,51,63]; conversely, women who have primary sleep disorders such as OSAS and RLS also have been reported to be diagnosed more frequently with depression or to be treated with antidepressants [9,10,13]. Because these sleep disorders may manifest with insomnia caused by depressive symptoms, delayed referral to a sleep clinic may have an adverse impact on health care utilization by women.

Gender differences of insomnia and health care use in women

Insomnia is more common in women than in men [64,65]. The gender differences in risk factors for insomnia and in clinical presentations of insomnia may affect health care use in women. Li and colleagues [64] reported that women were at about 1.6 times higher risk for insomnia than men. Gender differences in insomnia may include differences in the prevalence of psychiatric morbidities, symptom endorsement, gonadal steroids, socio-cultural factors, and coping strategies. Su and colleagues [65] reported that factors associated with insomnia for both genders were nocturia and regular use of hypnotics. Risk factors for men included pulmonary disease, single status, excessive daytime sleepiness, and mental illness, whereas lack of education and body pain were risk factors in women. Depression was strongly associated with insomnia in older women. A report by Chung and Tang [70] showed that somatic complaints, psychologic symptoms, and perceived stress were independent risk factors for sleep disturbance; women who had those symptoms had four to six times greater risk of reporting disturbed sleep. Women seem more likely than men to have insomnia, which is associated with psychiatric conditions.

Women who have insomnia may have more impact on health care systems than men who have insomnia. Rasu and colleagues [71] investigated health care use in patients who have insomnia and found that that men who had insomnia were less likely to receive a prescription for a medication than women who had insomnia (OR, 0.61; 95% CI, 0.45–0.81). Simon and VonKorff [72] investigated characteristics of outpatients who had insomnia in the United States and found that women were 1.5 times more likely to have insomnia-related physician visits ($P<.001$). Sleep disturbance was most frequently attributed to medical conditions (55.8%), depression and/or anxiety (27.3%), and primary insomnia (9.8%) ($P<.001$). In addition, they found that patients who had insomnia spent more on health care services during the 3 months before and the 3 months after a screening visit to a clinic than those who did not have insomnia ($2287 versus $1418, respectively) [72].

Insomnia is responsible for increased health care expenditure, but comprehensive cost-effectiveness analyses of different diagnostic and treatment strategies is challenging because of the variability in the definition of insomnia and methods of assessment for direct and indirect costs. Martin and colleagues [73] concluded that effective insomnia management holds promise as a cost-effective health care intervention. Some drugs for insomnia management have been reported to contribute to the reduction of health care cost in patients who have insomnia [74,75].

Summary

The different clinical presentations of OSAS and low suspicion for it in women may lead to delayed diagnosis. Women diagnosed as having OSAS tend to be more obese and to have depression more frequently than men. Women, in whom insomnia is more common, also have a higher incidence of anxiety and depression than men. Sleep disorders may impact women's health care expenditures. A cost burden is incurred by untreated and delayed sleep disorders. Increased awareness, and thus early diagnosis, of a sleep disorder may contribute to cost savings and improve the patient's quality of life.

References

[1] National Institutes of Health. National Institutes of Health State of the Science Conference Statement on Manifestations and Management of Chronic Insomnia in Adults, June 13-15, 2005. Sleep 2005;28(9):1049–57.

[2] Young T, Peppard PE, Gottlieb DJ. Epidemiology of obstructive sleep apnea: a population health perspective. Am J Respir Crit Care Med 2002; 165(9):1217–39.

[3] Tison F, Crochard A, Léger D, et al. Epidemiology of restless legs syndrome in French adults:

[4] Högl B, Kiechl S, Willeit J, et al. Restless legs syndrome: a community-based study of prevalence, severity, and risk factors. Neurology 2005; 64(11):1920–4.

[5] Taylor DJ, Mallory LJ, Lichstein KL, et al. Comorbidity of chronic insomnia with medical problems. Sleep 2007;30(2):213–8.

[6] Flemons WW, Douglas NJ, Kuna ST, et al. Access to diagnosis and treatment of patients with suspected sleep apnea. Am J Respir Crit Care Med 2004;169(6):668–72.

[7] Taylor DJ, Lichstein KL, Durrence HH, et al. Epidemiology of insomnia, depression, and anxiety. Sleep 2005;28(11):1457–64.

[8] Breslau N, Roth T, Rosenthal L, et al. Sleep disturbance and psychiatric disorders: a longitudinal epidemiological study of young adults. Biol Psychiatry 1996;39(6):411–8.

[9] Banno K, Delaive K, Walld R, et al. Restless legs syndrome in 218 patients: associated disorders. Sleep Med 2000;1(3):221–9.

[10] Smith R, Ronald J, Delaive K, et al. What are obstructive sleep apnea patients being treated for prior to this diagnosis? Chest 2002;121(1):164–72.

[11] Kryger MH, Walld R, Manfreda J. Diagnoses received by narcolepsy patients in the year prior to diagnosis by a sleep specialist. Sleep 2002; 25(1):36–41.

[12] Quintana-Gallego E, Carmona-Bernal C, Capote F, et al. Gender differences in obstructive sleep apnea syndrome: a clinical study of 1166 patients. Respir Med 2004;98(10):984–9.

[13] Shepertycky MR, Banno K, Kryger MH. Differences between men and women in the clinical presentation of patients diagnosed with obstructive sleep apnea syndrome. Sleep 2005;28(3):309–14.

[14] Valipour A, Lothaller H, Rauscher H, et al. Gender-related differences in symptoms of patients with suspected breathing disorders in sleep: a clinical population study using the sleep disorders questionnaire. Sleep 2007;30(3):312–9.

[15] Krishnan V, Collop NA. Gender differences in sleep disorders. Curr Opin Pulm Med 2006; 12(6):383–9.

[16] American Academy of Sleep Medicine. International classification of sleep disorders. In: Sateia MJ, editor. Diagnostic and coding manual. 2nd edition. Westchester (IL): American Academy of Sleep Medicine; 2005.

[17] Young T, Palta M, Dempsey J, et al. The occurrence of sleep-disordered breathing among middle-aged adults. N Engl J Med 1993;328(17): 1230–5.

[18] Banno K, Walld R, Kryger MH. Increasing obesity trends in patients with sleep-disordered breathing referred to a sleep disorders center. J Clin Sleep Med 2005;1(4):364–6.

[19] Banno K, Kryger MH. Sleep apnea: clinical investigations in humans. Sleep Med 2007;8(4): 400–26.

a nationwide survey: the INSTANT Study. Neurology 2005;65(2):239–46.

20] Al-Barrak M, Shepertycky MR, Kryger MH. Morbidity and mortality in obstructive sleep apnea syndrome 2: effect of treatment on neuropsychiatric morbidity and quality of life. Sleep Biol Rhythms 2003;1(1):65–74.

21] McCall WV, Harding D, O'Donovan C. Correlates of depressive symptoms in patients with obstructive sleep apnea. J Clin Sleep Med 2006; 2(4):424–6.

22] Shepertycky MR, Al-Barrak M, Kryger MH. Morbidity and mortality in obstructive sleep apnea syndrome 1: effect of treatment on cardiovascular morbidity. Sleep Biol Rhythms 2003;1(1): 15–28.

23] Peled N, Kassirer M, Shitrit D, et al. The association of OSA with insulin resistance, inflammation and metabolic syndrome. Respir Med 2007;101(8):1696–701.

24] Arzt M, Young T, Finn L, et al. The association of OSA with insulin resistance, inflammation and metabolic syndrome. Respir Med 2007;101(8): 1696–701.

25] Young T, Peppard P, Palta M, et al. Population-based study of sleep-disordered breathing as a risk factor for hypertension. Arch Intern Med 1997;157(15):1746–52.

26] Kryger MH, et al. Sleep disorders and cardiovascular disease. In: Zipes DP, Libby P, Bonow RO, editors. Braunwald's heart disease. 7th edition. Philadelphia: Elsevier Saunders; 2004. p. 1843–8.

27] Kryger MH, Roos L, Delaive K, et al. Utilization of health care services in patients with severe obstructive sleep apnea. Sleep 1996;19(9 Suppl): S111–6.

28] Ronald J, Delaive K, Roos L, et al. Health care utilization in the 10 years prior to diagnosis in obstructive sleep apnea syndrome patients. Sleep 1999;22(2):225–9.

29] Bahammam A, Delaive K, Ronald J, et al. Health care utilization in males with obstructive sleep apnea syndrome two years after diagnosis and treatment. Sleep 1999;22(6):740–7.

30] Albarrak M, Banno K, Sabbagh AA, et al. Utilization of healthcare resources in obstructive sleep apnea syndrome: a 5-year follow-up study in men using CPAP. Sleep 2005;28(10):1306–11.

31] Banno K, Manfreda J, Walld R, et al. Healthcare utilization in women with obstructive sleep apnea syndrome 2 years after diagnosis and treatment. Sleep 2006;29(10):1307–11.

32] Roos NP, Black C, Roos LL, et al. Managing health services: how the Population Health Information System (POPULIS) works for policymakers. Med Care 1999;37(6 Suppl):JS27–41.

33] Rana JS, Nieuwdorp M, Jukema JW, et al. Cardiovascular metabolic syndrome–an interplay of, obesity, inflammation, diabetes and coronary heart disease. Diabetes Obes Metab 2007;9(3): 218–32.

34] Bakris GL. Current perspectives on hypertension and metabolic syndrome. J Manag Care Pharm 2007;13(5 Supp):3–5.

[35] Otake K, Delaive K, Walld R, et al. Cardiovascular medication use in patients with undiagnosed obstructive sleep apnoea. Thorax 2002;57(5): 417–22.

[36] Tarasiuk A, Greenberg-Dotan S, Brin YS, et al. Determinants affecting health-care utilization in obstructive sleep apnea syndrome patients. Chest 2005;128(3):1310–4.

[37] Greenberg-Dotan S, Reuveni H, Simon T, et al. Gender differences in morbidity and health care utilization among adult obstructive sleep apnea patients. Sleep 2007;30(9):1173–80.

[38] Redline S, Kump K, Tishler PV, et al. Gender differences in sleep disordered breathing in a community-based sample. Am J Respir Crit Care Med 1994;149:722–6.

[39] Young T, Hutton R, Finn L, et al. The gender bias in sleep apnea diagnosis. Are women missed because they have different symptoms? Arch Intern Med 1996;25(156):2445–51.

[40] Bixler EO, Vgontzas AN, Lin HM, et al. Prevalence of sleep-disordered breathing in women: effects of gender. Am J Respir Crit Care Med 2001;163:608–13.

[41] Walker RP, Durazo-Arvizu R, Wachter B, et al. Preoperative differences between male and female patients with sleep apnea. Laryngoscope 2001;111:1501–5.

[42] Kapsimalis F, Kryger MH. Gender and obstructive sleep apnea syndrome, part 1: clinical features. Sleep 2002;15(25):412–9.

[43] Kapsimalis F, Kryger MH. Gender and obstructive sleep apnea syndrome, part 2: mechanisms. Sleep 2002;25(5):499–506.

[44] Jordan AS, McEvoy RD. Gender differences in sleep apnea: epidemiology, clinical presentation and pathogenic mechanisms. Sleep Med Rev 2003;7(5):377–89.

[45] Young T, Evans L, Finn L, et al. Estimation of the clinically diagnosed proportion of sleep apnea syndrome in middle-aged men and women. Sleep 1997;20:705–6.

[46] Larsson LG, Lindberg A, Franklin KA, et al. Gender differences in symptoms related to sleep apnea in a general population and in relation to referral to sleep clinic. Chest 2003;124(1): 204–11.

[47] Guilleminault C, Quera-Salva MA, Partinen M, et al. Women and the obstructive sleep apnea syndrome. Chest 1988;93(1):104–9.

[48] Leech JA, Onal E, Dulberg C, et al. A comparison of men and women with occlusive sleep apnea syndrome. Chest 1988;94(5):983–8.

[49] Collop NA, Adkins D, Phillips BA. Gender differences in sleep and sleep-disordered breathing. Clin Chest Med 2004;25(2):257–68.

[50] Thorpy MJ. Classification of sleep disorders. In: Kryger MH, Roth T, Dement WC, editors. Principles and practice of sleep medicine. 4th edition. Philadelphia: Elsevier Saunders; 2005. p. 615–25.

[51] Edinger JD, Means MK. Overview of insomnia: definitions, epidemiology, differential diagnosis, and

assessment. In: Kryger MH, Roth T, Dement WC, editors. Principles and practice of sleep medicine. 4th edition. Philadelphia: Elsevier Saunders; 2005. p. 702–13.

[52] Walsh JK, Engelhardt CL. The direct economic costs of insomnia in the United States for 1995. Sleep 1999;22(Suppl 2):S386–93.

[53] Leger D, Levy E, Paillard M. The direct costs of insomnia in France. Sleep 1999;22(Suppl 2): S394–401.

[54] Kapur VK, Redline S, Nieto FJ, et al. Sleep Heart Health Research Group. The relationship between chronically disrupted sleep and healthcare use. Sleep 2002;25(3):289–96.

[55] Novak M, Mucsi I, Shapiro CM, et al. Increased utilization of health services by insomniacs: an epidemiological perspective. J Psychosom Res 2004;56(5):527–36.

[56] Roth T. Prevalence, associated risks, and treatment patterns of insomnia. J Clin Psychiatry 2005;66(Suppl 9):10–3.

[57] Fullerton DS. The economic impact of insomnia in managed care: a clearer picture emerges. Am J Manag Care 2006;12(8 Suppl):S246–52.

[58] Hillman DR, Murphy AS, Pezzullo L. The economic cost of sleep disorders. Sleep 2006; 29(3):299–305.

[59] Ozminkowski RJ, Wang S, Walsh JK. The direct and indirect costs of untreated insomnia in adults in the United States. Sleep 2007;30(3):263–73.

[60] Rapkin AJ. Progesterone, GABA and mood disorders in women. Arch Womens Ment Health 1999;2:97–105.

[61] Parry BL, Newton RP. Chronobiological basis of female-specific mood disorders. Neuropsychopharmacology 2001;25(5 Suppl):S102–8.

[62] Katz DA, McHorney CA. The relationship between insomnia and health-related quality of life in patients with chronic illness. J Fam Pract 2002;51(3):229–35.

[63] Benca RM. Mood disorders. In: Kryger MH, Roth T, Dement WC, editors. Principles and practice of sleep medicine. 4th edition. Philadelphia: Elsevier Saunders; 2005. p. 1311–26.

[64] Li RH, Wing YK, Ho SC, et al. Gender differences in insomnia—a study in the Hong Kong Chinese population. J Psychosom Res 2002;53(1):601–9.

[65] Su TP, Huang SR, Chou P. Prevalence and risk factors of insomnia in community-dwelling Chinese elderly: a Taiwanese urban area survey. Aust N Z J Psychiatry 2004;38(9):706–13.

[66] Soares CN. Insomnia in women: an overlooked epidemic? Arch Womens Ment Health 2005; 8(4):205–13.

[67] Katz DA, McHorney CA. Clinical correlates of insomnia in patients with chronic illness. Arch Intern Med 1998;158(10):1099–107.

[68] Johnson EO, Roth T, Breslau N. The association of insomnia with anxiety disorders and depression: exploration of the direction of risk. J Psychiatr Res 2006;40(8):700–8.

[69] Lindberg E, Janson C, Gislason T, et al. Sleep disturbances in a young adult population: can gender differences be explained by differences in psychological status? Sleep 1997;20(6): 381–7.

[70] Chung KF, Tang MK. Subjective sleep disturbance and its correlates in middle-aged Hong Kong Chinese women. Maturitas 2006;53(4): 396–404.

[71] Rasu RS, Shenolikar RA, Nahata MC, et al. Physician and patient factors associated with the prescribing of medications for sleep difficulties that are associated with high abuse potential or are expensive: an analysis of data from the National Ambulatory Medical Care Survey for 1996–2001. Clin Ther 2005;27(12):1970–9.

[72] Simon GE, VonKorff M. Prevalence, burden, and treatment of insomnia in primary care. Am J Psychiatry 1997;154(10):1417–23.

[73] Martin SA, Aikens JE, Chervin RD. Toward cost effectiveness analysis in the diagnosis and treatment of insomnia. Sleep Med Rev 2004;8(1): 63–72.

[74] Jhaveri M, Seal B, Pollack M, et al. Will insomnia treatments produce overall cost savings to commercial managed-care plans? A predictive analysis in the United States. Curr Med Res Opin 2007;23(6):1431–43.

[75] Botteman MF, Ozminkowski RJ, Wang S, et al. Cost effectiveness of long-term treatment with eszopiclone for primary insomnia in adults: a decision analytical model. CNS Drugs 2007;21(4): 319–34.

SLEEP
MEDICINE
CLINICS

Sleep Med Clin 3 (2008) 141–146

Index

Note: Page numbers of article titles are in **boldface** type.

doi:10.1016/S1556-407X(08)00021-0
sleep.theclinics.com